Genetic Engineering in Eukaryotes

NATO Advanced Science Institutes Series

A series of edited volumes comprising multifaceted studies of contemporary scientific issues by some of the best scientific minds in the world, assembled in cooperation with NATO Scientific Affairs Division.

This series is published by an international board of publishers in conjunction with NATO Scientific Affairs Division

A	**Life Sciences**	Plenum Publishing Corporation
B	**Physics**	New York and London
C	**Mathematical and Physical Sciences**	D. Reidel Publishing Company Dordrecht, Boston, and London
D	**Behavioral and Social Sciences**	Martinus Nijhoff Publishers
E	**Applied Sciences**	The Hague, Boston, and London
F	**Computer and Systems Sciences**	Springer Verlag
G	**Ecological Sciences**	Heidelberg, Berlin, and New York

Recent Volumes in Series A: Life Sciences

Volume 56—Advances in Vertebrate Neuroethology
edited by Jörg-Peter Ewert, Robert R. Capranica, and David J. Ingle

Volume 57—Biochemical and Biological Markers of Neoplastic Transformation
edited by Prakash Chandra

Volume 58—Arterial Pollution: An Integrated View on Atherosclerosis
edited by H. Peeters, G. A. Gresham, and R. Paoletti

Volume 59—The Applications of Laser Light Scattering to the Study of Biological Motion
edited by J. C. Earnshaw and M. W. Steer

Volume 60—The Use of Human Cells for the Evaluation of Risk from Physical and Chemical Agents
edited by Amleto Castellani

Volume 61—Genetic Engineering in Eukaryotes
edited by Paul F. Lurquin and Andris Kleinhofs

Volume 62—Heart Perfusion, Energetics, and Ischemia
edited by Leopold Dintenfass, Desmond G. Julian, and Geoffrey V. F. Seaman

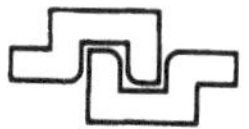

Genetic Engineering in Eukaryotes

Edited by

Paul F. Lurquin and
Andris Kleinhofs

Washington State University
Pullman, Washington

Plenum Press
New York and London
Published in cooperation with NATO Scientific Affairs Division

Proceedings of a NATO Advanced Study Institute,
held July 26–August 6, 1982,
at Washington State University, Pullman, Washington

Library of Congress Cataloging in Publication Data

NATO Advanced Study Institute (1982: Washington State University)
Genetic engineering in eukaryotes.

(NATO advanced science institutes series. Series A, Life sciences; v. 61)
"Proceedings of a NATO Advanced Study Institute, held July 26–August 6, 1982, at Washington State University, Pullman, Washington"—P.
Includes bibliographical references and index.
1. Genetic engineering—Congresses. 2. Eukaryotic cells—Congresses. I. Lurquin, Paul F. II. Kleinhofs, Andris. III. Title. IV. Series.
QH442.N36 1983 574.87′322 83-2296

DOI 10.1007/978-1-4684-4493-3

MyCopy version of the original edition 1983

A Division of Plenum Publishing Corporation
233 Spring Street, New York, N.Y. 10013

PREFACE

This book includes the proceedings of a NATO Advanced Study Institute held at Washington State University, Pullman, Washington from July 26 until August 6, 1982.

Although genetic engineering in eukaryotes is best developed in yeast and mammalian cells, the reader will find that some emphasis has been put on plant systems. Indeed, it was our position that the development of plant cell genetic transformation would benefit from the interactions between a comparatively smaller number of fungal and animal cell experts and a larger number of plant cell specialists representing various aspects of plant molecular genetic research. On the other hand, it is clear that the ultimate achievements of plant genetic engineering will have a tremendous impact on, among other things, food production without generating the problems of ethics encountered when one contemplates the genetic modification of human beings.

Therefore, this slight bias in favor of the plant kingdom simply reflects our belief that a "second green revolution" will benefit mankind to a greater extent than any other kind of genetic engineering.

The keynote lecture of the Institute was delivered by Dr. John Slaughter, Director of the National Science Foundation, whom we deeply thank for his words of encouragement and commitment to the genetic manipulation of plants.

This NATO Advanced Study Institute was hosted by the Program in Genetics and Cell Biology and was also sponsored by the National Science Foundation, Biogen, Chevron, the International Plant Research Institute and Monsanto. We thankfully acknowledge the financial assistance of the above mentioned.

Special thanks are also due to W. A. Becker, Program Chairman, and to E. C. Cocking, O. W. McBride and J. Schell for their help organizing this meeting. We also wish to thank F. Semingson and J.

Havens of the Washington State University Conference Office without whom the meeting may not have gone as smoothly as it has. Finally, we thank the faculty, staff and graduate students of the Program in Genetics and Cell Biology as well as all the spouses for their cooperation.

Paul F. Lurquin
Andris Kleinhofs

CONTENTS

TRANSFORMATION IN FUNGI

Mary E. Case

Department of Molecular and Population Genetics

University of Georgia; Athens, GA 30602

INTRODUCTION

Transformation has been a well established process for the transfer of genetic material in procaryotes for a number of years. Recently such a system for lower eucaryotes has been developed for yeast (Beggs, 1978; Hinnen et al., 1978; Beach and Nurse, 1981) and for the filamentous fungus *Neurospora crassa* (Case et al., 1979; Case, 1982). The development of efficient and reproducible systems for both of these organisms was made possible initially by the cloning of genes from both yeast and Neurospora which could be used as donor DNA.

Transformation in any organism involves two basic processes: first, a method to permeabilize the cell wall to permit the uptake of DNA into the cell and secondly, the integration of the DNA stably into a chromosome or its maintenance as a self-replicating entity. These two basic aspects of transformation will be described briefly for fungi.

TRANSFORMATION PROCEDURE

Conditions for DNA Uptake and for Spheroplast Regeneration

For DNA to be taken up by the cell, the cell wall must be permeabilized. In both yeast and Neurospora transformation glusulase is used in the presence of sorbitol as a stabilizing agent for spheroplast formation. Yeast workers have also used zymolyase and lyticase (Hinnen and Meyhack, 1982). Following spheroplast formation and the addition of donor DNA, procedures for both yeast and

Neurospora utilize the $CaCl_2$-polyethylene glycol 4000 (PEG) precipitation procedure developed by Hinnen et al. (1978). Since nuclease degradation of donor DNA seems to be a greater problem in Neurospora than in yeast, certain modifications in the yeast procedure were made to develop an efficient transformation procedure for Neurospora. These major changes in conditions for DNA uptake are listed as follows: a reduction in pH from 7.5 to 6.3 with MOPS buffer (4-morpholineporpane sulfonic acid), 50 mM $CaCl_2$, pretreatment of donor DNA with a nuclease inhibitor such as heparin, the addition of 50 µl of 40% PEG, and 5 µl of DMSO during incubation on ice. Then 40% PEG was added at 25° (Case, 1982). In yeast and Neurospora spheroplast regeneration and the expression of transformants takes place in 3% agar with 1 M sorbitol as an osmotic stabilizer.

Detection of Transformants and Integration of Donor DNA

Putative transformants are detected as colonies on a minimal medium. Although yeast transformation frequencies appear to depend largely on the type of donor plasmid DNA, data from crosses between yeast strains with high and low transformation frequencies suggest that several genetic loci may affect transformation frequencies (Hinnen and Meyhack, 1982). Comparable data are not available for Neurospora. However, the introduction of specific mutations -- a nuclease-less (nuc-1) mutation and two UV sensitive mutations (uvs-2 and uvs-3) -- into the standard recipient strain of Neurospora have no effect on transformation frequencies (Case, unpublished). When plasmids containing a yeast gene, such as $leu\text{-}2^+$, are utilized as donor DNA, transformation occurs at a low frequency of 1-4 transformants/µg DNA (Hinnen et al., 1978). High frequencies of transformation, 10^4 to 10^5 transformants/µg DNA, are observed when chimeric plasmids containing all or part of the yeast 2 µ circle are utilized, with selection for $leu\text{-}2^+$ transformants (Beggs, 1978). The low transformation frequencies are obtained when the donor DNA has integrated into the chromosome while high frequencies indicate the presence of some type of a self-replicating plasmid. In Neurospora experiments giving high transformation frequencies, 10^4 transformants/µg DNA, two types of transformants are observed: those which can continue to grow after transfer to fresh selective medium and those which cannot grow on transfer. The only transformants which have been recovered contain the donor DNA integrated into a chromosome. The high frequency of transformation observed in Neurospora would suggest that the transformants which cannot grow after transfer may be "abortive" transformants containing a slowly self-replicating plasmid which is subsequently lost.

Transformants have been analyzed genetically and by Southern hybridization in both yeast and Neurospora to determine the nature of the integration events (Hicks et al., 1978; Case et al., 1979). In both organisms donor DNA may (1) integrate and replace the recipient mutant gene, (2) integrate adjacent to the recipient gene (observed as a tandem duplication in yeast, Hicks et al., 1978), or (3) integrate at some other site within the genome. Southern hybridization studies indicate that none of the replacement types have plasmid pBR322 sequences integrated, while most of the linked insertion types and the unlinked duplication types frequently have pBR322 sequences integrated along with the donor DNA. Rescue experiments involving transformation back into E. coli with DNA from yeast or Neurospora transformants containing pBR322 sequences indicated that the donor DNA had probably inserted by a Campbell model event (Hicks, 1978; Schweizer, unpublished).

VECTOR SYSTEMS

Cloning Vectors

In the initial experiments in both yeast and Neurospora pBR322, or a close derivative, was used as a cloning vehicle. However pBR322 is not a self-replicating plasmid in either yeast or Neurospora. In yeast the major breakthrough in developing highly efficient cloning vectors was the construction of plasmids containing three different types of autonomously replicating sequences from yeast: a 2 μ circle (Beggs, 1978), an ars sequence (Struhl et al., 1979), and centromeric sequences (minichromosomes, Clark and Carbon, 1980). Although the transformation frequency in Neurospora is high enough to suggest that certain vehicles may contain ars sequences from Neurospora, no stable self-replicating plasmid has yet been constructed. An ars acting sequence from genomic Neurospora DNA has been selected for in yeast (Stinchcomb et al., 1981). However, when a chimeric plasmid containing this ars sequence was used to transform Neurospora, no stable self-replicating vehicle was recovered, as determined by Southern blot analyses (Huiet and Case, unpublished). Mitochondria isolated from some wild strains of Neurospora contain small plasmids (Collins et al., 1981). There is no evidence as yet that a chimeric plasmid containing mitochondrial plasmid sequences will be usable as a self-replicating vector in Neurospora (Lambowitz, personal communication). Mitochondrial plasmid-like DNA isolated from Podospora also has the potential use as a vector in the development of a transformation system for Podospora (Stahl et al., 1982). Since the qa gene cluster is tightly linked to the centromere, it might be possible to clone a centromere from Neurospora and to determine if a centromere vector would replicate in Neurospora as a minichromosome.

Expression of Yeast Genes in Neurospora

With the cloning of a number of yeast genes, it was hoped that these cloned genes (e.g. leu-2$^+$, hist-3$^+$, ura-3$^+$, or trp-1$^+$) might be used either as probes or would have the ability to complement the appropriate recipient strains of Neurospora in transformation experiments. However such experiments have proved to be unsuccessful (Huiet, personal communication).

Expression of Vector Genes in Eucaryotes

Two antibiotic resistance genes from E. coli are expressed in yeast, the chloramphenicol acetyl transferase gene which imparts resistance to chloramphenicol (Cohn et al., 1980) and the aminoglycoside phosphotransferase gene which imparts resistance to the 2-deoxystreptamine antibiotic G418 (Jimenez and Davis, 1980). A chimeric plasmid containing both of these resistance genes along with the $qa\text{-}2^+$ gene was used to transform Neurospora (Case and Vapnek, unpublished). Although transformants were recovered by selection for the $qa\text{-}2^+$ gene, none of these transformants was resistant to the antibiotics on growth tests. Southern hybridization analyses indicated that the plasmid genes are present and presumably unexpressed in the Neurospora transformants (Hughes and Case, unpublished).

SUMMARY

The development of efficient transformation systems for both yeast and Neurospora provides a foundation for the development of such systems for other, comparable organisms. The initial establishment of these systems was greatly aided by the cloning into E. coli plasmids of genes from both yeast and Neurospora which could be used as donor DNA. Cloning technology in Neurospora is not yet as advanced as it is in yeast because of the lack of suitable self-replicating cloning vectors. However, the ability to introduce exogenous DNA into either yeast or Neurospora by transformation will permit a greater understanding of gene organization and regulation in these eukaryotes.

REFERENCES

Beach, D. and Nurse, P., 1981, High frequency of transformation of the fusion yeast Schizosaccharomyces pombe, Nature 290:140-142.

Beggs, J.D., 1978, Transformation of yeast by a replicating hybrid plasmid, Nature, 275:104-108.

Case, M.E., 1982, Transformation of Neurospora crassa, in "Genetic Engineering of Microorganisms," A. Hollaender, R.D. DeMoss, S. Kaplan, J. Konisky, D. Savage, and R.S. Wolfe, ed., Plenum Publishing Corp., New York.

Case, M.E., Schweizer, M., Kushner, S.R., and Giles, N.H., 1979, Efficient transformation of Neurospora crassa utilizing hybrid plasmid DNA, Proc. Natl. Acad. Sci., USA, 76:5259-5263.

Clark, L. and Carbon, J., 1980, Isolation of yeast centromere and construction of functional small circular chromosomes, Nature, 287:504-509.
Cohen, J.D., Eccleshall, T.R., Needleman, R.B., Federoff, H., Buchferer, B.A., and Marmur, J., 1980, Functional expression in yeast of the Escherichia coli plasmid gene coding for chloramphenicol acetyltransferase, Proc. Natl. Acad. Sci., USA, 77: 1078-1082.
Collins, J. and Hohn, B., 1978, Cosmids: A type of plasmid genecloning vector that is packageable in vitro in bacteriophage lambda heads, Proc. Natl. Acad. Sci., USA, 74:4242-4246.
Collins, R.A., Stohl, L.L., Cole, M.D. and Lambowitz, A.N., 1981, Characterization of a novel plasmid DNA found in mitochondria of Neurospora crassa, Cell, 24:443-452.
Hicks, J.B., Hinnen, A., and Fink, G.R., 1978, Properties of yeast transformation, Cold Spring Harbor Symp., Vol. XLIII, 1305-1313.
Hinnen, A., Hicks, J.B., and Fink, G.R., 1978, Transformation of yeast, Proc. Natl. Acad. Sci., USA, 75:1929-1933.
Hinnen, A. and Meyhack, B., 1982, in: "Current Topics in Microbiology and Immunology," W. Henle, H. Koprowski, R. Rott, P.K. Vogt, eds., Springer-Verlag, Berlin Heidelberg, New York.
Jimenez, A. and Davies, J., 1980, Expression of a transposable antibiotic resistance element in Saccharomyces, Nature, 287:869-871.
Stahl, U., Tudzynski, P., Kuck, U., and Esser, K., 1982, Replication and expression of a bacterialmitochondrial hybrid plasmid in the fungus Podospora anserina, Proc. Natl. Acad. Sci., USA, 79: 3641-3645.
Stinchcomb, D.T., Thomas, M., Kelley, J., Selker, E. and Davis, R.W., 1980, Eucaryotic DNA segments capable of autonomous replication in yeast, Proc. Natl. Acad. Sci. USA, 77:4559-4563.
Struhl, K., Stinchcomb, D.T., Scherer, S., Davis, R.W., 1979, High frequency transformation of yeast: autonomous replication of hybrid DNA molecules, Proc. Natl. Acad. Sci., USA 76:1035-1039.

GENE ORGANIZATION AND REGULATION IN *NEUROSPORA CRASSA*. EVIDENCE FROM THE CLONING AND TRANSFORMATION OF THE *QA* GENE CLUSTER

Mary E. Case

Department of Molecular and Population Genetics

University of Georgia; Athens, GA 30602

INTRODUCTION

An analysis of the *qa* gene cluster in Neurospora offers an excellent opportunity for understanding the organization and regulation of a eukaryotic gene cluster. This cluster is involved in the catabolism of quinic acid and encodes three closely linked structural genes, *qa-2*, *qa-3*, and *qa-4*, and a positively acting regulatory gene, *qa-1*, Fig. 1 (Giles et al., 1978). The *qa* gene cluster is very tightly linked to *me-7* on the right arm of LG VII and so far has proved to be inseparable from the centromere. The *qa-2* gene encodes catabolic dehydroquinase; the *qa-3* gene, quinate dehydrogenase; and the *qa-4* gene, 5-dehydroshikimate dehydratase, Fig. 1. The *qa-2* gene was cloned by complementation of an $aroD^-$ strain of *E. coli* which lacks activity for the biosynthetic dehydroquinase (Vapnek et al., 1977). The entire *qa* gene cluster has been cloned on a 19 kb fragment utilizing the cosmid technique (Collins and Hohn, 1980) and selecting for $qa\text{-}2^+$ complementation in *E. coli* (Schweizer et al., 1981). In *E. coli*, only the $qa\text{-}2^+$ gene is expressed. The $qa\text{-}3^+$, $qa\text{-}4^+$ and $qa\text{-}1^+$ genes were detected on the basis of transformation back into Neurospora with these cosmid clones.

The cloning of the *qa-2* gene in *E. coli* permitted the development of an efficient and reproducible transformation system for Neurospora by modifying the $CaCl_2$-polyethylene glycol procedure developed for transformation of yeast by Hinnen et al., 1978. Further modifications of this procedure have resulted in high levels of transformation in Neurospora (Schweizer et al., 1981; Case, 1982). The transformation studies localizing the qa^+ genes on Neurospora DNA cloned into cosmids by selecting for $qa\text{-}2^+$ and $qa\text{-}1^+$ transfor-

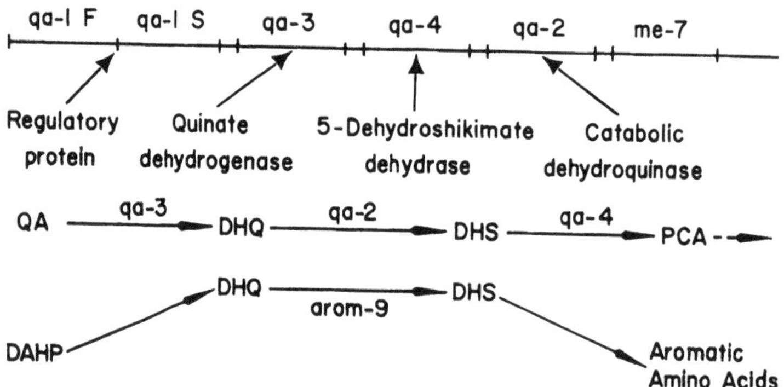

Fig. 1. Gene order in the qa gene cluster in linkage group VII. The methionine-7 (me-7) gene is very closely linked to the qa-2 locus. The relationships of the initial reactions in the inducible quinic acid catabolic pathway with the early reactions in the polyaromatic biosynthetic pathway in Neurospora are indicated below. Abbreviations: QA, quinic acid; DHQ, 5-dehydroquinic acid; DHS, 5-dehydroshikimic acid; PCA, protocatechuic acid.

mants have already been reported (Schweizer et al., 1981). In this discussion, a method selecting for $qa\text{-}3^+$ and $qa\text{-}4^+$ transformants in a liquid medium will be described.

Furthermore, results of transformation experiments with qa-1 and qa-2 mutants employing plasmid subclones containing various regions of the qa gene cluster will be described. This information provides further insights into the organization and regulation of the qa gene cluster in Neurospora. In addition, these studies provide evidence for the mechanism of integration of the donor DNA into the Neurospora genome and its subsequent behavior.

TRANSFORMATION STUDIES

Transformation of the Qa-3 and Qa-4 Genes

Qa mutations cannot grow on quinic acid as a carbon source. Qa-1 and qa-2 mutations, when coupled with an arom-9 mutation, have a requirement for the three aromatic amino acids because such double mutants are blocked in the conversion of DHQ to DHS (Fig. 1) in both the aromatic biosynthetic pathway and in the quinic acid catabolic pathway. The localization of the qa-3^{+} and qa-4^{+} genes was determined originally by selecting for qa-2+ transformants in a multiple mutant recipient strain with defects in each of the three genes, qa-2^{-}, qa-3^{-}, and qa-4^{-}. After recovery of qa-2^{+} transformants, complementation tests on liquid quinic acid medium employing appropriate qa-3^{-} and qa-4^{-} tester strains determined whether the different plasmids also contained the qa-3^{+} and qa-4^{+} genes. To be able to localize the qa-3^{+} and qa-4+ genes more accurately, it became desirable to develop a liquid transformation procedure in order to test plasmids which did not contain a qa-2^{+} gene. Since qa-3^{-} and qa-4^{-} mutants will utilize any carbon source for growth including agar, transformants cannot be selected for in these strains on the usual regeneration agar medium. Certain modifications of the transformation procedure were made to allow regeneration of the cell wall prior to incubation on selective media. After the addition of donor DNA and prior to plating on selective media, the spheroplasts were incubated overnight in a liquid regeneration medium, either 20% sucrose or 20% PEG sorbose-fructose-glucose minimal Fries medium, in order to allow the cell wall to regenerate. After regeneration of the cell wall, the spheroplast suspension was centrifuged, washed with water, added to quinic acid medium, and aliquoted into a number of 13 x 100 mm. test tubes to permit growth. Transformants were detected as cultures able to grow on quinic acid medium after two weeks at 25°. Under these conditions, positive results have been obtained with plasmids known to contain either the qa-4^{+} or qa-3^{+} genes; no transformants were obtained with plasmids known not to contain these genes. This liquid transformation procedure is qualitatative only, but it does permit the localization of these genes to specific regions of the restriction map of the qa gene cluster.

Transformation to Localize the Qa-1 Gene

The qa-1 has been characterized as a complex gene (Case and Giles, 1975). Two different types of qa-1 mutants have been detected on the basis of their complementation responses with qa-2^{-}, qa-3^{-}, and qa-4^{-} mutants. Qa-1^{F} mutants exhibit a rapid complementation response while qa-1^{S} mutants exhibit a very slow complementation response. In addition, certain qa-1^{S} mutants are temperature-sensitive constitutive mutations (qa-1^{C}). At 25° these mutants are unable to grow on quinic acid as a carbon source, but at 35° these mutants can grow in quinic acid and are constitutive for all three *qa* enzyme activities (i.e., they produce high levels of all three activities even in the absence of the inducer quinic acid). In addition, all *qa-1*^{S} mutants revert quite readily to *qa-1*^{C} mutations. The *qa-1*^{S} and *qa-1*^{F} mutations map in discrete regions of the *qa-1* locus (Case and Giles, 1975). It has been hypothesized that the amino acid sequence of the *qa-1*$^{+}$ gene product identified by *qa-1*^{S} mutations is involved in the binding of the *qa-1*$^{+}$ regulatory gene product (activator) to the DNA promoter regions of each of the three *qa* structural genes and that the *qa-1*^{F} mutations identify the amino acid sequence involved in binding the regulatory gene product to the inducer quinic acid. *Qa-1*^{C} mutations, which synthesize high levels of the three *qa* enzymes in the absence of inducer are dominant to wild type in heterokaryons suggesting that regulation of the *qa* gene cluster is positive. Recent DNA-RNA blot hybridization analyses (Patel et al., 1981) indicate that regulation of the *qa* gene cluster is at the level of transcription and that the *qa-1*$^{+}$ gene itself is autoregulated.

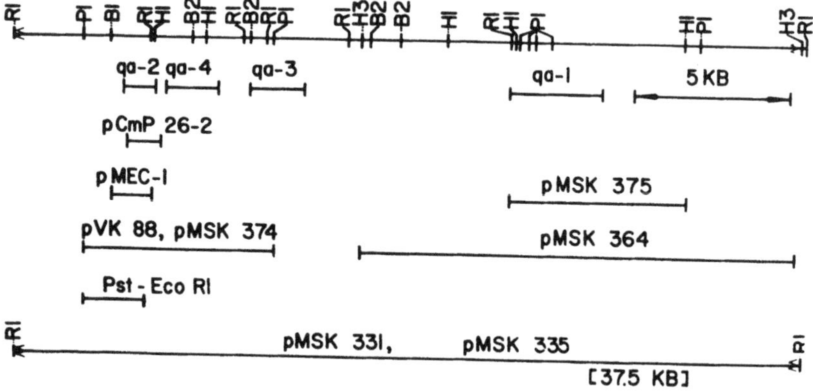

Fig. 2. Restriction endonuclease map of Neurospora DNA in the *qa* gene cluster region. The position of the plasmids used in these studies are indicated below the map. Restriction endonuclease abbreviations: B2, *Bgl* II; H1, *Bam* H1; H3, *Hind* III; P1, *Pst* 1; R1, *Eco* R1.

In the initial transformation experiments with cosmids pMSK331 or pMSK335 (Fig. 2) as donor DNA employing a $qa\text{-}1^F$ recipient strain (M158) many transformants were obtained. In later experiments, subclones of pMSK331 or pMSK335 (Fig. 2) were used in transformation experiments localizing the qa-1+ gene to a 5.5 kb Bam HI fragment (pMSK375 Fig. 2) to the right of the qa-3 gene (Schweizer et al., 1981).

Since all $qa\text{-}1^S$ mutants revert spontaneously to $qa\text{-}1^C$ mutants only $qa\text{-}1^F$ mutants mapping at opposite ends of the $qa\text{-}1^F$ region were used initially as recipients in transformation experiments employing a large 11 kb Hind III subcloned pMSK 364 (Fig. 2). Transformants were obtained with all of these $qa\text{-}1^F$ mutants. Despite the fact that $qa\text{-}1^S$ mutants revert spontaneously, four of $qa\text{-}1^S$ strains were used as recipient strains in transformation experiments with pMSK364 with the hope that transformants would occur at a frequency greater than spontaneous revertants. In these experiments, no transformants were detected. Genetic mapping data indicate that the $qa\text{-}1^S$ region should be adjacent to the qa-3 gene and should be present on this plasmid. This anomaly is being studied extensively by Huiet using additional subclones of this region in transformation experiments. These transformation results will be coupled with DNA base sequence analyses, S1 mapping to mRNA(s), and DNA-RNA blot hybridization analyses. These results should determine whether the $qa\text{-}1^S$ and $qa\text{-}1^F$ mutations occur in two adjacent genes involved in the regulation of the qa gene cluster or whether they occur in two discrete functional regions of the same gene, as originally hypothesized. If the qa-1 region comprises two discrete genes, then an attempt will be made to define more precisely the precise roles of these genes in the regulation of the qa gene cluster.

Transformation Experiments With Qa-2 Mutants Utilizing Plasmid DNA Containing a Qa-2 Gene Having A Terminal Deletion

A plasmid has been constructed (Tyler, personal communication) which contains the presumptive promoter region of the $qa\text{-}2^+$ gene which is in the region between the upstream Pst site and the 5' end of the qa-2 mRNA (Alton et al., 1981) but lacks the qa-2 coding region beyond the EcoRI site near the 3' end of the gene (Fig. 2). Although this plasmid does not complement an $aroD^-$ strain of E. coli, it was used in transformation experiments to determine whether such a plasmid would transform mutants located at opposite ends of the $qa\text{-}2^-$ gene. The assumption was made that positive results with mutants located at one end but not the other, would indicate the orientation of the qa-2 gene with respect to the other qa genes and me-7. No transformants were obtained with qa-2 mutations mapping at opposite ends or in the middle of the qa-2 gene. These results suggest that integration of donor DNA into the qa region of chromosome VII cannot occur by a mechanism that gives rise to a normal $qa\text{-}2^+$ gene (see later section).

Transformation of a Qa-2 Mutant (M246) with Plasmids pCmP26-1, pCmP26-2, and pCmP26-3 Lacking the Qa-2 Presumptive Promoter Region

Alton (personal communication) constructed three different plasmids in which a KpnI-Bam H1 fragment containing 772 bp of Neurospora DNA including the entire coding sequence of the qa-2$^+$ gene was cloned into the Hind III site in pCmP26 (a derivative of pBR322) adjacent to the chloramphenicol transacetylase (CAT) promoter (Fig. 2). This Neurospora DNA fragment is cut at the KpnI site 8 nucleotides proximal to the ATG qa-2$^+$ initiation codon removing the qa-2$^+$ presumptive promoter region. Three different plasmids were obtained -- pCmP26-1 and pCmP26-2 are in orientations A and B, respectively. pCmP26-3 is a tandem duplication of the fragment in orientation A (Alton, personal communication). In orientation A, the qa-2$^+$ gene fragment is inserted such that both the CAT promoter and the qa-2 coding sequence are transcribed in the same direction. In E. coli, only pCmP26-3 was able to complement an AroD$^-$ strain. This result suggested that this tandem repeat of the qa-2$^+$ gene permitted expression in E. coli either because of a ribosome binding sequence generated at the junction of the two qa-2$^+$ genes or because of a gene dosage effect (Alton, personal communication). These three plasmids were used in transformation experiments of the qa-2$^-$ recipient strain (M246) of Neurospora. All three plasmids transformed Neurospora at a relatively low frequency, although transformants occurred at a somewhat higher frequency with plasmid pCmP26-2 than with the other two. Although definitive genetic analyses are not yet complete, Southern hybridization indicates that some of these transformants are complex, and that some contain pBR322 sequences. The nature of the integration of the donor DNA into the N. crassa genome in these transformants should prove to be quite interesting.

GENETIC CHARACTERISTICS OF QA-2$^+$ TRANSFORMANTS DERIVED FROM PLASMID pVK88

How Does Donor DNA Integrate into the Neurospora Genome?

Transformants have been obtained utilizing donor DNA from a wide variety of plasmids and also utilizing several different recipient strains, e.g., qa-2$^-$ mutants, qa-1$^-$ mutants, and a multiple mutant strain qa-2$^-$, qa-3$^-$ qa-4$^-$. A discussion of studies on the integration and subsequent behavior of donor DNA in these transformants will be confined to transformants obtained with plasmid pVK88 DNA. pVK88 was one of the first qa-2$^+$ plasmids cloned in E. coli. This plasmid carries a 7.2 kb Pst-I fragment of Neurospora DNA which contains complete sequences for the qa-2$^+$ and qa-4$^+$ genes and partial sequences for the qa-3$^+$ and qa-x$^+$ genes (Patel et al., 1981). (Two additional messages, qa-x and qa-y, for genes under quinic acid regulation have been detected by RNA-DNA hybridization with poly(A)mRNA (Patel et al., 1981). No mutants have been isolated for these genes.) Although the qa-4$^+$ gene is apparently present on this plasmid, this gene is not expressed upon transformation into Neurospora. An identical Pst I subclone (pMSK374) obtained from wild type Neurospora (Fig. 2), does carry an active qa-4$^+$ gene detected by transformation into Neurospora (Schweizer et al, 1981). Studies of this plasmid and its integration into the genome of Neurospora will lay a foundation for later studies of other plasmids and recipient strains.

Since the conidia of Neurospora are often multinucleate, initial transformants are typically heterokaryotic. Hence all transformants were crossed to the closely linked gene me-7 to obtain homocaryotic isolates. Tetrad analyses have been performed on many of these crosses. Twenty-eight homokaryotic transformants obtained with donor DNA from plasmid pvK88 have been characterized genetically and by Southern hybridization analyses. These transformants were classified into three different types (Case et al., 1979): 1) replacement types in which the qa-2$^-$ gene was replaced by a qa-2$^+$ gene; 2) linked insertion types in which the qa-2$^+$ gene had inserted adjacent to the qa-2$^-$ gene and caused the inactivation of qa-4$^+$ gene; and 3) unlinked duplication types in which the qa-2$^+$ gene had inserted at a site in the genome either unlinked to, or not closely linked to, the qa-2 region. Southern hybridization analyses indicated that none of the replacement types, one of the two linked insertion types, and six of the seventeen unlinked insertion types contained pBR322 sequences integrated along with the qa-2$^+$ gene. pBR322 sequences integrated into the Neurospora genome replicate and segregate in a Mendelian manner.

When the original non-homokaryotic isolates were grown for Southern hybridization analyses, different results were obtained with respect to the presence of pBR322 sequences and to the presumptive classification of the transformants as replacement or unlinked duplication types. Of the nine replacement types, four were classified identically both as homokaryotic and heterokaryotic isolates. As heterokaryotic isolates, the other five replacement types not only contained pBR322 sequences, but would have been classified by Southern hybridization analyses as unlinked duplication types. One of the linked insertion types, as a heterokaryotic isolate, not only contained pBR322 sequences (transformant 6-2, Case et al., 1979) but also had multiple bands suggesting that this transformant could most easily be interpreted as having resulted from multiple transformation events. In the cross of the heterokaryotic transformant to me-7$^-$ more than one transformant type was obtained, i.e. a linked insertion type and an unlinked duplication type (Case unpublished). Five of the unlinked duplication types showed no differences between the homokaryotic and heterokaryotic isolates, while the other twelve transformants showed differences between heterokaryotic and homokaryotic isolates in the numbers and sizes of bands on Southern gels.

This variability of transformants as homokaryotic and heterokaryotic isolates had not been anticipated, in particular the variation in the presence of pBR322 sequences. All three types of homokaryotic transformants are mitotically stable. However, the differences observed between heterokaryotic and homokaryotic isolates suggest that there is instability following integration of donor DNA during either mitosis or meiosis. The homokaryotic replacement types may result from some type of "gene conversion" event or by a two-strand double crossover which occurred during mitosis or meiosis, changing an unlinked duplication type as a heterokaryotic isolate to a replacement type, as a homokaryotic isolate. Specific and frequent "conversion-like" events are known to occur during mitosis in the switching of the MAT genes in yeast whereby one or the other of the MAT genes is replaced by the silent mating type cassette with the replaced mating type gene being lost from the genome (Rine et al., 1980). One way to determine if gene conversion has occurred in the origin of replacement type transformants would be to clone the $qa\text{-}2^+$ gene from the heterokaryotic isolate of a replacement type transformant and to determine the restriction pattern of the flanking regions. If the restriction pattern in the flanking regions of the cloned $qa\text{-}2^+$ gene differs from the normal pattern observed for the recipient $qa\text{-}2^-$ gene, then these results would favor the "gene conversion" hypothesis for the origin of homokaryotic replacement type transformants. If two different types of $qa\text{-}2^+$ genes could be cloned from the heterokaryotic isolate, one having the normal restriction pattern of the qa-2 gene region (indicative of a replacement type transformant) and the other an altered restriction pattern (indicative of an unlinked duplication type transformant), then one could conclude that such heterokaryotic transformants probably resulted from multiple transformation events. Such multiple events are possible since the germinated spheroplasts contain several nuclei.

Previously, the origin of replacement type transformants in both yeast and Neurospora has been hypothesized to involve a two-strand double crossover event including pairing and subsequent recombination between the plasmid and the chromosome (Hinnen et al., 1978; Case et al., 1979). If a two-strand double crossover is involved in the origin of replacement type transformants, then why are $qa\text{-}2^+$ transformants not obtained with the Pst-EcoR1 plasmid containing a $qa\text{-}2^-$ gene with a partial terminal deletion, especially when mutants mapping near the middle of the qa-2 gene are used as recipient strains? Prototrophs are readily obtained in conventional genetic analyses of crosses between qa-2 mutants (Case et al., 1977). The origin of prototrophs in allelic crosses has been postulated to occur by gene conversion. However, if all prototrophs obtained in crosses of qa-2 mutants are the result of gene conversion events, then the fixed recombination points involved in the conversion event may be outside the qa-2 gene itself. The data with the Pst-EcoEl plasmid would support this hypothesis. If a two-strand double crossover event is involved in the origin of the replacement type transformants, then the two sites involved in the crossover event must be outside the qa coding region. If one of the sites for the recombination event had been within the qa-2 gene, then transformants should have been obtained with the Pst-EcoRl plasmid. If both sites are outside the coding region, then recombination between this Pst-EcoRl plasmid would have resulted only in a defective transformant (qa-2$^-$) which would not have been detected. If this plasmid had inserted by a single crossover, either as a linked insertion type or as an unlinked duplication type, no functional qa-2$^+$ gene would be obtained.

Another hypothesis for integration of donor DNA into a chromosome has been by the Campbell model. This model requires pairing between homologous regions of the cloned Neurospora DNA on the plasmid and the DNA of the recipient chromosome followed by insertion of the entire plasmid including the qa-2$^+$ gene into the Neurospora chromosome by a single crossover event. Evidence for this hypothesis comes from a plasmid rescue experiment of one of the unlinked transformant types containing pBR322 sequences (Schweizer et al., unpublished). The recombination event occurred in the region between qa-4 and qa-3. The linked insertion type transformants have been interpreted as resulting from insertion of the entire plasmid by a single crossover event near the qa-2$^-$ gene giving rise to a gene duplication. If pairing and recombination occurred between the qa-2$^+$ and qa-2$^-$ genes, then this could result in the loss of pBR322 sequences as well as sequences leading to the inactivation of the qa-4$^+$ gene. Tetrads which may have resulted from an event of the type just described, were obtained from the two linked insertion type transformants. One transformant contained isolates which were qa-2$^+$ qa-4$^-$, and the other transformant contained isolates which were qa-2$^-$ qa-4$^-$. In the second transformant the recombination event apparently eliminated the qa-2$^+$ gene and also inactivated the qa-4 gene. The origin of these two types of isolates from the transformants would depend on where the plasmid inserted near the qa-2$^-$ region, how the two qa-2 genes paired, and how the DNA, including the pBR322 sequences, was excised.

Does Donor DNA Integrate into Neurospora in the Same Manner as in Yeast?

In yeast and Neurospora donor DNA can integrate into the genome either at the same region as the recipient allele or at unlinked sites within the genome. Are then the same types of transformants observed in both of these organisms? Three different types of transformants have been obtained which probably originate by the same mechanisms and are comparable in both organisms (Hinnen et al., 1979; Case et al., 1979). Unlike yeast, however, the two unlinked insertion type transformants which have been obtained in Neurospora are stable and do not segregate out $qa\text{-}2^-$ isolates mitotically. This may be due to differences in the growth habit of the two organisms and to the fact that Neurospora transformants are heterokaryotic as isolated and require crossing before analysis.

Into How Many Different Sites Has the $Qa\text{-}2^+$ Gene Integrated During Transformation?

Integration of $qa\text{-}2^-$ donor DNA into various sites within the genome presumably involves some homology between the donor DNA cloned in *E. coli* and the Neurospora genomic sites at which integration occurs, either at the normal region on LG VII or at other sites within the genome. Neurospora DNA isolated from the transformants was cut with Xho and probed with the ^{32}P labeled plasmid pMEC1 DNA (Fig. 2). The following different band sizes in addition to the normal *qa-2* band at 7.9 kb were observed in Southern hybridization analyses: 2.5, 3.3, 4.8, 6.0, 7.1, 9.5, 10.2, 11.3, 13, and 15 kb. These results indicated that a minimum of five different integration sites are involved since the four largest bands and the 4.8 kb band contain pBR322 sequences in addition to the $qa\text{-}2^+$ gene. The other sites which do not contain pBR322 sequences may be derivatives of these five sites and result from the excision of pBR322 sequences. The 11.3 kb band is present in 11 of the transformants, suggesting that this is the predominant site for integration of donor DNA.

The insertion of pYeleu10 into various sites within the yeast genome has been interpreted on the basis of the presence of a repeated sequence in the $leu\text{-}2^+$ DNA on the plasmid which has homology to various regions in the genome (Kingsman et al., 1981). A similar interpretation presumably must be true in Neurospora to account for the ability of the $qa\text{-}2^+$ gene on pVK88 to integrate at several different sites within the Neurospora genome.

Further Evidence for Meiotic Instability and Gene Conversion in Tetrads

As indicated previously, tetrads from crosses of transformants to $me\text{-}7^-$ were dissected in order to obtain homokaryotic isolates. Tetratype asci obtained from crosses of unlinked duplication type transformants were analyzed further. The $qa\text{-}2^+$ $me\text{-}7^+$ isolates were crossed to $me\text{-}7^-$ to confirm that the $qa\text{-}2^+$ gene was still segregating independently of the *qa* region and methionine on LG VII. The $me\text{-}7^-$ isolates were crossed to either a $pan\text{-}2^-$ strain or to a qa-2^{-} strain to determine which of the me-7^{-} isolates contained a duplication of the qa-2 gene. If a me-7^{-} isolate contained a duplication of the qa-2^{+} gene then in crosses to the qa-2^{-} strain the me-7^{+} isolates should segregate in a 1:1 ratio of qa-2^{+} and qa-2^{-}, and all me-7^{-} isolates should be qa-2^{+}. However, in random ascospore analyses, certain of the me-7^{-} isolates segregated in a 1:1 ratio of me-7^{-} qa-2^{+} and me-7^{-} qa-2^{-}. The appearance of me-7^{-} isolates that were qa-2^{-} was totally unexpected because of the very tight linkage between the qa-2 and me-7 genes. Southern hybridization analyses and the genotype of the isolates from such a tetratype ascus (ascus number two from transformant 5-2) which showed unexpected segregation in further crosses are given on Table 1. Isolate 2.1 grows on quinic acid as a carbon source and contains a duplication of the qa-2 gene (qa-2^{+} unlinked and qa-2^{-}, in the normal region), indicated by bands 6 and 7.9, respectively. Isolate 2.4 cannot grow on quinic acid, contains only one qa-2 gene (qa-2^{-}) and has a single normal 7.9 band. Isolate 2.5 is methionine-requiring, and contains a duplication of the qa-2 gene (bands 6 and 7.9). Isolate 2.7 is methionine-requiring, contains only one qa-2 gene (qa-2^{+}), and has a normal band at 7.9. Southern hybridization analyses do not indicate whether a qa-2 gene is a functional qa-2^{+} gene. Subsequent genetic analyses with isolate 2.5 in crosses to a qa-2^{-} me-7^{+} strain indicated that the me-7^{-} isolate segregated in a 1:1 ratio of me-7^{-} qa-2^{+} and me-7^{-} qa-2^{-}. Further genetic analyses of the me-7^{-} qa-2^{-} isolates in crosses to a pan-2 allele (pantothenic acid-requiring) indicated that the qa-2^{-} gene

TABLE 1 Segregation Pattern in Ascus Number Two Isolated from a Cross of Unlinked Duplication Type Transformant 5-2 (qa-2^{+} me-7^{+}) x (qa-2^{+} me-7^{-}).

Ascus Isolate No.	Growth on Quinic Acid	No. Qa-2 Genes	Genotype of Isolates: Qa-2[a] Gene	Genotype of Isolates: Me-7[b] Gene	Band[c] Sizes
2.1	+	2	qa-2^{+}	qa-2^{-} me-7^{+}	6, 7.9
2.4	-	1		qa-2^{-} me-7^{+}	7.9
2.5	+	2	qa-2^{+}	qa-2^{-} me-7^{-}	6, 7.9
2.7	+	1		qa-2^{+} me-7^{-}	7.9

[a] qa-2 gene unlinked to me-7
[b] qa-2 gene linked to me-7
[c] Southern hybridization analyses. Neurospora DNA cut with Xho and hybridized with ^{32}P labeled plasmid pMEC1 DNA (Fig. 2).

was inseparable from the $me\text{-}7^-$ gene. Consequently, the band containing the functional $qa\text{-}2^+$ gene, which segregates independently from $me\text{-}7^-$, is the 6 kb band, and the band at the normal position at 7.9 is now a $qa\text{-}2^-$ gene.

The most reasonable interpretation for the origin of the $qa\text{-}2^-$ $me\text{-}7^-$ isolates is by a very specific "gene conversion" event which has changed the normal $qa\text{-}2^+$ gene adjacent to $me\text{-}7^-$ to a $qa\text{-}2^-$ isolate. This type of event is not rare and occurs frequently in tetratype ascus isolates derived from crosses of unlinked duplication type transformants (Case, unpublished). One further anomaly observed in Southern hybridization analyses of one of the $me\text{-}7^-$ $qa\text{-}2^-$ isolates (5-2-2.5-10), was the detection of two bands, one at the normal position, 7.9, and the other at 6 kb. Since this isolate is now $qa\text{-}2^-$, it was anticipated that only one band would be observed representing the $qa\text{-}2^-$ gene linked to $me\text{-}7^-$. The question now is whether the qa-2 gene at the 6 kb site is $qa\text{-}2^-$ also or is a silent gene. Genetically, it is not feasible to answer this question. In crosses to wild type having a normal $qa\text{-}2^+$ gene in LGVII $qa\text{-}2^+$ segregants would be dominant to any $qa\text{-}2^-$ gene segregating independently. In crosses to a $qa\text{-}2^-$ mutant in LG VII all segregants with two $qa\text{-}2^-$ genes would still be mutant in phenotype. If in a rescue experiment in E. coli, a $qa\text{-}2^+$ gene from such a transformant isolate can be cloned by complementation with an aroD mutant and the flanking regions indicate that this gene is unlinked to the qa gene cluster then the hypothesis that the unlinked $qa\text{-}2^+$ gene is silent would be correct. If a $qa\text{-}2^+$ gene cannot be cloned from such an isolate, then one can only conclude that the unlinked qa-2 gene is now $qa\text{-}2^-$ and may have arisen at the same time as the gene conversion event which gave rise to the $qa\text{-}2^-$ gene adjacent to $me\text{-}7^-$.

Ascus isolate 5-2-2.5 just described does contain a duplication of the qa-2 gene; however, genetic analyses indicate that one gene is qa-2 (linked to $me\text{-}7^-$) while the other is $qa\text{-}2^+$ (unlinked). On the basis of conventional meiotic segregation this isolate should contain two $qa\text{-}2^+$ genes. At the present time no ascus isolate has been found which does contain two $qa\text{-}2^+$ genes. Why are there no isolates with two $qa\text{-}2^+$ genes as expected? Why does some preferential type of "gene conversion" event apparently take place during meiosis which specifically changes one of the $qa\text{-}2^+$ genes (the one adjacent to me-7) to a $qa\text{-}2^-$ gene? These questions still remain to be answered. Perhaps additional genetic analyses of transformants with other plasmids will provide insight into this problem.

Will the Transformant Types Obtained from pVK88 Be Typical?

Since the $qa\text{-}2^+$ transformants obtained from pVK88 are the only transformants which have been analyzed extensively, only analyses of transformants from other $qa\text{-}2^+$-containing plasmids or from other cloned genes will determine whether the three types of transformants as classified by the nature of the integration events of donor pVK88 DNA will be the same for all plasmids and for all genes. It will be interesting to determine whether qa-2$^+$ transformants from pMEC-1 which contains a 1.2 kb fragment -- the smallest fragment which transforms the qa-2 gene -- will give rise to replacement type transformants only. Only replacement type transformants were obtained for the his-3 gene in yeast (Hicks et al., 1978). The only additional information concerning the integration of donor DNA into the Neurospora genome comes from tetrad analyses of transformants of an inositolless mutant from experiments utilizing total Neurospora DNA. These genetic analyses indicated that meiotic instability was common and that the integration of donor DNA could occur in more than one region of the genome (Szabo and Schablik, 1982).

These transformation experiments with qa mutants utilizing plasmids containing various regions of the qa gene cluster provide further information on the organization and regulation of the qa gene cluster. In addition genetic analyses of transformants have provided evidence for the mechanism of integration of the donor DNA into the Neurospora genome and its subsequent behavior.

ACKNOWLEDGEMENTS

The author thanks Joann Lay, Robert Geever, and Paulette Geever for valuable technical assistance with some of the experiments. I also thank Dr. Norman H. Giles for critical reading of the manuscript. This research was supported in part by grants from the National Institutes of Health Grant GM2877 (to Norman H. Giles) and by National Science Foundation Grant PCM-7910911 (M.E.C. and Norman H. Giles).

REFERENCES

Alton, N.K., Buxton, F., Patel, V., Giles, N.H., and Vapnek, D., 1982, 5' untranslated sequences of two structural genes in the qa gene cluster of *Neurospora crassa*, *Proc. Natl. Acad. Sci.*, 79:1955-1959.

Case, M.E., 1982, Transformation of *Neurospora crassa*, *in* "Genetic Engineering of Microorganisms," A. Hollaender, R.D. DeMoss, S. Kaplan, J. Konisky, D. Savage, and R.S. Wolfe, ed., Plenum Publishing Corp., New York.

Case, M.E. and Giles, N.H., 1975, Genetic evidence on the organization and action of the qa-1 gene product: a protein regulating the induction of three enzymes in quinate catabolism in *Neurospora crassa*, *Proc. Natl. Acad. Sci.*, USA, 72:553-557.

Case, M.E., Hautalia, J.A., and Giles, N.H., 1977, Characterization of qa-2 mutants in Neurospora crassa by genetics, enzymatic, and immunological techniques, Bacteriol. 129:166-172.

Case, M.E., Schweizer, M., Kushner, S.R. and Giles, N.H., 1979, Efficient transformation of Neurospora crassa utilizing hybrid plasmid DNA, Proc. Natl. Acad. Sci., USA, 76:5259-5263.

Giles, N.H., Alton, N.K., Case, M.E., Hautala, J.A., Jacobson, J.W., Kushner, S.R., Patel, V.B., Reinert, W.R., Strøman, P., and Vapnek, D., 1978, The organization of the qa gene cluster in Neurospora crassa and its expression in Escherichia coli, 1978 Stadler Genetics Symposia, 10:47-63.

Hicks, J.B., Hinnen, A., and Fink, G.R., 1978, Properties of yeast transformation, Cold Spring Harbor Symp., Vol. XLIII, 1305-1313.

Hinnen, A., Hicks, J.B., and Fink, G.R., 1978, Transformation of yeast, Proc. Natl. Acad. Sci., USA, 75:1929-1933.

Kingsman, A.J., Gimlich, R.L., Clarke, L., Chinault, A.C., and Carbon, J., 1981, Sequence variation in dispersed repetitive sequences in Saccharomyces cerevisiae, J. Mol. Bio. 145:619-632.

Patel, V.B., Schweizer, M., Dykstra, C.C., Kushner, S.R., and Giles, N.H.., 1981, Genetic organization and transcriptional regulation in the qa gene cluster of Neurospora crassa, Proc. Natl. Acad. Sci., 78:5783-5787.

Rine, J., Jensen, R., Hagen, D., Blair, L. and Herskowitz, I., 1980, Pattern of switching and fate of the replaced cassette in yeast mating-type interconversion, Cold Spring Harbor Symposium, 78: 951-960, Vol. 2.

Schweizer, M., Case, M.E., Dykstra, C.C., Giles, N.H. and Kushner, S.R., 1981, Identification and characterization of recombinant plasmids carrying the complete qa gene cluster from Neurospora crassa including the qa-1^{+} regulatory gene, Proc. Natl. Acad. Sci., 78:5086-5090.

Szabo, G. and Schablik, M., 1982, Behavior of DNA-induced inositol-independent transformants of Neurospora crassa in sexual crosses, Theor. Appl. Genet., 61:171-175.

Vapnek, D., Hautala, J.A., Jacobson, J.W., Giles, N.H., and Kushner, S.R., 1977, Expression in Escherichia coli K-12 of the structural gene for catabolic dehydroquinase of Neurospora crassa, Proc. Natl. Acad. Sci., 74:3508-3512.

USE OF TRANSFORMATION AND MEIOTIC GENE CONVERSION TO CONSTRUCT A YEAST STRAIN CONTAINING A DELETION IN THE ALCOHOL DEHYDROGENASE I GENE

V. M. Williamson*, D. Beier#, and E. T. Young#

*ARCO Plant Cell Research Institute
6560 Trinity Court
Dublin, California 94568

#Department of Biochemistry
University of Washington
Seattle, Washington

INTRODUCTION

Techniques have been developed using *in vitro* mutagenesis and yeast transformation to alter the genetic material of the yeast *Saccharomyces cerevisiae* (1). Features of the yeast system which make this possible include the following: the availability of selectable markers; the ease of transformation of yeast with exogenous DNA; the integration of DNA into yeast chromosomes by homologous recombination; and the ease of genetic manipulation of yeast cells. As an illustration of some of the features of the yeast system, we describe the construction of a yeast strain which contains a deletion of the 5' end of the alcohol dehydrogenase I (ADHI) gene (*ADC1*) of yeast. Deletions are, in general, rare events in yeast so the ability to introduce *in vitro* created deletions into the yeast genome is quite useful.

Alcohol dehydrogenase (E.C. 1.1.1.1. ADH) is responsible for the final step in the conversion of glucose to ethanol during fermentative growth of yeast. The three electrophoretically distinct isozymes of ADH in yeast, ADHI, ADHII, and mADH are coded for by three unlinked genes, *ADC1*, *ADR2* and *ADM*, respectively (2, 3). ADHI is the major activity present when cells are grown on glucose containing medium. ADHII is repressed in the presence of glucose and derepressed on nonfermentable carbon sources such as ethanol or glycerol. The third isozyme, mADH, is a minor species localized in the mitochodria. ADC1 and ADR2 proteins cross-react immunologically but can be distinguished by peptide cleavage (4). Cloning and sequencing of ADC1 and ADR2 (5, 6, 7, 8) reveal that the two genes are very homologous: about 95% of the amino acid sequence is concerved and about 90% of the nucleic acid sequence is identical. DNA sequence data indicates that a 150 bp stretch of identity exists between the two RNA's.

Because of the homology between ADC1 and ADR2, analysis of ADR2 regulation has been difficult. Dennis et al. (4) have used *in vitro* translation followed by immunoprecipitation and peptide cleavage to show that the level of translatable mRNA increases under derepression. The two mRNA species can also be distinguished by SI nuclease mapping which is described later in the text. However, both techniques are cumbersome and a strain which produces no ADC1 mRNA is very desirable. Mutations in ADC1 have been isolated by classical genetic techniques (2) but these are probably point mutations as ADC1 mRNA and inactive protein are detected (4).

Mutations at several loci affect ADR2 regulation and expression (2, 3, 9); also ADC1 and ADR2 containing plasmids which have been altered *in vitro* have been constructed (10). To allow us to measure ADR2 mRNA expression in mutant strains without interference from the homologous ADC1 mRNA, we report here construction of a yeast strain which has the 5' end of the ADC1 gene deleted and does not produce any ADC1 mRNA. Scherer and Davis (1) had developed an elegant technique called transplacement for the replacement of a chromosomal segment in yeast with an altered DNA sequence. This technique involves yeast transformation with integration of a plasmid containing the altered yeast sequence and a selective marker such as the URA3 gene by homologous recombination. Analysis of transformed yeast cells which have lost the marker after non-selective growth showed that about 50% of these strains contained the altered gene and had lost the vector sequences and the original chromosomal copy of the gene by recombination.

To produce an ADHI$^-$ yeast strain we first constructed a plasmid carrying a deletion of the 5' end of the ADC1 gene. This plasmid was used to transform yeast containing the wild-type ADC1 gene and directed to integrate at the wild-type ADC1 gene to yield yeast cells containing both the wild-type and altered ADC1 gene. Our attempts to excise vector and the intact ADC1, leaving behind the altered ADC1 gene, were not successful so an alternative strategy to isolate an ADC1-deletion was pursued as follows: Since transfer of information from one gene to a repeated copy of that gene on the same chromosome (i.e., intra-chromosomal gene conversion) occurs frequently during meiosis (11, 12), we crossed our transformed haploid yeast strain to another yeast strain containing the wild-type ADC1 gene. Analysis of the sporulation products of this diploid identified a yeast strain which contained two copies of the 5'-deleted gene. Meiotic gene conversion (11) is a frequent event and this technique may be useful for incorporating *in vitro* constructed mutations into the genome in cases where the mutation places the organism under a growth disadvantage or where recombination to delete the wild-type copy does not readily occur.

RESULTS

Construction of an ADC1 deletion in vitro

The ADC1 gene codes for the enzyme ADHI, the major isozyme of alcohol dehydrogenase which is present when yeast cells are grown in the presence of glucose (2). This gene has been cloned from a yeast genomic DNA pool in plasmid YRp7 by complementation of a mutation in the ADC1 gene (adc1-11) after transformation of yeast (5). We constructed a plasmid, YIpID36, containing the ADC1 region with a deletion extending from 1400 bp upstream from the ADC1 coding region to 40 bp within the structural gene. Two plasmids, pY9T5 (5) and pTF (10) containing yeast DNA inserts from the ADC1 region were used to construct this deletion. Figure 1 outlines the construction of plasmid YIpID36. Briefly the DNA fragment which extends from 1400 to about 4000 bp upstream from the ADC1 structural gene was modified and isolated as described in the legend to Figure 1. A second fragment which extends downstream from a SalI site 40 bp within the structural gene for ADC1 and includes the 3' end of the gene as well as some non-coding region 3' to the structural gene was prepared as described in the legend to Figure 1. These two fragments were ligated together to produce a DNA fragment which contains a modified ADC1 region. This yeast DNA fragment was inserted into the vector plasmid YIP5 (1) to produce the plasmid YIpID36 shown in Figure 1. Plasmid YIP5, which contains bacterial plasmid pBR322 sequences and a yeast fragment containing the URA3 gene, is capable of complementing a yeast mutation in URA3 after transformation of the defective yeast strain, but only if integrated into the yeast genome.

Yeast transformation and meiotic gene conversion

Plasmid YIpID36 described above was used to transform a yeast strain (M12) containing a deletion of the ura3 gene (1). Transformed yeast strains become URA^+ when the plasmid is

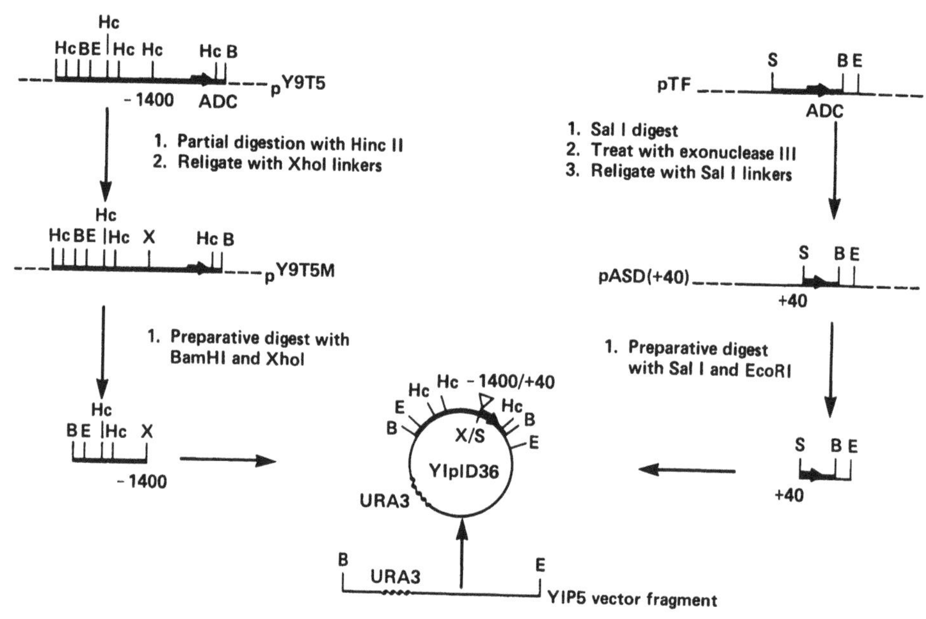

Figure 1. Construction of the ADC1-deletion mutation *in vitro*. The heavy arrow represents the ADC1 gene and the arrow indicates the direction of transcription. The heavy lines represent yeast sequences, thin lines represent bacterial vector sequence and the jagged line represents the yeast URA3 gene. Restriction enzyme cleavage sites are designated as follows: HincII (Hc); BamHI (B); EcoRI (E); XhoI (X); and SalI (S). The ADC1 containing plasmid pY9T5 (4) was partially digested with the restriction enzyme HincII to produce about one cut per molecule. The molecules were ligated in the presence XhoI linkers and used to transform *E. coli*. *E. coli* containing plasmid pY9T5M were identified as described by Beier and Young (10). The fragment extending from about 1400 to about 4000 bp upstream from the ADC1 structural gene was preparatively isolated from this plasmid. Plasmid pTF which also contains ADC1 (10) was cut at a SalI site upstream from the gene, treated with exonuclease III to delete from this restriction site. The molecules were ligated in the presence of SalI linkers and used to transform *E. coli*. Plasmid pASD (+40) which is deleted about 40 bp into the structural gene for ADC1 was isolated. Conditions for creation of this deletion are detailed elsewhere (10). The BamHI-EcoRI fragment of plasmid YIP5 (1) was isolated and ligated with the two DNA fragments described above to produce plasmid YIpID36.

integrated into the yeast genome by homologous recombination. Since restriction enzyme cleavage of a site within the region of plasmid DNA homologous to chromosomal DNA greatly increases the frequency of plasmid integration and directs integration into the homologous chromosomal sequence (13), we transformed the yeast with plasmid YIpID36 which had been linearized by partial digestion with the enzyme HindIII (see Figure 2). DNA was isolated from six stable URA+ transformants by the method of Denis (14), cleaved with BamHI, and analyzed by Southern transfer and hybridization with an ADC1 containing probe (Figure 3). In each case at least one copy of the plasmid has integrated into the yeast genome. Comparison of the intensity of the bands indicates that in four out of six cases, more than one copy of the plasmid has become integrated into the yeast genome. The conserved sizes of the fragments suggests that these are tandem copies at the ADC1 locus.

A general method for replacement of chromosomal segments with altered DNA sequences constructed *in vitro* has been described by Scherer and Davis (1). In their experiments, Ura- colonies were produced at a relatively high frequency (about 1% after 10 generations of growth) due to deletion of the plasmid by homologous recombination between adjacent yeast sequences. The recombination event is accompanied by loss of either the wild-type or *in vitro* mutated DNA sequences. Attempts to isolate ADC1 deletion mutants from the YIpID36 integrants by this process were not successful. Because yeast strains which are defective in ADC1 expression grow much more slowly on medium containing a fermentable carbon source such as glucose, Ura- strains were selected after growth on medium containing the non-fermentable carbon source glycerol. Ura- colonies appeared at a much lower frequency than 1%. Of 1800 colonies screened, only four were Ura-. All four were positive for ADC1 activity. Furthermore, ureido-succinic acid selection (15) for Ura- cells was not successful. The reasons for the failure to obtain adc1-deletions by this method were not clear but possibilities include: 1) homologous recombination is inhibited in this region of the genome or 2) the growth rate of the deletion is so poor that even on a non-fermentable carbon source such as glycerol it is out-competed by the strain carrying the wild-type gene.

To circumvent the two problems mentioned above we decided to attempt to convert the wild-type ADC1 gene to the copy containing the mutated gene by intrachromosomal gene conversion as illustrated in Figure 2. Intrachromosomal gene conversion, in which information from one gene is non-reciprocally transferred to a repeated copy of that gene on the same chromosome, has been shown to occur in yeast (11, 12). The frequency of meiotic

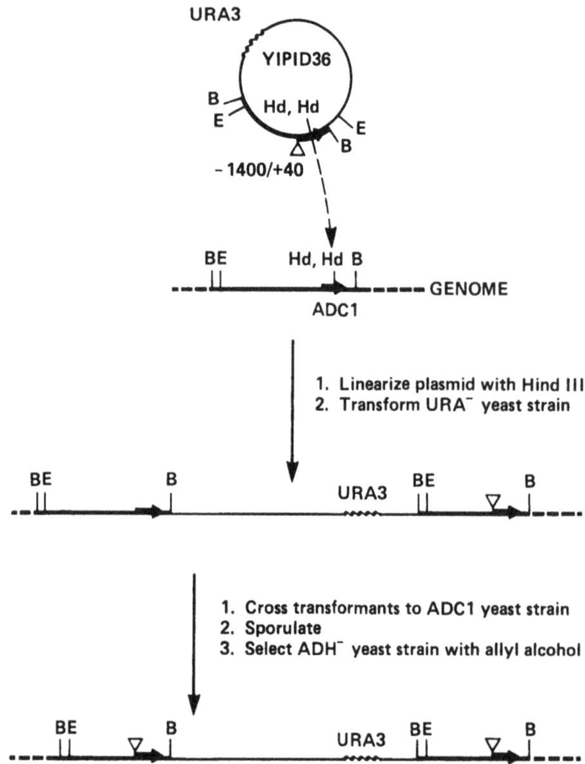

Figure 2. Construction of the deletion-containing yeast strain using gene conversion. Symbols used here are the same as those described in the Figure 1 legend. Plasmid YIpID36 was linearized by partial cleavage with the restriction enzyme HindIII. This linearized plasmid was used to transform an $ADHI^+$ Ura^- yeast strain essentially as described by Beggs (19). Stable transformants were shown to contain the wild-type ADC1 gene, the vector, and the deletion-containing ADC1 gene. Transformants were mated to ADC1-containing yeast strains (309-51 or 309-108) to produce diploids. After meiosis, a strain in which the wild-type ADC1 gene was converted by non-reciprocal DNA exchange to the deleted form was isolated by its ability to grow on allyl alcohol containing plates (2).

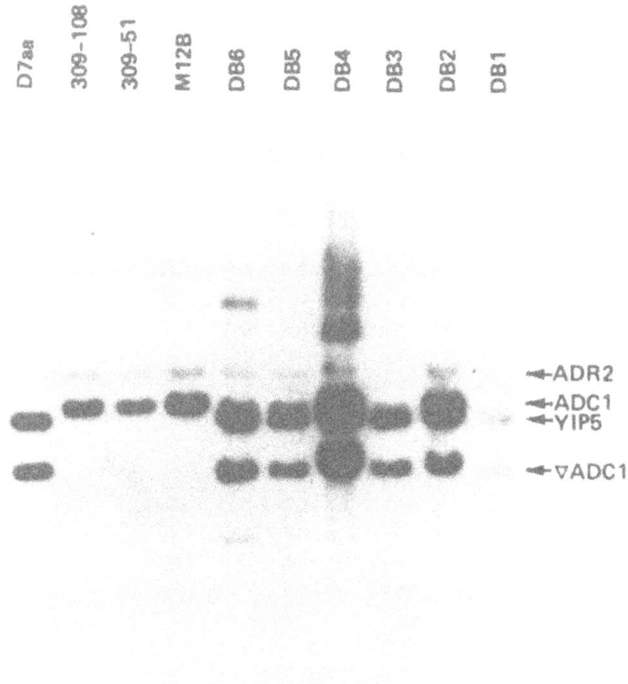

Figure 3. Southern blot analysis of yeast genomic DNA. DNA was isolated from the following yeast strains: six transformants which had become Ura$^+$ due to integration of plasmid YIpID32 (DB1-DB6); the Ura$^-$ parent before transformation (M12B); the strains used for the meiotic gene conversion (309-51 and 309-108); and D7aa. DNA from these strains was cleaved with BamHI, electrophoresed in an agarose gel, transferred to nitrocellulose and hybridized with a cloned ADC1 fragment in pBR322 (JD14, Ref. 7). Shown is an autoradiograph of the labeled bands. The identity of the bands is indicated on the right.

intrachromosomal gene conversion has been determined for an arrangement of two LEU2 genes, one mutant and one wild-type, separated by plasmid sequence. Analysis of unselected yeast tetrads indicated that in about 2% of the tetrads intrachromosomal gene conversion resulting in two mutant leu2 genes had occurred (11). A similar conversion frequency was observed with a simlar construct of HIS4 genes at the HIS4 locus (12). We hoped that this high frequency would allow us to select for strains carrying two copies of the adc1 deletion as shown in Figure 2. Individual spores from tetrads can be separated and grown individually to produce single colonies. Thus the problem of competition with non-converted cells would be avoided.

The yeast strains carrying the integrated deletion were crossed to strains which carried wild-type ADC1 gene but have the opposite mating type from the transformants. The diploids from the cross were sporulated to form tetrads then treated with gluculase to separate individual spores. The spores, which had undergone meiosis and were haploid, were allowed to germinate and form individual colonies on non-selective plates. These were then replica-plated onto allyl alcohol-containing plates which permit growth of only those strains which express no ADH activity (2). Such strains appeared at a frequency of about one percent. One such colony which we called D7aa was analyzed further. DNA was isolated from this strain which resulted from a cross of DB1 to a strain (309-51; unpublished) with a wild-type ADC1 gene. Southern analysis of the DNA from this strain revealed that the fragment containing the wild-type ADC1 gene was missing from this strain, but one or more copies of the vector and ADC1 deletion containing DNA segment were still present (Figure 3).

Properties of adc1-deletion strain, D7aa

ADH activity assays (4) of D7aa extracts showed no detectable ADH activity under any conditions. Parent 309-51 of the yeast cross used to obtain D7aa lacks ADHII activity due to a mutation in the structural gene ADR2, and this adr2 allele appears to be present in D7aa. D7aa grows very slowly on glucose containing medium with a generation time of about six hours as compared to about two hours for wild-type strains. Cell morphology appears normal and the strain has a Ura^+ phenotype. As mentioned earlier, ADC1 and ADR2 mRNA's share homology and are approximately the same size. We have used SI nuclease protection experiments as described below to differentiate between ADC1 and ADR2 mRNA's (16, 17, 18). This procedure involves hybridization of a 5' end labeled single-stranded DNA fragment containing the

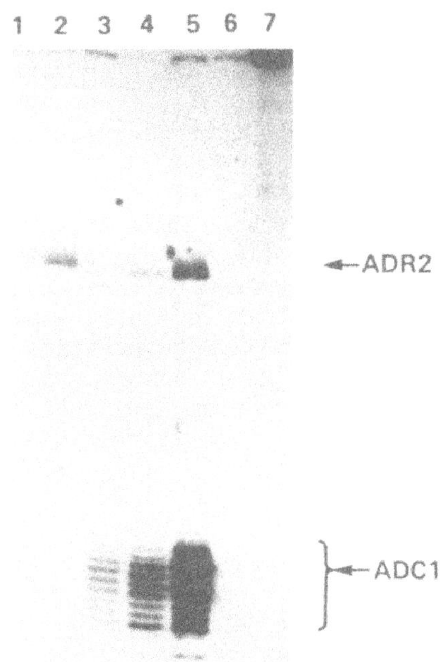

Figure 4. Determination of ADC1 and ADR2 transcripts by SI nuclease mapping. A single stranded DNA fragment (17) with its 5'-end within the structural gene for ADR2 and its 3' end 170 bp upstream from the ADR2 coding region was labeled at its 5'-end with P^{32} and hybridized to total yeast RNA. Molecules were hybridized and treated with SI nuclease as described by Nasmyth et al. (18), denatured in 90% formamide and analysed on an 8% polyacrylamide sequencing gel. Lane 1 uses 5μg of total RNA from strain D7aa grown on glucose. Lane 2 uses 5μg of D7aa RNA from cells grown on ethanol. Lanes 3, 4 and 5 contain 2.5, 5, and 20μg, respectively, of RNA from a wild-type strain grown on ethanol containing medium. Lane 6 is a no RNA control and Lane 7 shows the labeled DNA fragment before treatment with SI nuclease.

5' flanking region and some coding region of the ADR2 gene to total yeast RNA. Hybridization is followed by digestion with the single-strand specific nuclease SI and the sizes of the protected fragments are analysed on a DNA sequencing gel. The size of the fragment protected by ADR2 mRNA is longer than that protected by ADC1 mRNA due to non-homology of ADR2 DNA with regions in the 5' untranslated portion of the ADC1 RNA. Results of this type of SI analysis indicate that as expected no RNA is produced corresponding to the 5' coding region of ADC1 in strain D7aa. Northern gel analysis which would detect any mRNA transcripts hybridizing to ADC1 also showed no transcripts from this gene (C. Denis, unpublished).

Strain D7aa, which lacked both ADHI and ADHII activities, was crossed to strain 7972C which contained both activities. Tetrad analysis of the progeny from this cross showed 2:2 segregation of $ADHI^+$:$ADHI^-$. This indicated that the converted gene segregated normally. Also 2:2 segregation also occurred at the ADR2 locus. Thus strains which contain the adc1 deletion and a wild-type copy of the ADR2 gene can be obtained.

DISCUSSION

By *in vitro* mutagenesis, yeast transformation, and meiotic gene conversion we were able to produce a yeast strain which has a deletion and therefore lacks detectable ADC1 transcripts. This mutant strain contains at least two, and probably more, copies of the defective gene as well as at least one integrated copy of vector YIP5. Nevertheless, this strain will be very useful for studying ADR2 gene regulation without interference from homologous ADC1 gene products. The effects of a true ADHI-null i.e., a strain completely lacking ADHI protein, on yeast growth and metabolism are also under investigation.

The method described here should be of general interest to others who wish to create yeast strains containing alterations which would or may cause them to compete poorly with strains carrying the wild type gene. Unlike the transplacement procedure where cells are grown non-selectively for many generations, the altered cells (in this case spores) are separated immediately after the alteration event and are not required to compete with cells containing the wild-type genes. If the recombination event required to delete the wild-type copy is restricted in some regions of the chromosome, meiotic gene conversion would also be a useful alternative technique. The frequency of meiotic gene conversion is high enough (approximately 2%) so that _in vitro_ mutations which carry an unknown phenotype could be screened for directly in cases where restriction site polymorphism or deletions are produced. For example, when deletions are produced, the convertants could be detected by yeast colony hybridization (20) using the deleted fragment as a probe and screening for non-hybridizing colonies.

ACKNOWLEDGEMENTS

We thank Bob Simpson for critical reading of this manuscript and Karen Long for typing.

This work was partially done while V. M. Williamson was a National Institutes of Health Postdoctoral Fellow at the University of Washington. This research was also supported by a Research Grant from the National Institutes of Health (GM-26079) at the University of Washington. D. Beier is a predoctoral student in the University of Washington Medical Scientist Training Progam (GM-07266).

REFERENCES

1. S. Scherer and R. W. Davis, Replacement of chromosomal segments with altered DNA sequences constructed _in vitro_, _Proc. Nat. Acad. Sci._, USA 76:4951-4955(1979).
2. M. Ciriacy, Genetics of alcohol dehydrogenase in _Saccharomyces cerevisiae_. I. Isolation and genetic analysis of _adh_ mutants, _Mutation Research_ 29:315-326(1975).
3. M. Ciriacy, Genetics of alcohol dehydrogenase in _Saccharomyces cerevisiae_. II. Two loci controlling synthesis of the glucose repressible ADHII. _Mol. Gen. Genet._ 138:157-164(1975).
4. C. L. Denis, M. Ciriacy, and E. T. Young, A positive regulatory gene is required for accumulation of the functional messenger RNA for the glucose-repressible alcohol dehydrogenase from _Saccharomyces cerevisiae_, _J. Mol. Biol._ 148:355-368(1981).
5. V. M. Williamson, J. Bennetzen, E. T. Young, K. Nasmyth, and B. D. Hall, Isolation of the structural gene for alcohol dehydrogenase by genetic complementation in yeast. _Nature_ 283:214-216(1980).

6. V. M. Williamson, E. T. Young, and M. Ciriacy, Transposable elements associated with constitutive expression of yeast alcohol dehydrogenase II, Cell 23:605-614(1981).
7. J. L. Bennetzen and B. D. Hall, The primary structure of the Saccharomyces cerevisiae gene for alcohol dehydrogenase I, J. Biol. Chem. 257:3018-3025(1982).
8. D. W. Russell, V. M. Williamson, E. T. Young, and M. Smith, Nucleotide sequence of the yeast alcohol dehydrogenase II gene, manuscript in preparation.
9. M. Ciriacy, Isolation and characterization of further cis- and trans-acting regulatory elements involved in the synthesis of glucose-repressible alcohol dehydrogenase (ADHII), Mol. Gen. Genet. 176:427-431(1979).
10. D. R. Beier and E. T. Young, Characterization of a regulatory region upstream of the ADR2 locus of S. cerevisiae, submitted.
11. H. L. Klein and T. D. Petes, Intrachromosomal gene conversion in yeast, Nature 289:144-148(1981).
12. J. A. Jackson and G. R. Fink, Gene conversion between duplicated genetic elements in yeast, Nature 292:306-311(1981).
13. T. L. Orr-Weaver, J. W. Szostak, and R. J. Rothstein, Yeast transformation: a model system for the study of recombination, Proc. Nat. Acad. Sci. USA 78:6354-6358(1981).
14. M. Ciriacy and V. M. Williamson, Analysis of mutations affecting Ty-mediated gene expression in Saccharomyces cerevisiae. Mol. Gen. Genet. 182:159-163(1981).
15. C. T. Korch, F. Lacroute, F. Exinger, A regulatory interaction between pyrimidine and purine biosynthesis via ureido succinic acid, Mol. Gen. Genet. 133:63-75(1974).
16. A. J. Berk and P. A. Sharp, Spliced early mRNAs of similar virus 40, Proc. Nat. Acad. Sci. U.S.A., 75:1274-1278(1978).
17. V. M. Williamson, D. Cox, E. T. Young, D. W. Russell, and M. Smith, Characterization of transposable element-associated mutations that alter yeast alcohol dehydrogenase II expression, submitted.
18. K. A. Nasmyth, K. Tatchell, B. D. Hall, C. Astell, and M. Smith, Physical analysis of mating-type loci in Saccharomyces cerevisiae, Cold Spring Harbor Symp. Quant. Biol. 45:961-981(1980).
19. J. D. Beggs, Transformation of yeast by a replicating hybrid plasmid, Nature 275:104-108(1978).
20. A. Hinnen, J. B. Hicks, and G. R. Fink, Transformation of yeast, Proc. Nat. Acad. Sci. USA, 75:1929-1933(1978).

TRANSFORMATION AND STORAGE OF COMPETENT YEAST CELLS

M. R. Altherr[1], L. A. Quinn[1], C. I. Kado[2] and R. L. Rodroguez[1]

Davis Crown Gall Group[2]
Departments of Genetics[1] and Plant Pathology[2]
University of California
Davis, California 95616 USA

Since the transformation of yeast was first demonstrated using hybrid plasmids[1], several procedures have been developed which allow yeast to be transformed with plasmid DNA[1,2,3]. A new transformation procedure has been recently developed (K. Murata, in press) which represents a radical departure from previously published methods. This procedure employs lithium acetate instead of exogenous enzymes (i.e. glusulase, lyticase, zymolyase) to make yeast cells competent for transformation. As a result of this and other changes, yeast can be transformed more rapidly and more reproducibly. Furthermore, the time required for the detection of transformants is dramatically reduced. We have adapted this procedure to allow the storage of competent yeast cells for up to 2 weeks at -70°C without significant loss of transformation efficiency.

MATERIALS AND METHODS

Strains. The *Saccharomyces cerevisiae* strains 21D and 2490-6d were used in this study. Strain 21D (*mat* α *leu*2-3 *leu*2-112 *his*4 *lys*1) was obtained from J. D. Cohen. Strain 2490-6D (*mat* α *ura*3 *leu*2-3 *leu*2-112 *his*3) was obtained from S. R. Snow.

Plasmid DNA. Purified pEP101 DNA (Close et al. in preparation) was a generous gift of T. J. Close. Plasmid pEO201 contains a 600 bp fragment containing the yeast 2 μ origin of DNA replication[4] and the yeast *leu*2 gene cloned into the EcoRI and HindIII sites of pBR329[5], respectively. This plasmid allows the detection of both yeast and *E. coli* transformants.

Plasmid DNA was prepared for transformations by the Triton mini-screen[6] or the alkaline-SDS Froman method[7].

Transformation or yeast. The following has been adapted from the procedure of K. Murata.

1. Yeast were grown to stationary phase in 5 ml of YEPD medium (1% Difco Yeast Extract, 2% Difco peptone, 2% glucose). A fresh 50 ml culture was innoculated with 0.05 ml of the stationary phase culture. This culture was incubated at 30 C with aeration until an A_{600} of 1.5 to 2 was reached.

2. Cells were harvested by centrifugation in a table-top centrifuge and the cell pellet washed twice with 10 ml of TE buffer (10 mM TRIS-HCl, 0.1 mM EDTA, pH=7.5).

3. The cells were resuspended in 5 ml of a 0.1 M solution of lithium acetate in TE. The cell suspension was incubated 1 hour at 30°C with agitation.

4. The competent cells were harvested by centrifugation and resuspended in an equal volume of 0.1 M lithium acetate in TE containing 15% glycerol. The cells were dispensed in 0.5 ml aliquots into sterile plastic tubes and stored at -70°C. When needed, aliquots were thawed and the transformation continued.

5. 0.3 ml of competent cells was added to a sterile eppendorf tube containing 10 µl (0.1-10 µg) of plasmid DNA.

6. 0.7 ml of a 50% solution of polyethylene glycol (PEG4000) was added, the tube was inverted three times, then incubated at 30°C for 1 hour.

7. Following this incubation, the cells were heated to 42°C for 5 minutes and then plated directly on minimal medium (Difco Yeast Nitrogen Base without amino acids, supplemented with auxotrophic requirements). Yeast transformants were selected as leucine prototrophs.

RESULTS AND DISCUSSION

The viability and transformation efficiency of the competent cells was examined after 1, 3, 5, 7, and 14 days of storage at -70°C. No loss of viability was observed over this period, and the efficiency of transformation remained relatively constant ($>10^2$ transformants per µg of pEP101 DNA for strain 2490-6d). When plasmid DNA was purified from the transformed yeast cells and analyzed with restriction endonucleases, the DNA was indistinguishable from the DNA used in the transformation. These results indicate that yeast cells made

Table I. Transformation Efficiency

Strain	Plasmid DNA	Source	μgs	Transformation Frequency[a]
21 D	pEP101	Pure[b]	0.1	$>10^3$
2490-6d	pEP101	Pure[b]	1.0	$>10^2$
2490-6d	pEO201	Miniscreen[c]	<1.0	$>10^1$
2490-6d	pEO201	Miniscreen[d]	<1.0	10^1

[a]Transformation frequency was determined as the number of prototrophic colonies growing after 72 h per μg plasmid DNA used in the transformation.

[b]Plasmid DNA was prepared by the cleared lysate/phenol-neutral chromatography procedure described by Close and Rodriquez (in press).

[c]Triton-miniscreen procedure (6).

[d]Froman-miniscreen procedure (7).

competent with lithium acetate can be stored for up to 2 weeks without altering the nature of the transformation or reducing the efficiency of transformation.

While developing this method for storing competent yeast cells, several other parameters were examined. We examined the effects of dimethylsulfoxide (DMSO) and $CaCl_2$ on the transformation efficiency by including these compounds in the PEG solution. While the presence of DMSO had little effect on the transformation efficiency, $CaCl_2$ appeared to inhibit transformation slightly. DNA purified by several different methods was also used with this transformation procedure, and although transformation efficiencies were highest with purified supercoiled plasmid DNA, transformants were obtained with DNA purified by two miniscreen methods (see Table I). As shown in Table I, the efficiency of transformation may vary with the strain of yeast being transformed. The strain 21D consistently exhibited a 10-fold greater transformation efficiency than the strain 2490-6d.

The lithium acetate transformation procedure as modified to allow the storage of the competent cells has several advantages over previous yeast transforamtion procedures. Competent cells can be easily prepared and stored to allow routine transformations of yeast. Transformants can be detected as small colonies after only 36 hours of incubation at 30°C. Transformation efficiencies are relatively high, although there is a definite strain dependency, and it is not necessary to use extensively purified DNA for transformation.

We would like to acknowledge K. Murata, whose work on the lithium acetate transformation method was originally presented as a poster at the Fourth Internation Symposium on Genetics of Microorganisms.

REFERENCES

1. A. Hinnen, J. B. Hicks, and G. R. Fink, Proc. Natl. Acad. Sci. (USA) 75:1929-1933 (1978).
2. J. D. Beggs, Nature 275:104-109 (1978).
3. K. Struhl, D. T. Stinchcomb, S. Scherer, and R. W. Davis, Proc. Natl. Acad. Sci. (USA) 76:1035-1039 (1979).
4. J. R. Broach, and J. B. Hicks, Cell 21:501-508 (1980).
5. L. Covarrubias, and F. Bolivar, Gene 17:79-89 (1982).
6. R. B. Meagher, R. C. Tait, M. Betlach, and H. W. Boyer, Cell 10:521-536 (1977).
7. R. C. Tait, R. C. Lundquist, and C. I. Kado, Mol. Gen. Genet. 186:10-15 (1982).

DNA TRANSFER INTO ANIMAL CELLS

Axel C. Garapin and Florence Colbère-Garapin

Biologie Moléculaire du Gène et Virologie Médicale

Institut Pasteur - 75724 Paris Cédex 15 - France

The introduction or the reintroduction of cloned genes into eukaryotic recipients is somewhat of a paradox. It is often necessary to check the functional integrity of a cloned cDNA or chromosomal gene, or to study the expression of a gene normally in the repressed state. The complementation of defective animal cells can be studied *in vitro* by gene transfer.

OBTENTION OF GENE TRANSFER INTO ANIMAL CELLS

Several methods are available to transfer DNA into cells of higher eukaryotes. We will briefly describe some of them.

Liposomes, phospholipids bilayer membrane vesicles encapsulate a water phase which can trap RNA or DNA. The liposomes fuse their lipid membrane to the cell membrane and the genetic material can penetrate inside the cell (Papahadjopulos et al., 1974). Fraley et al. (1980) have succesfully introduced SV 40 DNA into animal cells. The efficiency will have to be optimized for its use in animal cells.

The calcium-phosphate technique (Graham and Van der Ebb, 1973) allows, by gravity sedimentation of the nascent calcium precipitate, the trapping of DNA and its cellular penetration. The transformation efficiency (T.E.) is very much cell dependent. The T.E. varies for the high efficiency LM TK^- from 1000-5000 colonies/μg of plasmid, when using carrier DNA, to 25-100 colonies/μg of plasmid without carcier, for 10^6 cells.

The DEAE-dextran method according to Milman and Herzberg (1981) would allow the transient expression of thymidine kinase at a much higher efficiency than the permanent expression.

The fusion of bacterial protoplasts (Schaffner, 1980 ; Sandri-Goldin et al., 1981 and Rassoulzadegan et al., 1982) to eukaryotic cells with polyethylene glycol (PEG) is a high efficiency system. The T.E. may be as high as 10 % of the cells and more. One does not have to extract the plasmid DNA and choramphenicol can be used to amplify the plasmids in the bacteria. It is obviously a method of choice that can be used on plant cells, for PEG has already been used to fuse plant spheroplasts.

Finally, it has been shown that the microinjection of DNA (Graessmann and Grausman, 1980 ; Capecchi, 1980) is also a powerful method. The DNA material can be delivered in known amounts into the nuclei and the transient expression of herpes simplex virus thymidine kinase (HSV TK) can vary from 50 % to 100 % of the injected cells. The permanent expression is a 100 times lower (Capecchi, 1980). It should also be a system usable to transfect plant cells once immobilized (by surface antisera p.e.).

VECTORS

In many cases, the transfected DNA is merely a recombinant plasmid with little or no replication autonomy. However, a higher efficiency of expression is obtained by linking a gene to the regulating sequences of papovavirus DNA. Small DNA fragments (about 2500 bp) can be linked to the promoter of the late region of SV 40, the splice region and the polyeadenylation signal sequence. The expression can thus be amplified in this lytic system 100.000 times and a progeny virus can be obtained if a helper virus is provided (Mulligan and Berg, 1979 ; Gruss and Khoury, 1981).

Larger segments of DNA can also be inserted precluding encapsidation. This system then uses the high expression level promoter born by SV 40 DNA. The recombinant plasmid can thus be expressed in murine cells or in simian cells at will. A maximum efficiency of expression will however be attained in *Cos* cells. They are simian cells transformed by an origin defective SV 40 DNA and they produce the T antigen (Gluzman, 1981). *Cos* cells replicate plasmid carrying an SV 40 origin or replication.

An elegant system has been established by Mocarski et al. (1980) whereby the gene to be studied is inserted in the TK gene of an HSV-TK bearing plasmid. After cotransfection with HSV DNA and the now TK^- plasmid, recombination takes place in the cell and HSV-TK^- viruses are selected in the presence of ara T. Most of the TK^- viruses thus selected have recombined through the TK sequences. In theory this HSV vector could carry 7-8000 bp.

Lastly one form of viral vector, the bovine papilloma virus (BPV) DNA exists in the cell as a circular autonomous form (10-120 copies/cell) (Sarver et al., 1981). In this vector, the size of the integrated is not critical (Law et al., 1981). The recombinant vectors are not integrated and can be used to transform E. coli if they have the proper bacterial plasmid properties (Shuttle vector : Di Maio et al., 1982).

SELECTABLE MARKERS

Kit and Dubbs (1963), Munyon et al. (1971), Wigler et al. (1977) have been active in demonstrating the existence of HSV TK and the feasibility of transfecting mouse TK^- cells to the TK^+ phenotype. The TK gene has been cloned in pBR322 (Colbère-Garapin et al., 1979). This marker has been used extensively for selecting cells that have been transformed to the TK^+ phenotype and have also acquired a new phenotype (cotransfection, see below).

The dominant selectable markers have the great advantage to allow the selection of transformed cells of any kind or species devoid or not of genetic defect. Mulligan and Berg (1980) have linked a bacterial gene for xanthine-guanine phosphoribosyl transferase (XGPRT or Eco gpt) onto SV 40 early promoter, leader and intron region and have cloned $XGPRT^+$ cells of different animal species in the presence of mycophenolic acid which blocks the purine biosynthesis pathway leading to the xanthine monophosphate formation. This forces the cells to use the added xanthine if the bacterial enzyme is expressed. O'Hare et al. (1981) have similarly cloned a bacterial dihydrofolate reductase on an SV 40 plasmid. The high level of enzyme produced allows a resistance to methotrexate in LTK^- cells.

We have cloned (Colbère-Garapin et al., 1981) a bacterial transposon which codes for the resistance to an antibiotic (G-418). The gene coding for the enzyme is under the dependance of the HSV TK promoter (see chapter in this volume).

A third type of selectable markers exists : it consist in an amplifiable dominant selectable marker. Dihydrofolate reductase is such a marker. Such an enzyme is blocked by methotrexate and to escape the block the cell increases the gene copy number (Alt et al., 1978). The eukaryotic gene itself cannot be used (40 kb) but its cDNA (Lee et al., 1981) linked to the 5' of the long terminal repeat of MMTV and born or an SV 40 plasmid is regulated by glucocorticoids and is amplifiable in chinese hamster ovary cells (CHO) $DHFR^-$. It has not been shown to be a dominant marker as yet. The amplifiable gene coding for the multifunctional enzyme aspartate transcarbamylase (CAD) is 25 kb in length and behaves as a dominant marker by selection in one step at high concentration of the inhibitor N-(phosphonacetyl-L-aspartate) (PALA) (Wahl et al., 1979). Its mRNA is 8500 nucleotides long which is a little cumbersome for a plasmid. Moreover, hamster cells become spontaneously resistant to PALA at a frequency of 10^{-5}, some more convenient marker or plasmid has to come.

DISCUSSION

It is now widely accepted that foreign genes introduced into eukaryotic are integrated into the chromosomal DNA. There are two consecutive phases if expression takes place. First, a transient phase which is usually operative 1-4 days after transfection. This may, or may not, be followed by a permanent expression if integration has occurred. The permanent expression can be fairly stable even in the absence of selection pressure (our unpublished experiments).

Perucho et al. (1980) have shown that cotransfection in murine cells of two different genes is usually followed by the formation of a "pekalasome" which is integrated in one locus with the result that the two genes will be closely linked on the same chromosomal segment. The consequence of this discovery has been widely used to screen for cells doubly transformed by a selectable and a non selectable genes. As a general rule, the regulating sequences of a DNA (sequences for glucocorticoid regulation, for cadmium regulation, promoter, etc.) are kept in a functional state and can be used to improve expression (Lee et al., 1981).

Another promising aspect of gene transfer is that of the transplantation of genetic material into the male pronucleus of mouse zygote. Evidence has been obtained that genes (TK, β-globin) can be introduced by microinjection in the male pronucleus and integration takes place. If the zygote develops into a full adult, the foreign gene is expressed and can be transmitted to the offspring in a mendelian distribution (Wagner et al., 1981 ; Costantini and Lacy, 1981 ; Brinster et al., 1981 ; Rusconi and Schaffner, 1981).

Besides the reasons alluded to in the introduction, a future direction of work should be the establishment of recombination to the locus of foreign gene to help to promote complementation of genetic defects in cells or in the animal.

REFERENCES

Alt, F., Beatino, R. and Schink R.T., 1978, Selective multiplication of dihydrofolate reductase genes in methrothrexate resistant variants of cultured murine cells - J. Biol. Chem., 253 : 1357.

Brinster, R.L., Chen, H.Y., Trumbauer, M., Senear, A.W., Warren, R. and Palmiter, R.D., 1981, Somatic expression of herpes thymidine kinase in mice following infection of a fusion gene into eggs - Cell, 27 : 223

Capecchi, M.R., 1980, High efficiencyl transformation by direct micro-injection of DNA into cultured mammalian cells - Cell, 22 : 479.

Colbère-Garapin, F., Hordonicean, F., Kourilsky, P. and Garapin, A.C., 1981, A new dominant hybrid selective marker for higher eukaryotic cells - J. Mol. Biol., 150 : 1.

Colbère-Garapin, F., Chousterman, S., Horodniceanu, F., Kourilsky, P. and Garapin, A.C., 1979, Cloning of the active thymidine kinase gene of herpes virus simplex type I in <u>E. coli</u> K12 - Proc. Natl. Acad. Sci., U.S.A., 76 : 3755.

Costantini, F. and Lacy, E., 1981, Introduction of a rabbit β-globin gene into the mouse germ line - Nature (London) 294 : 92.

Di Maio, D., Treisman, R. and Maniatis, L., 1982, Bovine papilloma-virus vector that propagates as a plasmid in both mouse and bacterial cells - Proc. Natl. Acad. Sci., U.S.A., 79 : 4030.

Fraley, R., Subramani, S., Berg, P., and Papahadjopoulos, D., 1980, Introduction of liposome encapsulated SV 40 DNA into cells - J. Biol. Chem., 255 : 10431

Gluzman-Yakov, 1981, SV 40 transformed simian cells support the replication of early SV 40 mutants - Cell : 23 : 175.

Graessmann, M. and Graessmann, A., 1976, Early simian virus 40 specific RNA contains information of tumor antigen formation and chromatin replication - Proc. Natl. Acad. Sci., U.S.A., 77 : 7380.

Graham, F.L. and Van der Eb, A., 1973, A new technique for the assay of infectivity of human adenovirus 5 DNA - Virology, 52 : 456.

Gruss, P. and Khoury, G., 1982, Gene transfer into mammalian cells : use of viral vectors to investigate regulatory signals for the expression of eukaryotic genes - Current Topics in Microbiol. and Immunol., 96, Henk, W., Ed. - Springer Verlag, Berlin.

Kit, P. and Dubbs, D.R., 1963, Acquisition of thymidine kinase activity by herpes simplex infected mouse fibroblast cells - Biochem. Biophys. Res. Commun., 11 : 55.

Lee, F., Mulligan, R., Berg, P. and Ringold, G., 1981, Glucocorticoids regulate expression of dihydrofolate reductase cDNA in mouse mammary tumor virus chimaeric plasmids - Nature (London) 294 : 228.

Millman, G. and Herzberg, M., 1981, Efficient DNA transfection and rapid assy for thymidine kinase activity and viral antigenic determinants - Somat. Cell. Genet., 7 : 161.

Mulligan, R.C., Howard, B.H. and Berg, P., 1979, Synthesis of rabbit β-globin in cultured monkey kidney cells following infection with a SV 40 β-globin recombinant genome - Nature (London) 277 : 108.

Munyon, W., Kraiselburd, E., Davis, D. and Mann, J., 1971, Transfer of thymidine kinase to thymidine kinaseless L cells by infection with ultraviolet irradiated herpes simplex virus - J. Virol., 7 : 1971.

Mocarski, E., Post, L.E. and Roizman, B., 1980, Molecular engineering of the herpes simplex virus genome insertion of a second L-S function into the genome causes additional genome inversions. Cell, 22 : 243.

Papahadjopoulos, D., Mayhow, E., Poste, G., Smith, and Vail, W.J., 1974, Incorporation of lipid vesicles by mammalian cell provides a potential method for modifying cell behavior - Nature (London) 252 : 163.

Perucho, M., Hanahan, D. and Wigler, M., 1980, Genetic and physical linkage of exogeneous sequences in transformed cells - Cell, 22 : 309.

O'Hare, K., Benoist, C. and Breathnach, R., 1981, Transformation of mouse fibroblasts to methrotrexate resistance by a recombinant plasmid expressing a prokaryotic dihydrofolate reducatase - Proc. Natl. Acad. Sci., U.S.A., 78 : 1527.

Rassoulzadegan, M., Binetruy, B. and Cuzin, F., 1982, High frequency of gene transfer after fusion between bacteria and eukaryotic cells - Nature (London) 295 : 257.

Rusconi, S. and Schaffner, 1981, Transformation of frog embryos with a rabbit β-globin gene - Proc. Natl. Acad. Sci., U.S.A., 78 : 5051.

Sandri-Goldin, R., Goldin, A., Levine, M. and Glorioso, J.C., 1981, High frequency transfer of cloned herpes simplex virus type 1 sequences to mammalian cells by protoplast fusion - Mol. Cell. Biol., 1 : 743.

Schaffner, W., 1980, Direct transfer of cloned genes from bacteria to mammalian cells - Proc. Natl. Acad. Sci., U.S.A., 77 : 2163.

Sarver, N., Gruss, P., Law, M.F., Khoury, G. and Howley, P.M., 1981, Bovine papillomavirus deoxyribonucleic acid : a novel eukaryotic cloning vector - Mol. Cell. Biol., 1 : 486.

Wagner, E.F., Stewart, T.A. and Mintz, B., 1981, The human β-globin gene and a functional viral thymidine kinase gene in developing mice - Proc. Natl. Acad. Sci., U.S.A., 78 : 5016.

Wahl, G.M., Padjett, R.A. and Stark, G.R., 1979, Gene amplification causes overproduction of three enzymes of UMP in N-(phosphonacetyl)-L-aspartate resistant hamster cell - J. Biol. Chem., 254 : 8679.

Wigler, M., Silverstein, S., Lee, L.S., Pellicer, A., Cheng, Y.C. and Axel, R., 1977, Transfer of purified herpes virus thymidine kinase gene to cultured mouse cells - Cell, 11 : 223.

THE DOMINANT SELECTIVE MARKER APH 3' AND THE STUDY OF THE EXPRESSION OF THE COTRANSFECTED GENE

Axel C. Garapin, Philippe Kourilsky, Florian Horodniceanu and Florence Colbère-Garapin

Biologie Moléculaire du Gène et Virologie Médicale
INSTITUT PASTEUR - 75724 Paris Cédex 15 - France

Molecular cloning and genetic engineering often lead to the assay of the biological properties and of the molecular integrity of purified clones of DNA. The reintroduction of cloned DNA material into a living eukaryotic cell should allow such a verification. Once the methodology for amplifying the DNA (usually through a bacterial plasmid) and for insuring the penetration of the DNA into the cell (transfection of a bacterial plasmid only or of a vectored eukaryotic recombinant) has been achieved, the discrimination of the cells that harbour or express the foreign gene must be brought about. A certain number of selective markers have been developed. The herpes simplex virus thymidine kinase (HSV TK) cloned in pBR322 (Colbère-Garapin et al., 1979 ; Bolivar et al., 1977) has been the first of such markers to be expressed in thymidine kinase defective (TK^-) cells. An important aspect of such transfection has been the discovery, by Perucho et al. (1980) that when two genes are transfected together into a cell, they are integrated via a "pekalasome" at the same locus on a chromosome. This allows, with the help of a selective medium, the survival of cells which often coexpress the marker gene and the recombinant gene.

One of the drawbacks of the HSV TK marker is the obligation of using TK^- cells. The use of the dominant selective markers recently engineered can solve this problem. O'Hare et al. (1981) have cloned a prokaryotic dihydrofolate reductase and used it to induce resistance to methotrexate in mouse cells. Another bacterial gene, coding for the enzyme xanthine : guanine phosphoribosyl transferase was cloned in a simian virus 40 vector and transfected into different cell lines as a dominant marker (Mulligan and Berg, 1980). Jimenez and Davis (1980) have shown that yeasts are sensitive to the aminoglycoside antibiotic G-418. However, if yeasts are transfected with the transposon Tn 601 before exposure to G-418, some cells become resistant to the killing drug. The transposon codes for an aminoglycoside 3'-phosphotransferase (APH 3') which inactivates the drug.

We have used the transferase activity of a related transposon Tn 5 to engineer a hybrid molecules fit to be expressed in the cells of higher eukaryotes by linking the APH 3' gene to the promoter region of the HSV TK gene. This constructed molecule has been optimized to give high transformation efficiencies and shown to be cotransfected with other genes (the total HSV TK or the human hepatitis B surface antigen (S) gene). A different pattern of synthesis of the latter antigen takes place if one uses mouse as opposed to other animal species cells.

THE APH 3', A DOMINANT SELECTIVE MARKER

Construction

Random integration of a prokaryotic gene into eukaryotic cellular DNA followed by its expression is a rare event (10^{-7} to 10^{-8}). The bacterial promoter is not active in the animal cell and only a rare event can allow the linkage of the gene close to an active eukaryotic promoter region (EPR). We decided to link the coding region of the APH 3' to the EPR of HSV thymidine kinase gene. This region had already been sequenced (Garapin et al., 1981). This segment of DNA is contained in a plasmid pAGO (Colbère-Garapin et al., 1979) which contains pBR322 + the HSV TK gene. A HincII-HincII DNA segment from the Tn 5 transposon (Jorgensen et al., 1979) was flush ligated to a partial HincII digest of pAGO. Colonies having acquired the resistance to kanamycin were selected and the orientation of the coding sequence was determined. The recombinant segment of DNA has kept its bacterial promoter and can thus be expressed in both orientations in bacteria. One recombinant plasmid pAG40 (in which the bacterial promoter is close to the EPR region of the TK gene) was used for further studies.

In order to reduce the distance (some 1500 bp) between the EPR and the first AUG of the gene coding for the resistance to kanamycin or G-418 (both are related aminoglycosides) a BglII fragment of DNA was resected from pAG40 and transferred anew into pAGO linearized by the same enzyme. The resultant plasmid pAG50 harbors the coding section close to the eukaryotic EPR and the APH 3' has lost its bacterial promoter.

The AATAAA regulatory sequence which is found at the 3' end of most eukaryotic genes and is responsible for the addition, some 10 bp downstream of the poly A sequence on the mRNA, is also found at the end of the TK gene. In order to bring together what we believe is the 3' end of the APH 3' coding segment (no sequence for the 3' end of the coding sequence is yet available) and the TK polyadenylation site, a new plasmid, pAG60 was constructed. The purpose of these operations was to optimize the expression level of the resistance factor in the cell and the efficiency of transfection that we believed to be connected.

It has been shown that most genes in eukaryotes are segmented. However, some of them -the TK gene belongs to this group- have no intron (MacKnight, 1980 ; Wagner et al., 1981). It was thought that the grafting of an intron could reinforce the level of expression and possibly the transformation efficiency. The large intron of rabbit β-globin (plasmid 2-pCRI/R chr βG-1, a kind gift of Dr. P. Dierks) (Dierks et al., 1981) was resected by a double cut BamHI and BglII and grafted into the plasmid pAG60 at the BglII site upstream of the sequence coding for the APH 3' gene. The resulting plasmid pAG90 harbors in line the TK EPR and the cap site, the rabbit intron, the APH 3' coding sequence and TK polyadenylation site. Finally, in order to test a different EPR, the coding sequence of the APH 3' genes was grafted onto the promoter region of hepatitis S antigen gene (this gene has a high level of expression) to give the recombinant pAG110.

Transformation efficiency (T.E.)

The aminoglycoside G-418 is one of the rare antibiotics that kill the eukaryotic cells *in vitro* (Jimenez and Davies, 1980 ; Colbère-Garapin et al., 1981). At doses in the range of 50 to 500 μg/ml no spontaneously resistant colony was ever seen. However, eventhough chemically related to G-418, kanamycin at a concentration of 10 mg/ml does not kill cells.

Assayed in the 1 D clone of LM TK^- cells (Kit and Dubbs, 1963) (a cell line highly susceptible to transfection (Wigler et al., 1978)), the plasmid in which the construction had been optimized (pAG60) had an efficiency of about 100 colonies/μg of plasmid DNA, the parent pAG50 being at a level of about 40 colonies/μg of DNA while pAG40 stood around 5 colonies/μg of DNA. The optimisation of the construction thus had a real effect on the T.E. Surprisingly, the addition of an intron (pAG90) did not modify the T.E., neither did the addition of a different promoter (pAG110).

This is probably due to the existence of a liminal level of APH 3' in the cell which is sufficient to insure the cell survival. It is likely that only a modification of the level of integration would enhance the T.E. This efficiency does not depend on the drug concentration (between 100-300 μg/ml) nor on the time of G-418 addition after transfection. Other cells have been successfully transformed : the human HeLa, the simian VERO, CV1, OMK (owl-monkey kidne line), LL-MK2 and a rabbit skin fibroblast line. However, the highes T.E. were always attained in the murine LM TK⁻ line while for the other animal species the T.E. were lower by a factor of 10-1000.

Eukaryotic APH 3' activity

After chromatography on Sephadex G-200 of an extract of mouse cells transformed by the plasmids pAG50 and pAG60, the levels of enzyme expressed in cts/min of phosphorylated kanamycin per µg of protein correlated roughly with the degree of optimization of the plasmid. The substrate specificity of the eukaryotic enzyme for three different aminoglycosides (kanamycin, G-418 and tobramycin) were the same as that of the bacterial enzyme. These results connected to the absolute absence of spontaneous resistance and the 100 % killing of the cells by G-418 alone are ample proofs of the expression of the hybrid gene in the animal cells. However, by molecular sieving, the eukaryotic enzyme elutes as a protein of Mr 45.000 while the bacterial enzyme elutes as a protein of Mr 25.000. The glycosylation inhibitor, tunicamycin, does not change this behaviour but chromatogra phy on Sephadex G-200 in the presence of 50 mM dithiothreitol (DTT) brings the eukaryotic enzyme to a molecular weight closer to that of the bacterial one. There is apparently a binding of the enzyme to some cellular material which is detached in the presence of 50 mM DT (Colbère-Garapin et al., 1981).

Molecular configuration of the gene in transformed cells

The cellular DNA of several mouse clones transformed by pAG50 or pAG60 were cut by the XbaI endonuclease (which does not cut the plas mids) and blotted against a probe resected from the coding sequence. In all cases the hybridization bands were found at a higher level than the APH 3' hybrid gene indicating the integration in a high molecular weight cellular DNA.

Coexpression of the TK gene transferred along with the hybrid gene

In order to demonstrate the feasibility of cotransfection and co expression of the APH 3' gene along with another gene, we chose the TK gene. We then used a mass ratio of 5(pAG60) to 8(pAGO coding for TK) and cotransfected LM TK⁻ cells by the calcium phosphate technique. After selection in G-418 alone, 20 clones were isolated. Nine out of 20 clones were able to grow in the selective medium for TK and expressed high levels of thymidine kinase.

TRANSFER AND EXPRESSION OF THE HUMAN HEPATITIS B VIRUS SURFACE (HBVS) ANTIGEN GENE

Charnay et al. (1979) and Galibert et al. (1979) have cloned the entire genome of the human hepatitis B virus (subtype ayw) and sequenced the entire 3182 pb DNA. Dubois et al. (1980) have constructed a two EcoRI HBV DNA fragment plasmid (inserted in a head-to-tail tandem in pBR322). The resultant plasmid (pCP10) was cotransfected along with pAGO (TK) into LM TK^- cells by the same authors. The result was that, in the cell clones, the surface antigen (S) is not only expressed but is also excreted in the medium at high levels (2.4×10^6 polypeptides/cell/24 hrs) (Dubois et al., 1980).

We decided to study the expression of the surface antigen gene in primate cells (human and simian) with the help of the dominant selective marker APH 3'.

Expression in mammalian cells after cotransfection with pAG60

When transfected into LM TK^- along with pAG60, the pCP10 plasmid elicits not only the expression but also the excretion of the S antigen which can be detected two weeks after transfection. The S synthesis was followed in the transformation plate and in the resulting clones for up to 6 months. It showed a high level of expression stable with time.

However, when the same experiment is done with the simian VERO cells, the pattern of expression is different. The excretion is significant at the 5th day after transfection (while it is barely detectable at day 15 in murine cells) and increases up to 3 weeks where it plateaus for a week and levels off to zero between 5-12 weeks after transfection. This totally unexpected result was obtained several times.

After the S antigen expression shut off, no antigen could be detected by radioimmunoassay in the cell culture medium, even after a 10 times concentration. The block was not at the level of excretion since no antigen was found in cell extracts.

An increased toxicity of the antibiotic G-418 in conjonction with the excretion of the S antigen has been eliminated by the lowering of the antibiotic concentration. It has not been possible to trigger the S synthesis by induction of the transformed cells with BudR, cyclic AMP, glucocorticoids or oestradiol.

The expression of an other viral antigen "e" antigen was detected in cells transfected with pCP10 and its kinetics of synthesis and excretion follows that of the S antigen.

The presence of "e" antigen in human serum has often been associated with HBV infectivity. Moreover, the pCP10 plasmid has two complete viral genomes in a head-to-tail arrangement which could, upon recombination, liberate a circular viral genome capable of full expression and infectivity. This situation could eventually lead to the cell lysis (even though HBV is not a lytic virus when it infects the human liver). To eliminate this possibility, the S gene was isolated. Moreover, in order to bypass a possible regulatory region responsible for the shutt off of S synthesis in VERO cells, we have constructed plasmids in which the S coding sequence is under the control of herpes virus promoters.

Two plasmids pAG83 and pAG85 were thus obtained by transferring a BglII-BglII fragment of pCP10 into the pAGO (TK) linearized by BglII. pAG85 has the 5' end of the coding sequence under the control of the TK promoter and pAG83 has the coding sequence in the opposite orientation. Two conclusions were brought up by this experiment. First, both plasmids transform TK^- mouse cells to the TK^+ phenotype. (The transformation efficiency is only of an order of magnitude lower than with the pAGO parent plasmid). This result is surprising in view of the insertion of a 2325 bp fragment between the TK EPR and the TK AUG. Secondly, both plasmids elicited the expression of S antigen and pAG83 was even 2-3 times more efficient. The explanation of this unexpected result is that a more efficient promoter (P3) exists downstream of the BglII site of the TK gene and that it works at counter-current. This hypothesis is in agreement with *in vitro* transcription experiments (Beck and Millett, 1981). Despite this change of promoter, the S synthesis and excretion peaked around 10 days after transfection and levelled off 3 weeks after transfection in simian cells.

Is the 3' end of the S gene responsible for the shut off ?

The previous results showed that the regulatory sequences, including the TATA box, found usually upstream of the coding region do not seem to be involved in the disappearance of the S expression.

In order to study a possible role of the distal segment of the 3' end of the S gene, several plasmids were constructed in which this distal segment was clipped off. This study showed that at least 700 bp after the stop codon are necessary to obtain the transient expression but that the next 600 bp do not allow a permanent and stable synthesis when cleaved off. This is in agreement with the results of Pourcel et al. (1981) which indicate that the BamHI site which lies downstream of the S coding region is necessary for the synthesis of S. The mRNA studies of Pourcel et al. (1982) have shown that no splicing takes place on the mRNA coding for S. Thus, the possibility of abnormal splicing at the 3' end of the gene is ruled out.

Is cointegration deficient in primate cells ?

It has been mentionned in the first part of this paper that the T.E. of APH 3' coding plasmids is 10-1000 times lower in primate than in murine cells. It is agreed that in most cases a stable expression is linked to the integration of the foreign gene into the chromosomal DNA of the recipient cell. One could hypothesize that, if cointegration at the same locus is absent in primate cells, it would be very difficult in view of the low transformation efficiency to find a doubly transformed cell when the marker and the S antigen gene are unlinked. We, therefore, constructed the pAG66 plasmid which bears both the APH 3' coding gene and an RsaI-TaqI segment of the HBV genome (2600 bp). We have tested this recombinant in the murine and in the simian cells. There again expression is stable in the mouse cells and transient in the simian cells.

In addition, we have shown that coexpression of two genes cotransfected on separate molecules into simian cells may occur. We have cotransfected by the calcium technique the plasmid (Mulligan and Berg, 1980) coding for xanthine : guanine phosphorybosyl transferase and pAG60 into simian VERO cells. Three cell clones out of 15 were doubly resistant to mycophenolic acid and G-418.

State of the HBV DNA in the simian cells

VERO cells transfected by the HBVS gene and the APH 3' gene born on separate plasmids were selected on the basis of their resistance to G-418. Clones were isolated and grown to confluence. The cellular DNA was extracted and cut by the EcoRI endonuclease which cleaves once in the HBV DNA. The DNAs were hybridized on Southern blots to an HBV probe. In 7 out of 8 clones tested, no HBV DNA was found. The same blot hybridization was repeated with DNAs extracted from simian cells transformed with pAG66. There again the S gene was not found intact at the chromosomal level.

Is a stable expression of HBVS antigen possible in other cells ?

We have tested the expression of the S antigen on a limited number of other cells. We have used the human HeLa and the GM 4312/SV 40 cells. These two cell lines express the S antigen transiently. The same phenomenon is observed on rabbit skin fibroblasts even when the marker and the S gene are born on the same plasmid (pAG66).

Discussion

In our study on the expression of the HBVS in eukaryotic cells in conjonction with the APH 3' marker, we have confirmed the previously published results in mouse LM TK^- (Dubois et al., 1980) which show a stable synthesis of the antigen with the cellular doublings. We have demonstrated that the synthesis and the excretion of S takes place in other animal species and in other cell lines, but that in all cells tested the synthesis is transient and that the HBV DNA is not stably integrated at least in the simian VERO cells. We do not know whether this phenomenon is due to an excision of the DNA or if rearrangements take place after integration. It is also possible that some restriction analogous to what occurs in bacteria happens in animal cells and that only restriction fragments are integrated. In view of the apparent specific interaction between the cells and the HBV DNA, it might be possible that only some types of differentiated cells could stably express the S antigen. Experiments are in progress to study the expression in human hepatoma cell lines. In primates, the liver is the only organ in which the virus is replicated at high titer. It is then possible that the state of differentiation of the recipient cell influences not only the replication but also the expression of the viral protein S. Patients who have contracted the disease can carry the S antigen in their sera for many years after recovery. Most of the mouse lines carry retroviruses which might derepress some cellular function responsible of the block in the non murine cells. This shall also be tested.

In conclusion, the development of dominant selective marker has been indispensable to study the expression of non marker genes for which the expression can not be studied easily.

ACKNOWLEDGEMENTS

We thank Dr. P. Daniels (Schering Corporation) for providing G-418, Dr. P. Tiollais for the pPCP10 plasmid and Dr. J. Pillot for anti-HBVS antisera. We acknowledge Dr. C. Tram for PPLO testing. We are grateful to J. Lavolé and P. Brisset for excellent technical help and V. Caput for typing the manuscript.

This work was supported by grants from I.N.S.E.R.M. (72.79.104 contrat 012, P.R.C. 124006 and 124031, S.C. 20) and C.N.R.S. (95. 5097 and 95.5039 and E.R. 201).

REFERENCES

Beck, T. W., Millett, R. L., 1981, In vitro transcription of herpes simplex type I DNA by RNA polymerase II from Hep-2 cells. In : "International Workshop on Herpes Viruses", Esculapio Ed., Bologne.

Bolivar, F., Rodriguez, R.L., Green, P.J., Betlach, M. C., Heyneker, H. L., Boyer, H. W., Crona, J. H. and Falkow, S., 1977, Construction and characterization of new cloning vehicles II a multipurpose cloning system. Gene, 2 : 95.

Charnay, P., Pourcel, C, Louise, A., Fritsch, A. and Tiollais, P., 1979, Cloning in E. coli and physical structure of hepatitis B virion DNA, Proc. Natl. Acad. Sci., U.S.A., 76 : 2222.

Colbère-Garapin, F., Chousterman, S., Horodniceanu, F., Kourilsky, P. and Garapin, A., 1979, Cloning of the active thymidine kinase gene of herpes virus simplex type 1 in E. coli K.12, Proc. Natl. Acad. Sci., U.S.A., 76 : 3755.

Colbère-Garapin, F., Horodniceanu, F., Kourilsky, P. and Garapin, A., 1981, A new dominant hybrid selective marker for higher eukaryotic cells. J. Mol. Biol., 150 : 1.

Dierks, P., Van Ooyen, A., Mantei, M. and Weissmann, C, 1981, DNA sequences preceding the rabbit β-globin gene are required for formation in mouse L cells of β-globin RNA with the correct 5' terminus. Proc. Natl. Acad. Sci., U.S.A., 78 : 1411.

Dubois, M. F., Pourcel, C., Rousset, S., Chany, C. and Tiollais, P., 1980, Excretion of hepatitis B surface antigen particles from mouse cells transformed with cloned viral DNA. Proc. Natl. Acad. Sci., U.S.A., 77 : 4549.

Galibert, F., Mandart, E., Fitoussi, E., Tiollais P. and Charnay, P., 1979, Nucleotide sequence of the hepatis B virus genome (subtype ayw) cloned in E. coli. Nature (London) 281 : 646.

Garapin, A. C., Colbère-Garapin, F., Cohen-Solal, M., Horodniceanu, F. and Kourilsky, P., 1981, Expression of the herpes simplex virus type I thymidine kinase in E. coli, Proc. Natl. Acad. Sci., U.S.A., 78 : 815.

Jimenez, A. and Davies, J., 1980, Expression of a transposable antibiotic resistance element in saccharomyces. Nature (London) 287 : 869.

Kit, S. and Dubbs, D.R., 1963, Acquisition of thymidine kinase activity by herpes simplex infected mouse fibroblast cells. Biochem. Biophys. Res. Commun., 11 : 55

McKnight, S. L., 1980, The nucleotide sequence and transcript map of the herpes simplex thymidine kinase gene. Nucl. Acids. Res., 8 : 5949.

Mulligan, R. A. and Berg, P., 1980, Expression of a bacterial gene in mammalian cells. Science, 209 : 1423.

O'Hare, K., Benoist, C. and Breathnach, R., 1981, Transformation of mouse fibroblasts to methotrexate resistance by a recombinant plasmid expressing a prokaryotic dehydrofolate reductase. Proc. Natl. Acad. Sci., U.S.A., 78 : 1527

Perucho, M., Hanahan, D. and Wigler, M., 1980, Genetic and physical linkage of exogeneous sequences in transformed cells. Cell, 22 : 309.

Pourcel, C, Charnay, P., Dubois, M. F., Brechot, C., Louise, A., Gervais, M. and Tiollais, P., 1981, Expression du gène S du virus de l'hépatite B. "Hepatitis B Vaccine INSERM Symposium" No. 18, Maupas, P. and Guesny, P., Eds., Elservier/north hollan(Biomedical Press.

Pourcel, C., Louise, A., Gervais, M., Chenciner, N., Dubois, M. F. and Tiollais, P., 1982, Transcription of the hepatitis B surfac(antigen gene in mouse cells transformed with cloned viral DNA. J. Virol., 42 : 100.

Wagner, M. J., Sharp, J. A. and Summers, W., 1981, Nucleotide sequence of the thymidine kinase gene of herpes simplex virys type I. Proc. Natl. Acad. Sci., U.S.A., 78 : 1441.

Wigler, M., Pellicer, A., Silverstein, S. and Axel, R., 1978, Biochemical transfer of single copy eukaryotic genes using total cellular DNA as donor, Cell, 14 : 725.

CLOSE LINKAGE OF TRANSFERRED GALACTOKINASE AND THYMIDINE KINASE GENES IN A TRANSFORMANT AFTER DNA-MEDIATED GENE TRANSFER

Jane L. Peterson* and O. Wesley McBride

Laboratory of Biochemistry, National Cancer Institute
National Institutes of Health, Bethesda, MD 20205

INTRODUCTION

There are many similarities and some differences between DNA- and chromosome-mediated gene transfer. The cellular uptake of both DNA[1] and metaphase chromosomes[2] involves phagocytosis and there is a requirement for co-precipitation of the donor DNA[3] or chromosomes[4] with calcium phosphate to achieve optimal frequencies of gene transfer. In either method, transformants usually initially exhibit an unstable phenotype, and stabilization ultimately occurs through covalent integration of the donor DNA with recipient chromosomal DNA at multiple non-homologous sites. The optimal frequency for gene transfer is dependent upon many factors but a higher frequency of transfer has been reported for chromosome- than DNA-mediated gene transfer under similar conditions.[5]

A major difference between these two gene transfer procedures may involve the size of DNA fragments which are transferred. Following chromosome-mediated gene transfer, donor chromosome fragments as large as 1% of the haploid genome (i.e. about 3×10^7 base pairs) have been detected in transformants.[6,7] To compare the size of fragments incorporated following both DNA- and chromosome-mediated gene transfer, we determined the frequency of cotransfer of two linked genes, *thymidine kinase* (*tk*) and *galactokinase* (*galk*). We previously reported DNA-mediated co-transfer of Chinese hamster *galk* in one of 100 transformants selected for *tk* transfer.[8] Cosegregation of these two markers was also demonstrated after transfer, indicating that the *galk*

*Present address: National Science Foundation, 1800 G Street, N.W. Room 332, Washington, D.C.

and tk genes were physically linked in the transformant. Based on these results, two mechanisms of cotransfer were considered: 1) the two genes were cotransferred on a single large DNA fragment or 2) that a deletion had occurred between the two genes, thereby permitting cotransfer on a much smaller fragment. Subsequently, Perucho et al.[9] reported that DNA fragments undergo ligation to form large concatamers after entry into a recipient cell. This indicated a third potential mechanism for cotransfer which involves entry of the tk and galk genes into the cell on separate fragments with ligation of the fragments later in the transformation process.

We have now examined serial transfer of the tk gene using donor DNA isolated from the cotransformant cell line to evaluate the linkage of tk and galk in these cells. We found that the Chinese hamster tk and galk markers were both serially transferred at a high frequency indicating close linkage of these genes in the primary transformant. Hence, a rearrangement of these two genes must have occurred either prior or subsequent to the original gene transfer event.

MATERIALS AND METHODS

Cells

Mouse LMTK$^-$ clone 1D cells[10] were used as recipients in all experiments. DE4-3 was a primary transformant line resulting from transfer of Chinese hamster tk and galk into an LMTK$^-$ cell as previously described.[8] Chinese hamster cells (CHV79) were used as the DNA donor in the original tk-galk transfer.[8] Culture conditions and media have been described.[11,12]

DNA Transformation

DNA was isolated according to the method of Pellicer et al.[13] and DNA-mediated transformation was performed by the method of Wigler et al.[14] with modifications described earlier.[8] The preparation of cell extracts and starch gel electrophoresis have been described.[8]

DNA Shearing

DNA, at a concentration of 20 μg/ml in 0.2M sodium acetate, was sheared in a Virtis 60 homogenizer at 1000 or 3000 RPM for 5 minutes to yield DNA fragments in the size ranges of 15-100 kilobase pair (Kb) and 6-15 Kb, respectively.

Agarose Gel Electrophoresis

Electrophoresis of DNA in 0.2% agarose gels was performed by the method of Fangman.[15]

RESULTS

Serial Transfer of tk and galk genes

To distinguish between the various mechanisms proposed to explain cotransfer of Chinese hamster tk and galk, we performed DNA mediated transfer using DNA isolated from DE4-3, a primary transformant resulting from cotransfer of hamster tk and galk genes to a $LMTK^-$ cell.[8] We reasoned that a frequency of serial cotransfer similar to that for the original cotransfer (i.e. about 1%) would indicate that the two genes had not been rearranged. However, a significantly higher frequency of cotransfer than observed originally could be most readily explained by a DNA rearrangement resulting in the two genes being in closer proximity to each other. The TK^+ colonies were isolated in selective medium, expanded, and extracts were examined for the presence of Chinese hamster galactokinase. The results (Table 1B)

Table 1 TK transfer and TK-GalK Cotransfer

Expt.	A. TK^+ plates (positive/total) DNA[b]			B. TK^+-$GalK^+$ colonies ($GalK^+$/TK^+)[a] DNA[b]			DNA size (Kb)
	0K	1K	3K	0K	1K	3K	
1	10/10	10/10	1/7	3/10	6/10	1/1	7-13[c] 23-100[d]
2	2/5	7/8	3/8	1/1	5/6	1/2	---
3	2/5	6/6	6/8	0/1	5/5	0/2	---
4	5/10	5/6	2/6	2/4	1/3	0/2	7-12[c] 14-84[d]
5	10/10	10/10	4/10	8/8	4/10	0/2	6-22[c] 21-92[d]
6	6/10	9/10	3/10	5/5	3/6	0/1	6-22[c] 24->100[d]
1C	18/21[e]			0/17[e]			

[a] TK^+ colonies which exhibited Chinese hamster type galactokinase divided by total TK^+ colonies examined.

[b] DNA (20 μg) isolated from primary transformant DE4-3 cells was incubated with $LMTK^-$ cells (10^6) in each petri dish. Unsheared DNA (0K) and DNA sheared at 1000 RPM (1K) and 3000 RPM (3K) was used in each experiment.

[c] DNA size after shearing at 3000 RPM

[d] DNA size after shearing at 1000 RPM

[e] Donor DNA was isolated from CHV79 Chinese hamster cells.

indicate that 65% of the TK^+ colonies produced by transformation with unsheared DNA also expressed Chinese hamster GalK. The high frequency of serial cotransfer (65% versus 1 % in the original cotransfer) strongly suggests that the two genes are much more closely linked in the primary transformant (DE4-3) than they were linked in the original donor DNA isolated from Chinese hamster cells.

A control experiment (Experiment 1C) again revealed no galk cotransfer in 17 TK^+ primary transformants. In contrast, the frequency of tk transfer was similar in the primary and serial (Table 1A) transformation assays. This indicates that differences in the DNA preparations (or DNA size) or copy number of the tk and galk genes in Chinese hamster cells and primary transformants are improbable explanations for these results.

Serial Transformation with Sheared DNA

To determine the approximate distance between the hamster tk and galk genes in the primary transformant, DNA mediated transfer was performed with DE4-3 DNA which had been sheared to the 15-100 Kb range and less than 15 Kb size. The size range of each DNA preparation was determined by agarose gel electrophoresis (Fig. 1).

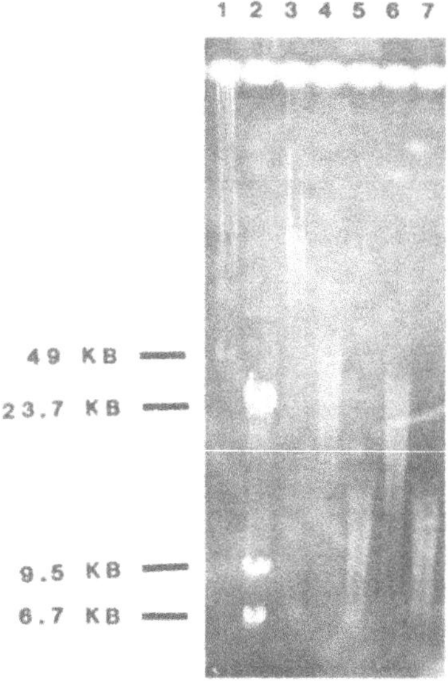

Figure 1: DNA size estimates from agarose gel electrophoresis and ethidium bromide staining. ORI = origin and numbers on abseissa = lane numbers; numbers along ordinate = DNA size in Kilobases. The DNAs applied to the lanes were: 1, λ (49Kb); 2, HinD3 digested λ; 3, unsheared DE4-3; 4 and 6, DE4-3 DNA after shearing at 1000 RPM; 5 and 7, DE4-3 DNA after shearing at 3000 RPM.

Resulting TK^+ colonies were isolated and cell extracts were examined for the presence of Chinese hamster Galk. The frequency of tk transfer, tk-galk cotransfer, and the DNA size in each preparation is shown (Table 1). Between 70 and 94% of the plates transformed with unsheared DNA or DNA of 15-100 Kb size range contained TK^+ colonies compared to 39% TK^+ plates after transformation with DNA sheared to less than 15 Kb length. 65% of the TK^+ colonies appearing after transformation with unsheared DNA and 60% of those produced by transformation with DNA sheared to 15-100 Kb also expressed Chinese hamster GalK. Only 20% of the TK^+ colonies arising after transformation with DNA sheared to less than 15Kb length contained both genes (Table 1B). Variation in the fraction of colonies containing galk in different experiments many reflect slight differences in the size of the sheared transforming DNA. Some variation in the approximate size distribution of sheared DNA preparations was observed (Table 1).

DISCUSSION

As previously noted, several potential mechanisms could be used to explain the cotransfer of Chinese hamster tk and galk genes at a very low frequency (~1%) in the original DNA-mediated gene transfer experiments. We have performed serial transfer of these linked genes to provide additional information relative to these alternatives and specifically to determine whether rearrangements of the genes has occurred. A similar low frequency for primary and serial cotransfer of tk and galk would have been expected if cotransfer involved occasional uptake of a very large DNA fragment or it represented a smaller intergenic distance than previously estimated. The very high frequency (i.e. 60-65%) of serial cotransfer is incompatible with these explanations and it strongly suggests a DNA rearrangement involving tk and galk.

It is presently impossible to ascertain whether the DNA rearrangement resulted from the original transformation process or preceded it, but we strongly favor the latter alternative. The tk and galk genes are known to be linked and the distance between these genes in humans[8] has been estimated to be about 1200-6000 Kb (i.e. 0.04-0.2% of the haploid genome). The similar frequency (i.e. about 25%) for cotransfer of these markers by chromosome-mediated transfer[2] using either human or hamster chromosomes suggests that the tk-galk intergenic distance does not differ greatly in these two species. If the donor Chinese hamster fibroblasts (CHV79) contained a small subpopulation of cells with a large deletion between tk and galk, cotransfer of these genes would be anticipated at a frequency corresponding to the fraction of the total cell population which contained this deletion. Serial transfer of both genes would then occur at a high frequency determined only by the rearranged intergenic distance and average size of the transforming DNA.

We consider it exceedingly unlikely that the observed high frequency of serial cotransfer of the *tk* and *galk* genes could have resulted from their uptake on separate DNA fragments and subsequent ligation in the primary transformant. If this mechanism was responsible, the frequency of serial cotransfer would be proportional to the product of two relatively low frequency events. One event, or factor, is the probability of uptake of two separate and specific DNA fragments by a cell (i.e. the primary transformant). This probability is directly proportional to the fraction of the donor genome incorporated by each recipient cell. Perucho et al.[9] and Robins et al.[16] have reported that the exogenous DNA present in transformed cells can represent as much as 0.1-0.2% of the haploid genome of the host. This calculation was based on the copy number of a specific incorporated sequence in the transformed cells, and it could represent an overestimate due to amplification of incorporated DNA fragments after transfer. Using 0.1% as a reasonable estimate for the fraction of incorporated host sequences, the probability for the original independent transfer of both genes (10^{-3}) is roughly compatible with the observed frequency for primary cotransfer (10^{-2}). However, the second factor is the statistical probability that these two specific genes would have become juxtaposed during ligation. Assuming that ligation of incorporated fragments is a random process, this probability is inversely proportional to the quantity of donor DNA (i.e. fraction of the donor genome) in each transformed cell. The product of these two factors is no longer dependent on assumptions concerning the quantity of donor DNA incorporated by a cell, but it is merely equal to the size of transferred DNA fragments divided by the genome size or approximately 10^{-5}. These considerations indicate that a DNA rearrangement following the primary transformation event is not a plausible explanation for our observations.

Our data also indicates that the *tk* and *galk* genes are relatively small since both can be transferred on a DNA fragment about 15 Kb in length. Previous evidence (unpublished) from our laboratory has demonstrated that DNA sheared to 10-15 Kb is capable of *tk* transfer. The original cotransfer of *tk* and *galk* probably represented a fortuitous event, resulting from transfer of DNA from a small fraction of the donor Chinese hamster cells that contained rearranged, and thus closely linked, *tk* and *galk* genes. However, this transformed cell line could be useful in cloning the *galk* gene. Isolation of the hamster *tk* gene might permit "chromosome walking" to the closely linked *galk* gene in a recombinant DNA library prepared from DE4-3.

SUMMARY

A single transformant containing donor thymidine kinase and galactokinase genes was previously isolated at low frequency (1%)

after DNA-mediated gene transfer. A high frequency of serial cotransfer of these genes has now been demonstrated indicating that a rearrangement of these genes has occurred and it probably preceded the original transfer.

REFERENCES

1. A. Loyter, G. Scangos, D. Juricek, D. Keene and F.H. Ruddle, Mechanisms of DNA entry into mammalian cells. II Phagocytosis of calcium phosphate DNA co-precipitate visualized by electron microscopy, Exp. Cell Res. 139:223 (1982).
2. O.W. McBride and J.L. Peterson, Chromosome-mediated gene transfer in mammalian cells, Ann. Rev. Genet. 14:321 (1980).
3. F.L. Graham and A.J. van der Eb, A new technique for the assay of infectivity of human adenovirus 5 DNA, Virology 52:456 (1973).
4. C.L. Miller and F.H. Ruddle, Co-transfer of human X-linked markers into murine somatic cells via isolated metaphase chromosomes, Proc. Natl. Acad. Sci. USA 75:3346 (1978).
5. W.L. Lewis, P.R. Srinivasan, N. Stokoe and L. Siminovitch, Parameters governing the transfer of the genes for thymidine kinase and dihydrofolate reductase into mouse cells using metaphase chromosomes or DNA, Somatic Cell Genet. 6:333 (1980).
6. A.S. Olsen, O.W. McBride and D.E. Moore, Number and size of human X chromosome fragments transferred to mouse cells by chromosome-mediated gene transfer, Mol. Cell. Biol. 1:439 (1981).
7. O.W. McBride, A.S. Olsen, G.S. Aulakh and R.S. Athwal, Measurement of transcribed human X-chromosomal DNA sequences transferred to rodent cells by chromosome-mediated gene transfer, Mol. Cell. Biol. 2:52 (1982).
8. J.L. Peterson and O.W. McBride, Cotransfer of linked eukaryotic genes and efficient transfer of hypoxanthine phosphoribosyltransferase by DNA-mediated gene transfer, Proc. Natl. Acad. Sci. USA 77:1583 (1980).
9. M. Perucho, D. Hanahan and M. Wigler, Genetic and physical linkage of exogenous sequences in transformed cells, Cell 22: 309 (1980).
10. S. Kit, D.R. Dubbs, L. Piekarski and T.C. Hsu, Deletion of thymidine kinase activity from L cells resistant to bromodeoxyuridine, Exp. Cell Res. 31:297 (1963).
11. O.W. McBride and H.L. Ozer, Transfer of genetic information by purified metaphase chromosomes, Proc. Natl. Acad. Sci. USA 70:1258 (1973).
12. J.W. Burch and O.W. McBride, Human gene expression in rodent cells after uptake of isolated metaphase chromosomes, Proc. Natl. Acad. Sci. USA 72:1797 (1975).

13. A. Pellicer, M. Wigler, R. Axel and S. Silverstein, The transfer and stable integration of the HSV thymidine kinase gene into mouse cells, Cell 14:133 (1978).
14. M. Wigler, A. Pellicer, S. Silverstein and R. Axel, Biochemical transfer of single-copy eucaryotic genes using total cellular DNA as donor, Cell 14:725 (1978).
15. W.L. Fangman, Separation of very large DNA molecules by gel electrophoresis, Nucleic Acids Res. 5:653 (1978).
16. D.M. Robins, S. Ripley, A.S. Henderson and R. Axel, Transforming DNA integrates into the host chromosome, Cell 23:29 (1981).

TRANSFER OF DNA INTO HIGHER EUKARYOTIC CELLS USING RECOMBINANT VECTORS BASED ON SIMIAN VIRUS 40 AND CHLORAMPHENICOL ACETYLTRANSFERASE GENES

Cornelia M. Gorman, Raji Padmanabhan and
Bruce H. Howard

Laboratory of Molecular Biology
Division of Cancer Biology and Diagnosis
National Cancer Institutes
National Institutes of Health
Bethesda, Maryland

INTRODUCTION

Over the past few years considerable progress has been made in the development of eukaryotic vectors. There have been reports describing improved methods for introduction of DNA into mammalian cells [1-3], more sensitive assays for vector function [4,5], and new selectable markers for stable transformation of tissue culture cells [6-8]. In this article we present recent work from our laboratory relating to these areas.

Early efforts in eukaryotic vector construction made use of simian virus 40 (SV40) as a model replicon [9,10]. The detailed knowledge of SV40 structure, including the DNA sequence of the genome, together with extensive mapping data on viral transcripts, greatly facilitated construction of recombinants [11-13]. Expression of recombinant genes in mammalian cells was first demonstrated using SV40 lytic vectors. SV40-rabbit-β-globin hybrids were shown to direct synthesis of rabbit β-globin polypeptide in monkey kidney CV-1 cells [14,15]. The results of those experiments established that mammalian cell mRNA processing and transport mechanisms were compatible, in most instances, with efficient expression of novel hybrid transcripts. Subsequently, investigators have used SV40 as a vector to achieve expression of such diverse products as *E. coli* xanthine guanine phosphoribosylsyltransferase [16], rat preproinsulin [17], Harvey sarcoma virus transforming protein p21 [18], mutant human tRNA [19], and influenza hemagglutinin [20]. In studies where high levels of RNA or protein synthesis are required, the gene copy amplification afforded by SV40 lytic infection continues to be extremely useful.

There are of course several limitations imposed by propagating recombinants in eukaryotic cells as defective SV40 viruses. First, viral packaging requirements severely restrict the size of gene segments that can be cloned. Since recombinant viruses must carry an essential viral function to prevent overgrowth by complementing helper virus, the maximum length of inserted non-viral DNA segments is only about 2.5 kilobase pairs. Second, cells permissive for viral replication must be used, in the case of SV40 usually a continuous line such as CV-1 African Green monkey kidney cells. Third, host cell lysis resulting from replication of recombinant and helper viruses precludes genetic analysis by stable complementation of host cell functions.

Non-lytic mammalian vectors were originally based on the Herpes simplex thymidine kinase (tk) gene. M. Wigler et al. [21] demonstrated that a 3.4 kilobase pair fragment carrying the Herpes tk gene could be taken up by mouse Ltk$^-$ cells, integrated into high molecular weight DNA, and constitutively expressed to permit growth of transformants in hypoxanthine-aminopterin-thymidine (HAT) selective medium [21]. This process was shown to occur with the surprisingly high efficiency of 1 transformant/ng tk DNA/10^6 mouse Ltk$^-$ cells [22]. It has been further established that non-selected genes may be integrated intact in a high percentage of tk$^+$ transformants [23]. Human and Chinese hamster ovary tk$^-$ cell lines also take up and express the Herpes tk gene, although efficiencies are 50 to 100 times lower than with mouse Ltk$^-$ cells [24,25].

Although the Herpes tk system has provided a model for stable transfer of genes into mammalian cells, the requirement for tk$^-$ recipient cell lines represents a serious deficiency. Frequently the appropriate tk$^-$ cell type to study regulation of a cloned gene locus does not exist; alternatively, if a tk$^-$ derivative is created, the mutagenesis required to generate the tk mutation often yields a cell line that manifests slow growth or poor transformation competence. To circumvent this problem considerable effort has been expended to create mammalian vectors that carry dominant selectable markers.

One approach to the development of dominant markers has been to construct novel recombinant genes that are constitutively expressed following introduction into the host cell. For example, coding sequences from *E. coli* or prokaryotic plasmid resistance elements may be inserted into a mammalian gene that contains appropriate transcription initiation, processing, and termination signals. Unlike markers based on mutant mammalian genes, such *in vitro* constructed markers have the potential to provide enzymatic activities that mammalian cells have no demonstrable potential to reproduce. With this goal in mind, the recombinant genome pSV2-βG was constructed (B. Howard and P. Berg, unpublished results).

pSV2-βG is composed of the pBR322 ampicillin-resistance cistron and replication origin linked to a modified SV40 early region transcription unit. The SV40 moiety consists, in 5' to 3' orientation, of fragments containing the following components: SV40 early promoter/origin of replication, rabbit β-globin cDNA, SV40 small t intron, and SV40 polyA addition site. The β-globin cDNA segment is flanked on the 5' end by a HindIII site and on the 3' end by a BglII site; since these are unique sites within the pSV2-βG recombinant, the cDNA segment is readily excised to generate a vector component, termed pSV2 (Fig. 1) Other amino acid coding regions may be inserted into pSV2 place of the β-globin sequence; this is usually accomplished by addition of mixed HindIII and BamH1 synthetic oligonucleotide linkers to the coding region fragment of interest.

A number of pSV2 derivatives have been constructed that serve as selectable markers. pSV2-dhfr, which carries a mouse dihydrofolate reductase cDNA fragment, complements the dihydrofolate reductase mutation in dhfr-negative CHO cells isolated by Urlaub and Chasin [26,27]. Similarly, pSVK-gal, which carries an *E. coli* galactose kinase coding region, complements a galK-negative CHO line [4]. pSV2-gpt, which carries the *E. coli* xanthine-guanine phosphoribosyltransferase (gpt) gene, complements the gpt^- mutation in human Lesch-Nyhan cells [16]. In addition, pSV2-gpt confers upon mammalian cells the capacity to use xanthine as a purine salvage substrate; thus in mycophenolic acid-xanthine-HAT selective medium it may be used as a dominant selectable marker [6]. Finally, pSV2-neo, which carries the *E. coli* Tn5 aminoglycoside phosphotransferase (neo) gene, functions as a dominant selectable marker by protecting mammalian cells from the toxic aminoglycoside G-418 [8].

Eukaryotic vectors such as pSV2-gpt and pSV2-neo that provide dominant markers are extremely useful in mammalian gene transfer experiments. With or without covalently linked non-selected genes they may be introduced and stably carried in many permanent mammalian cell lines. In principle, virtually any permanent line and most primary cell lines could be used as recipients. In practice, the competence of cell types other than fibroblastic lines to take up DNA by standard techniques is quite variable. It is frequently necessary to vary parameters in the calcium phosphate-DNA coprecipitation procedure or to test alternate transfection procedures to obtain a reasonable DNA uptake efficiency. In other cases it is necessary to alter the vector, e.g., by substituting a different promoter or by inserting a transcription enhancer sequence, to ensure adequate expression of the selectable marker. For these reasons we have developed a set of eukaryotic expression vectors based on the E. coli chloramphenicol acetyltransferase (CAT) gene [28]. CAT vectors can greatly facilitate the accumulation of information required to achieve efficient introduction of DNA into mammalian, avian or other eukaryotic cells.

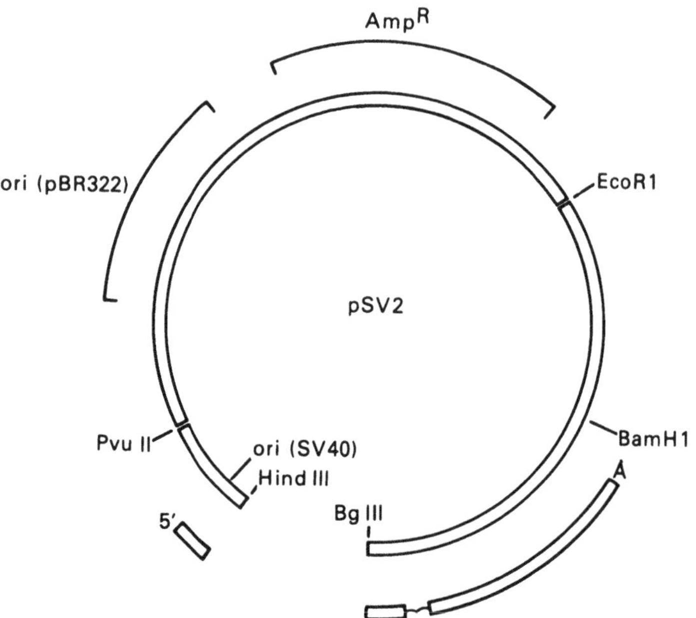

Fig 1. Schematic of pSV2. The SV40 early region transcription unit is composed of the following elements (see Buchman et al [36], for nucleotide numbers associated with restriction sites): early promoter/ origin of replication from a 400 bp fragment limited by PvuII (253) and HindIII (5154) sites; small t intron from a 610 bp fragment limited by MboI sites (4083 and 4693); polyA addition signal from a 988 bp fragment limited by BclI (2753) and EcoR1 (1765) sites. Positions of the SV40 promoter, small t intron, and polyA signal are indicated by 5' and 3' flanking segments of the early region transcript. The region between unique EcoR1 and BamH1 sites is nonessential.

PSV2-CAT AND ITS DERIVATIVES

Our selection of chloramphenicol acetyltransferase as the basis for eukaryotic expression vectors was based on the following considerations:

1) The CAT gene, derived from the E. coli transposable element Tn9, has a relatively small coding region (657 bp) that is contained within in a 773 bp TaqI fragment [29]. Since the nucleotide sequence of this fragment is known, its manipulation within the context of eukaryotic vectors is considerably simplified.

2) CAT activity does not occur, to our knowledge, in higher eukaryotic cells. The absence of this activity in recipient cells is important, since it eliminates the need to distinguish vector from host gene function.

3) Rapid and sensitive assays for CAT have been developed. [30] In the assay that we have adopted, acetylation of commercially available 14-C chloramphenicol is monitored by thin layer chromatography on silica gel plates. Localization of radioisotopic label in the chloramphenicol substrate rather than in acetyl-coenzyme A allows specific assay in crude extracts without interference by unrelated metabolic reactions that involve acetyl group transfer.

4) CAT enzyme is commercially available (P.L. Biochemicals); thus it is a simple matter to set up the assay and run appropriate controls.

The prototype vector in the CAT family is pSV2-cat [28] (Fig. 2). In this construct expression in mammalian cells is, as described earlier, under control of a modified SV40 early region transcription unit.

We have introduced pSV2-cat into a variety of cultured cells by the DNA-calcium phosphate coprecipitation method. In our standard experimental protocol, cells are incubated for 48 hours after DNA introduction to allow vector expression, then extracts are prepared by sonication and CAT activity is assayed. Fig. 3 shows results obtained when pSV2-cat, pSV2-cat^R, calf thymus, or pBR322-Tn9 DNA is introduced into monkey kidney CV-1 cells. pSV2-cat^R is identical to pSV2-cat, except that the CAT insert includes the bacterial promoter region. pBR322-Tn9, which carries Tn9 inserted between the origin of replication and ampicillin resistance cistron of pBR322 (L. Rosner, unpublished results), serves as a control to show that CAT expression in CV-1 cells requires SV40 early region transcription signals. Other cell types in which pSV2-cat expression has been demonstrated include human HeLa, mouse NIH/3T3 hamster CHO, and chicken embryo fibroblasts.

Results obtained using pSV2-cat indicate that the calcium phosphate-DNA coprecipitation method is sensitive many variables. For example, the procedure by which plasmid DNA has been prepared strongly affects expression. In our experience, plasmid DNA isolated by double cesium chloride/ethidium bromide equilibrium centrifugation is reproducibly active material. Conditions for growth of tissue culture cells also influence transfection efficiency. Cells should be passaged frequently, e.g. every 4-5 days, so that they do not reach and remain at complete confluence. It is necessary to select an active lot of fetal bovine serum; in addition it is important to monitor the pH of the tissue culture medium (optimum for CO_2-equilibrated cell-free medium is usually pH 7.3-7.4). Even under favorable conditions the competence of cultured cells to take up DNA steadily decreases during continuous passaging; thus it is generally good practice to thaw cells from frozen stocks at regular intervals, e.g. after 10-15 passages.

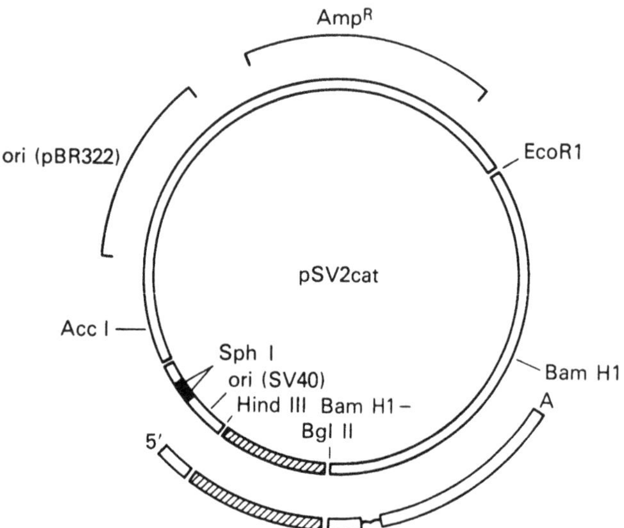

Fig 2. Schematic of pSV2cat. Striped segment represents the 773 bp CAT coding region insert. Solid segment denotes repeated 72 bp enhancer sequences of the SV40 early promoter.

In addition to its usefulness for optimizing transfection conditions, the CAT assay has permitted us to compare the apparent strengths of several eukaryotic promoter regions. Of the promoters that we have inserted into pSV2-cat in place of the SV40 early promoter, the 3' long terminal repeat (LTR) from the Schmidt-Ruppin D strain of Rous sarcoma virus directs the highest levels of CAT synthesis in our transient expression assays [31]. This Rous LTR promoter, subcloned into the plasmid pRSV-cat, yields 3-10 fold higher levels of CAT in human HeLa cells, monkey CV-1 cells, mouse

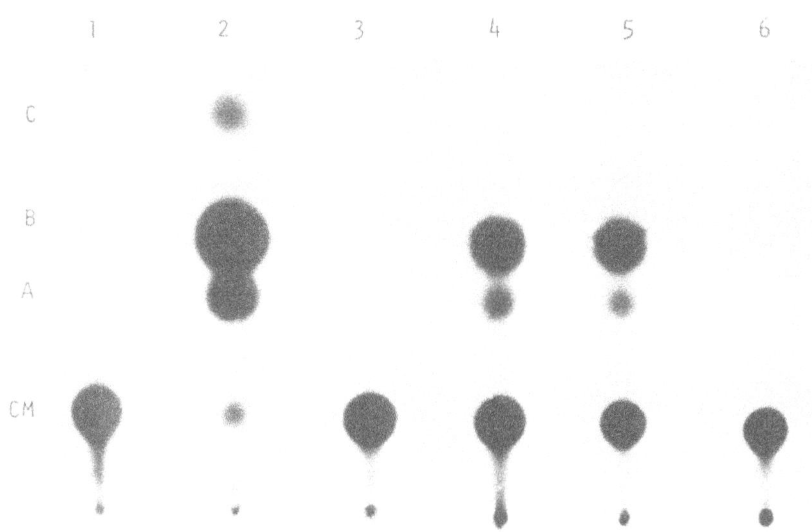

Fig 3. Assay of CAT activity in monkey kidney CV-1 cells. Extracts (100 µl final volume) were prepared following transfection of 5x10^5 cells with 20 µg DNA. Reactions contained in a final volume of 180 µl: 100 µl 0.25 M Tris HCl pH 7.5, 1 µCi ^{14}C chloramphenicol (50 µCi/mmole; New England Nuclear), 10-50 µl extract (where indicated), and 20 µl acetyl-coenzyme A. After extraction with ethyl acetate, samples were applied to silica gel thin layer plates and developed in chloroform: methanol (95:5; ascending). The autoradiograph shows products from reactions containing: no enzyme, lane 1; chloramphenicol acetyltransferase (P.L. Biochemicals), lane 2; extract from calf thymus DNA transfected cells, lane 3; extract from pSV2cat transfected cells, lane 4; extract from pSV2cat^R transfected cells, lane 5; extract from pBR322-Tn9 transfected cells, lane 6.

NIH/3T3 cells, and chick embryo fibroblasts than the SV40 early promoter. In Chinese hamster ovary cells the LTR appears to be about 50% less active than the SV40 promoter. The results obtained from such experiments have led us to construct pRSV-gpt, a vector in which the Rous LTR controls transcription of the E. coli xanthine guanine phosphoribosyltransferase coding region, and pRSV-neo, in which the LTR controls the Tn5 aminoglycoside phosphotransferase gene. Function of these vectors as dominant selectable markers is currently under investigation.

We of course hope that the CAT assay will prove useful to other researchers, particularly in the study of transcription control regions. To provide a vehicle for insertion of alternate promoters adjacent to the CAT coding region, we have therefore constructed the vector pSV0-cat [28]. An initial version of pSV0-cat was derived from pSV2 by excision of the the entire SV40 early promoter region, addition of HindIII synthetic oligonucleotide linkers, and recircularization. Using HindIII-SmaI oligonucleotide adaptors, a second version of pSV0-cat was then constructed in which two HindIII sites flank a SmaI site (C. Gorman et al, unpublished results). The HindIII and SmaI sites for promoter insertion into this latter construct are located about 70 bp upstream from the CAT translation initiation codon.

A final comment on the CAT system concerns its application as a selectable marker in eukaryotic cells. Both mammalian and avian cells in tissue culture are sensitive to chloramphenicol, the degree of sensitivity being determined by the choice of sugar and certain other substituents in the culture medium [32,33]. It has been proposed that toxicity results from inhibition of mitochondrial protein synthesis and subsequent loss of mitochondrial function [34,35]. We have found that some cell types may be protected from chloramphenicol-induced growth inhibition following introduction of pRSV-cat. Experiments in progress should determine whether pRSV-cat or similar CAT vectors will prove to be as useful for isolating stable mammalian transformants as are the more established dominant selectable markers pSV2-gpt and pSV2-neo.

REFERENCES

1. B. Parker and G. Stark, Regulation of simian virus 40 transcription: sensitive analysis of the RNA species present early in infections by virus or viral DNA, J. Virol. 31:360 (1979).

2. W. Schaffner, Direct transfer of cloned genes from bacteria to mammalian cells, Proc. Natl. Acad. Sci. USA 77:2163 (1980).

3. L.M. Sompayrac and K.J. Danna, Efficient infection of monkey cells with DNA of simian virus 40, Proc. Natl. Acad. Sci. USA 78:7575 (1981).

4. D. Schumperli, B.H. Howard, and M. Rosenberg, Efficient expression of Escherichia coli galactokinase gene in mammalian cells, Proc. Natl. Acad. Sci. USA 79:257 (1982).

5. B. Fong and M. Scriba, Use of 125-I deoxycytidine to detect Herpes simplex virus specific thymidine kinase in tissues of latently infected guinea pigs, J. Virol. 34:644 (1980).

6. R.C. Mulligan and P. Berg, Selection for animal cells that express the Escherichia coli gene coding for xanthine-guanine phosphoribosyl transferase, Proc. Natl. Acad. Sci. USA 78:2072 (1981).

7. F. Colbere-Garapin, F. Horodniceanu, P. Kourilsky, and A.C. Garapin, A new dominant hybrid selective marker for higher eukaryotic cells, J. Mol. Biol. 150:1 (1981)

8. P.J. Southern and P. Berg, Transformation of mammalian cells to antibiotic resistance with a bacterial gene under control of the SV40 early region promoter, J. Molec. Appl. Genet. 1:327 (1982).

9. S.P. Goff and P. Berg, Construction of hybrid viruses containing SV40 and lambda phage DNA segments and their propagation in cultured monkey cells, Cell 9:695 (1976).

10. G. Ganem, A.L. Nussbaum, D. Davoli, and G.C. Fareed, Propagation of a segment of bacteriophage lambda DNA in monkey cells after covalent linkage to a defective simian virus 40 genome, Cell 7:349 (1976).

11. W. Fiers, R. Contreras, G. Haegeman, R. Rogiers, A. van de Voorde, H. van Heuverswyn, J. van Herreweghe, G. Volckaert, and M. Ysebaert, Complete nucleotide sequence of SV40 DNA, Nature, 273:113 (1978).

12. V.G. Reddy, B. Thimmappaya, R. Dhar, K.N. Subramanian, B.S. Zain, J.Pan, P.K. Ghosh, M.L. Celma, and S.M. Weissman, The genome of simian virus 40, Science 200:494 (1978).

13. V.G. Reddy, P.K. Ghosh, P. Lebowitz, M. Piatak, and S.M. Weissman, Simian virus 40 early mRNAs, J. Virol. 30:279 (1979).

14. R.C. Mulligan, B.H. Howard, and P. Berg, Synthesis of rabbit β-globin in cultured monkey kidney cells following infection with a SV40 β-globin recombinant genome, Nature 277:108 (1979).

15. D.H. Hamer, K.D. Smith, S.H. Boyer, and P. Leder, SV40 recombinants carrying rabbit β-globin gene coding sequences, Cell 17:725 (1979).

16. R.C. Mulligan and P. Berg, Expression of a bacterial gene in mammalian cells, Science 209:1422 (1980).

17. P. Gruss and G. Khoury, Expression of simian virus 40-rat preproinsulin recombinants in monkey kidney cells: use of preproinsulin RNA processing signals, Proc. Natl. Acad. Sci. USA 78:133 (1981).

18. P. Gruss, R.W. Ellis, T.Y. Shih, M. Konig, E.M. Scolnick, and G. Khoury, SV40 recombinant molecules express the gene encoding p21 transforming protein of Harvey murine sarcoma virus, Nature 293:486 (1981).

19. M. Zasloff, T. Santos, and D.H. Hamer, tRNA precursor transcribed from a mutant human gene inserted into a SV40 vector is processed incorrectly, Nature 295:533 (1982).

20. M.M. Sveda and C.J. Lai, Functional expression in primate cells of cloned DNA coding for the hemagglutinin surface glycoprotein of influenza virus, Proc. Natl. Acad. Sci. USA 78:5488 (1981).

21. M. Wigler, S. Silverstein, L.S. Lee, A. Pellicer, Y. Cheng, and R. Axel, Transfer of purified Herpes virus thymidine kinase gene to cultured mouse cells, Cell 11:223 (1977).

22. A. Pellicer, M. Wigler, R. Axel, and S. Silverstein, The transfer and stable integration of the HSV thymidine kinase gene into mouse cells, Cell 14:133 (1978).

23. M. Wigler, R. Sweet, G.K. Sim, B. Wold, A. Pellicer, E. Lacy, T. Maniatis, S. Silverstein and R. Axel, Transformation of mammalian cells with genes from prokaryotes and eukaryotes, Cell 16:777 (1979).

24. T. Grodzicker and D.F. Klessig, Expression of unselected adenovirus genes in human cells co-transformed with the HSV-1 tk gene and adenovirus 2 DNA, Cell 21:453 (1980).

25. I. Abraham, J.S. Tyagi, and M.M. Gottesman, Transfer of genes to Chinese hamster ovary cells by DNA-mediated transformation, Somat. Cell. Genet. 8:23 (1982).

26. R. Subramani, R. Mulligan, and P. Berg, Expression of the mouse dihydrofolate reductase complementary deoxyribonucleic acid in simian virus 40 vectors, Mol. Cell. Biol. 1:854 (1981).

27. G. Urlaub and L.A. Chasin, Isolation of Chinese hamster cell mutants deficient in dihydrofolate reductase activity, Proc. Natl. Acad. Sci. USA 77:4216 (1980).

28. C.M. Gorman, L.F. Moffat, and B.H. Howard, Recombinant genomes which express chloramphenicol acetyltransferase in mammalian cells, Molec. Cell Biol. 2:1044-1051 (1982).

29. N. Alton and D. Vapnek, Nucleotide sequence analysis of the chloramphenicol resistance transposon Tn9, Nature 282:864 (1979).

30. J. Cohen, T. Eccleshall, R. Needleman, H. Federoff, B. Buchferer, and J. Marmur, Functional expression in yeast of the Escherichia coli plasmid gene coding for chloramphenicol acetyltransferase, Proc. Natl. Acad. Sci. USA 77:1078 (1980).

31. C.M. Gorman, G.T. Merlino, M.C. Willingham, I. Pastan, and B.H. Howard, The Rous sarcoma virus long terminal repeat is a strong promoter when introduced into a variety of eucaryotic cells by DNA mediated transfection, Proc. Natl. Acad. Sci. U.S.A. (in press).

32. I. Fettes, D. Haldar, and K. Freeman, Effect of chloramphenicol on enzyme synthesis and growth in mammalian cells, Can. J. Biochem. 50:200 (1972)

33. M. Ziegler and R. Davidson, The effect of hexose on chloramphenicol sensitivity and resistance in Chinese hamster cells, J. Cell Physiol. 98:627 (1979).

34. K. Freeman, Inhibition of mitochondrial and bacterial synthesis by chloramphenicol, Can. J. Biochem. 48:479 (1970).

35. S. Kearsey and I. Craig, Altered ribosomal RNA genes in mitochondria from mammalian cells with chloramphenicol resistance, Nature 290:607 (1981).

36. A.R. Buchman, L. Burnett, and P. Berg, Appendix A, The SV40 nucleotide sequence, in: "Molecular Biology of Tumor Viruses," Part 2, J. Tooze, ed., Cold Spring Harbor Laboratory, Cold Spring Harbor, N.Y. (1980).

CONSTRUCTION AND TRANSFER INTO MAMMALIAN CELLS OF A VECTOR CONTAINING INSECT HISTONE GENES

Raymond Reeves*, Cornelia M. Gorman†, and
Bruce H. Howard†

*Biochemistry/Biophysics Program
Washington State University
Pullman, Washington 99164

†Laboratory of Molecular Biology
National Cancer Institute
Bethesda, Maryland 20205

INTRODUCTION

As illustrated by other articles in this volume, with the advent of recombinant DNA technology and methods for introducing functional foreign genes into many types of eukaryotic cells, a revolution has occurred in the level of our understanding of the way genes are regulated in living cells. Nonetheless, in spite of the impressive progress made concerning the role of DNA sequence in functions such as promotion, enhancement, initiation of transcription, splicing, polyadenylation and termination, much remains to be learned. It is worth considering, for example, whether such information, by itself, will enable us to understand the subtleties of gene expression and regulation known to occur during complex cellular processes such as development and differentiation. For, in addition to the obvious importance of DNA sequence in the regulation of gene activity in eukaryotic cells, it is very likely that genomic function is also regulated by the structure and composition of the chromatin itself[1-4]. Thus, it seems reasonable to predict that a complete knowledge of the mechanisms regulating genomic activity in eukaryotic cells will only come when we understand both the structure and function of all the various components of chromatin.

In addition to DNA, the primary components of chromatin are basic histone proteins and various types of nonhistone proteins.

The histones are present in about equal amounts with the DNA in chromatin and, since they are among the most evolutionarily conserved of the known proteins[5], they are believed to be stable structural components of chromosomes. There are within most cells five main classes of histones designated H1, H2a, H2b, H3 and H4. In different cell types, and in different organisms, several different variants of each type of the main classes of histones are found which vary in only a few amino acids from the other members in the group[5-7]. Most of the chromatin is organized in a periodic subunit structure called a nucleosome[8]. Nucleosomes are composed of about 145 base pairs of DNA wrapped around a protein "core" composed of two each of the histones H2a, H2b, H3 and H4[2,3,8]. Although nucleosomes are found on both inactive and active genes[2-4,8], those found on active genes have a distinctive structure and composition suggesting that these properties of chromatin may play a major role in the control of gene expression and cell differentiation in eukaryotes. Until now investigations aimed at eludicating the role of chromatin structure in genomic function have been based on indirect techniques and correlations. However, with the new technologies now available we may be in a better position to investigate these same problems by directly modifying the types of chromatin found in living cells.

We report here the results of preliminary experiments whose eventual goal is to remodel chromatin in vivo by the introduction into mammalian cells of foreign genes coding for various protein components of the chromatin itself. We have chosen as a model system the histone genes of the insect Drosophila melanogaster which we have introduced into monkey tissue culture cells using the hybrid prokaryotic/eukaryotic vector pSV2•cat[9]. Additionally, we report a protocol which we have found useful for introducing various plasmid DNAs into both monolayer and suspension cultures of mammalian cells by means of bacterial protoplast fusion. Together these techniques may prove useful for studying the relationships between chromatin structure and function.

MATERIALS AND METHODS

Published recombinant DNA technology procedures have been used for these experiments[10-12]. Restriction and other enzymes, as well as synthetic oligonucleotide linkers, were obtained from either New England Biolabs or Bethesda Research Laboratory and used according to the manufacturers' instructions. The col E1 plasmid cDM500 containing the Drosophila melanogaster histone gene repeat sequence [13,14] was generously supplied by Dr. George Spiegelman, University of British Columbia. The construction of the hybrid virus/plasmid expression vectors pSV2 and pSV2•cat have been described in detail [9,15]. Exogenously supplied plasmid DNAs were introduced into either CV-1 monkey kidney cells or Friend erythroleukemia mouse cells as calcium phosphate precipitates by described procedures [9,16]. Additionally, as outlined in the APPENDIX of this paper, plasmid DNAs have been introduced into both suspension and monolayer cultures of mammalian cells by modifications of protoplast fusion techniques described by others[17,18]. Assays for the expression of bacterial chloramphenicol acetyltransferase enzyme activity in transfected mammalian cells were by rapid thin layer chromatographic techniques described by Gorman et al[9]. Analysis of histones by acid-urea polyacrylamide gel electrophoresis[19] and by triton-acid-urea gel elelctrophoresis[20] were by published protocols. Drosophila histone marker proteins were isolated from either early embryos (generously supplied by Peter Cserjesi) or from permanent tissue culture cell lines (K_c or Schneider line 2). Radioisotopes were obtained from New England Nuclear or from Amersham.

RESULTS

In order to successfully develop an experimental system for artificially "remodelling" mammalian cell chromatin *in vivo*, a number of conditions must be met. Among these are: i) A means must be found for introducing isolated foreign genes coding for specific chromosomal proteins into mammalian cells and have these genes fully functional in the host cells; ii) Experimental means must be available for unambiguously distinguishing the products of the introduced genes from the endogenous host cell chromosomal proteins; and, iii) It must be demonstrated that the protein products coded for by the foreign genes are indeed incorporated into the host cell chromatin and, if possible, to demonstrate that the incorporated proteins affect in some way either the structure or the function of the host cell chromatin. We have made some progress on the first two aspects of this problem but the third is awaiting future work.

The group of hybrid SV40/pBR322 expression vectors produced by Howard, Mulligan and Berg[12,15] have proven to be useful for introducing a number of different genes (of both bacterial and eukaryotic origin) into a number of different types of mammalian tissue culture cells[9,12,15,21-26]. In particular, the plasmid pSV2•cat which contains the bacterial gene coding for the enzyme chloramphenicol acetyltransferase (CAT) placed under the control of SV40 early promoter region of the vector has proven to be a useful vehicle for studies of transfection of cells with foreign inserted DNAs. The main advantages of this plasmid as a vector are: 1) endogenous CAT activities in mammalian cells are very low or nonexistant; 2) the CAT enzyme assay itself is extremely sensitive, very rapid and simple to use; and, 3) the pSV2•cat vector has a number of additional cloning sites where foreign genes can be inserted and thus the CAT gene can act as an internal control standard for plasmid expression of the other foreign genes present on the same vector. We, therefore, decided to use this expression vector for introducing foreign histone genes into mammalian cells.

The next problem was to select a foreign histone protein species which could be unambiguously and easily distinguished from the endogenous histones of mammalian cells. As already mentioned, histones are evolutionarily very conserved proteins and, therefore, experimentally determining whether a given histone is derived from one organism or another is often quite difficult, if not impossible. For example, on standard one dimension acid-urea polyacrylamide electrophoretic gels routinely used for separating histone protein species the mobilities of the nucleosome "core" histones of monkey CV-1 cells and of Drosophila embryo cells are quite similar. Therefore, by simply observing relative mobilities, it is difficult to distinguish the species of origin of a given histone protein band using this electrophoretic separation technique (see Figure 1, Panel A). Fortunately, the resolution of various histone species on acid-urea

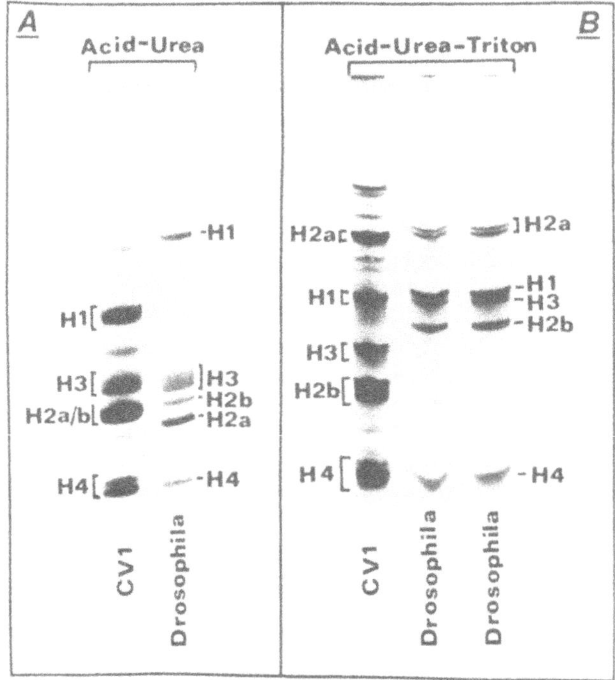

Fig. 1. Separation of Drosophila embryo and CV-1 monkey kidney cells histones on 15% polyacrylamide gels containing acid-urea (Panel A) or acid-urea-triton X-100 (Panel B).

gels is greatly increased when the nonionic detergent Triton X-100 is added to the gels[20]. Panel B in Fig. 1 shows that on such gels it is relatively easy to distinguish some of the CV-1 histones from their *Drosophila* counterparts (see, for example, histones H2a and H2b). Additionally, it is possible to distinguish *Drosophila* histone H2a from the mammalian H2a histone by differentially labeling this histone with isotopically labeled methionine since the insect histone contains this amino acid residue internally whereas the monkey histone does not[5,13,27] (see Table I). Furthermore, since the *Drosophila* histone gene repeat had already been molecularly cloned by Goldberg and Hogness [13,14], we decided to introduce the genes coding for *Drosophila* histones H2a and H2b into CV-1 cells using the pSV2·cat vector and determine whether these insect histones could be synthesized in monkey cells.

Figure 2 diagrams the construction of plasmid pSV2·CAT·DmH2a/b used for the transfection of mammalian tissue culture cells. Briefly, the 4.8 kb DNA fragment cut from plasmid cDM500 by Hind III contains a single copy of each of the five main *Drosophila* histone genes (H1, H2a, H2b, H3 and H4). Purified preparations of this fragment were digested with the enzyme Hinf I. A 1.85 kb fragment of DNA containing the entire coding sequences of histones H2a and H2b (along with their promoter and terminator regions) and part of

Table I. Internal Methionine Residues in *Drosophila* and Mammalian Histones

Histone	Calf[a] moles %	*Drosophila*[b] moles %
H1	0	0 (0.4)[c]
H2a	0	1 (1.0)[c]
H2b	2	2 (1.4)[c]
H3	2	1 (1.5)[c]
H4	1	1 (0.8)[c]

[a]Reference (5).
[b]Reference (13).
[c]Reference (27).

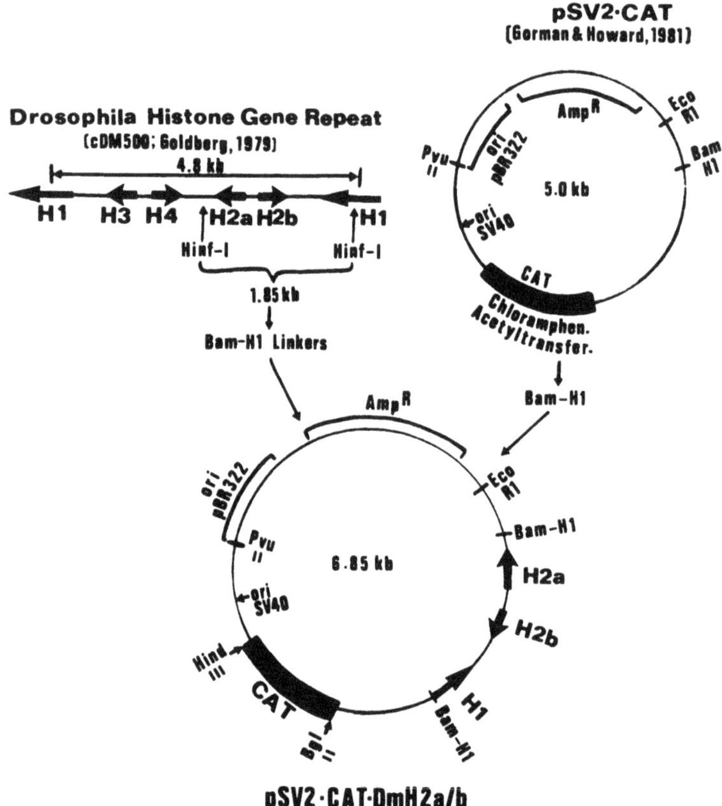

Fig. 2. Diagram showing the construction of plasmid pSV2·CAT·DmH2a/b.

the 3' end of the histone H1 sequence was isolated from the Hinf 1 digest by agarose gel electrophoresis and DNA band electroelution. The ends of the fragment were blunted by filling in with E. coli DNA polymerase I and the four deoxynucleotide triphosphates. Synthetic Bam H1 oligonucleotide linkers were added to the blund ends by means of the T4 ligase reaction and the reaction product digested with Bam H1 enzyme. The 1.85 kb DNA fragment with the Bam H1 tails was then purified by agarose gel electrophoresis and elution and ligated into the Bam H1 site of the appropriately cut pSV2·cat vector. The resulting recombinant plasmid, pSV2.CAT. DmH2a/b, was then isolated from ampicillin-resistant clones on the basis of size (the vector is 6.85 kb in length). Recombinant vectors with both orientations of the inserted histone H2a and H2b histone genes were recovered and the gene orientation of the inserts determined, relative to the CAT gene, by restriction mapping using various endonuclease enzymes.

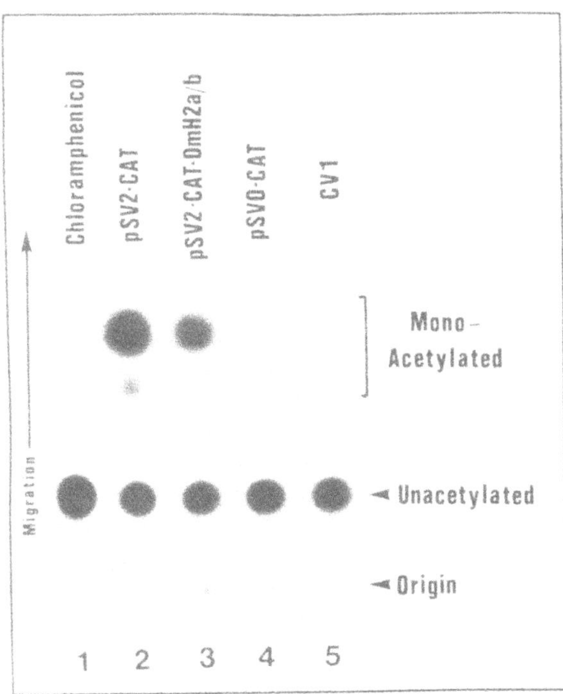

Fig. 3. Chloramphenicol acetyltransferase enzyme assays of extracts of CV-1 cells transfected with various plasmid DNAs.

Purified pSV2.CAT.DmH2a/b plasmid DNA, along with various control plasmid DNAs, was used to transfect CV-1 monkey tissue culture cells using the calcium phosphate precipitation method. Forty-eight hours after transfection, extracts of the cells were prepared and assayed for CAT enzyme activity to monitor for intracellular vector function. Figure 3 shows the results of such an assay. From this figure it is evident (as judged by the appearance of the monoacetylated forms of chloramphenicol) that both the parental vector pSV2.cat and the recombinant vector pSV2.CAT.DmH2a/b induce readily detectable amounts of CAT activity in transfected cells whereas another control vector, pSV0.cat (which lacks the SV40 early promoter sequences) does not. Thus, we conclude that the vector containing the histone gene sequences is functional for at least one of its expressible genes.

We next analyzed transfected cells for the presence of insect histones. Forty-eight hours after transfection the cells were labeled with high concentration of (^{14}C)-methionine (20 μCi/ml) for 8 hours, nuclei were isolated, histones extracted and the proteins separated by electrophoresis on long acid-urea-triton polyacrylamide gels. The gels were cut into equal sections, dissolved, and counted for radioactivity. As shown in Figure 4 (Panel A) CV-1 cells transfected with pSV2.CAT.DmH2a/b unambiguously contain (^{14}C)-labeled, acid-soluble proteins migrating in the region of the gels were authentic _Drosophila_ H2a histones migrate. On the other hand, CV-1 control cells transfected with the parental plasmid pSV2.cat do not (Fig. 4, Panel B). The region of the gels where _Drosophila_ H2b histones migrate is very close to the region of migration of the histone H3 species of CV-1 cells and thus it is unclear which proteins the radioactive labeled peaks represent in this region of the gel. These results suggest, but obviously do not prove, that the pSV2.CAT.DmH2a/b transfected cells are synthesizing an acid-soluble, methionine containing, basic nuclear protein closely resembling _Drosophila_ H2a histone. Whether this putative protein is indeed authentic insect H2a histone and, if it is, whether it is incorporated into the mammalian cell chromatin, remains to be demonstrated.

In conjunction with the above experiments on the introduction of insect histone genes into mammalian cells by calcium phosphate precipitation methods, we also explored the possibility of introducing plasmids containing these and other foreign genes into cells by means of bacterial protoplast fusion techniques. We based our procedures on modifications of the techniques described by Schaffner [17] and by Sandri-Goldin et al[18]. The APPENDIX to this paper gives our protocol for the introduction of bacterial plasmids into both monolayer tissue culture cells (such as CV-1s) as well as mammalian

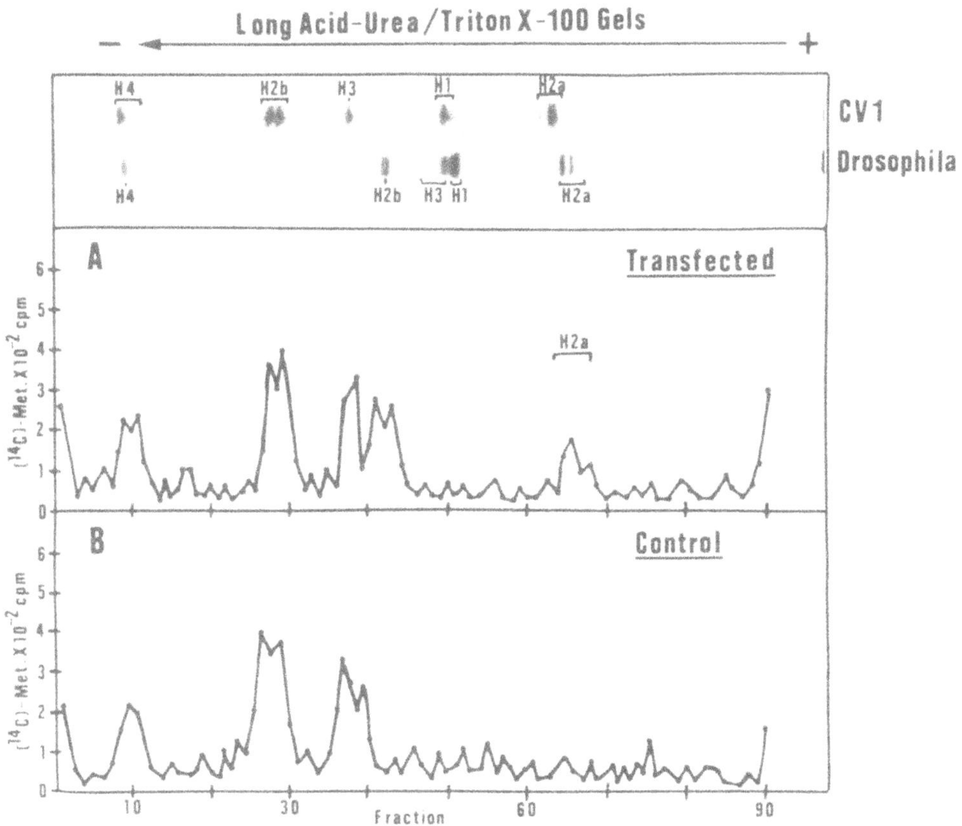

Fig. 4 Long acid-urea-triton polyacrylamide gel electrophoretic separation of histones from control CV-1 cells transfected with pSV2.cat (Panel B) and cells transfected with pSV2.CAT/DmH2a/b (Panel A). Stained reference gels at top.

cells which grow in suspension culture (such as Friend erythroleukemic mouse cells). Using these bacterial protoplast fusion techniques we have been able to introduce pSV2.cat and pSV2.CAT.DmH2a/b into both CV-1 and Friend cells and have demonstrated that the cells express appreciable amounts of CAT enzyme activity. Furthermore, using this technique we have introduced the plasmid pSV2.gtp[21,23] into CV-1 cells and demonstrated that the transfected cells can, in the presence of aminopterin and mycophenolic acid, utilized exogenously supplied xanthine as their sole source of purine. In our hands the protoplast fusion technique seems to be at least as efficient as the calcium phosphate method of transfecting CV-1 cells and may prove to be a useful alternative to this procedure.

DISCUSSION

Results reported here demonstrate that the vector pSV2.cat is a useful vehicle for carrying foreign genes into mammalian cells in short-term transfections of cells with exogenous DNA. Its main advantage as a vehicle is that the covalently attached CAT gene allows for an exquisitely sensitive "internal standard" assay for the function of the vector inside cells. For example, if during a transfection it can be demonstrated that the CAT gene is very active within the cells but some other foreign gene attached to the same plasmid is not, then the reasons for this inactivity can be investigated knowing that the vector is at least getting into the cells and capable of some expression. This consideration was of importance in the experiments reported here. Initial transfections of CV-1 cells with pSV2.CAT.DmH2a/b showed unequivocally that the vector was functioning and that large amounts of CAT activity were present. However, in the same experiments, when the cells were labeled with (^{14}C)-methionine (at 1-2 μCi/ml) for 4 hours and then nuclear histones extracted and analyzed, no labeled proteins migrating in the position of *Drosophila* H2a histones were seen on the gels. Only when much higher concentrations of isotopic label, and/or longer labeling times, were used were proteins resembling the *Drosophila* H2a histones found in transfected cells.

Possible reasons for the relatively low activity of the *Drosophila* genes (if indeed they are functional) compared to the bacterial CAT gene found on the same plasmid are plentiful. For example, in these plasmid constructs the CAT gene is driven by the SV40 early promoter region of the plasmid whereas, most probably, the *Drosophila* genes are under the control of their own insect promoter regions which might not be very active in CV-1 cells. Furthermore, most mammalian cell histone synthesis normally occurs in the S-phase of the cell cycle[28] and the transfecting plasmids most likely enter cells in all phases of the cycle; thus, the histone promoters might be inhibited in many of the transfected cells, lowering the apparent activity of these genes. Additionally, preliminary hybridization data suggest that Drosophila histone messenger RNAs are synthesized in transfected cells but much of it may be degraded rapidly--again possibly leading to lower levels than expected of the histone proteins (unpublished data). Numerous other possibilities also exist, of course, some rather trivial, such as the possibility that the CAT protein has had 48 hours to accumulate before assays are done on cell extracts whereas the labeling experiments only detect proteins made in a fairly short period of time.

In any event, the preliminary results strongly suggest that transfected CV-1 cells are synthesizing nuclear proteins closely resembling *bona fide Drosophila* H2a histones. It must be stressed, however, that considerably more evidence (for example, peptide maps of the putative insect histones) must be accumulated before it can be stated with certainty that authentic *Drosophila* histones are being synthesized in mammalian cells.

The results obtained using bacterial protoplast fusions to introduce functional plasmid genes into cells suggests that this method of cell transfection may be a viable alternative to the calcium phosphate preciptation method. In some ways it has certain advantages over the older method in that the plasmid DNA does not have to be extensively purified prior to transfections (as it does in the calcium phosphate method); this has the practical benefit of allowing the researcher, within a relatively short time period, to screen large numbers of possible recombinant plasmids for a particular gene that is functional in mammalian cells

REFERENCES

1. B. Lewin, "Gene Expression 2: Eucaryotic Chromosomes," John Wiley & Sons, New York (1980).
2. G. Felsenfeld, Chromatin, *Nature*, 271:115 (1978).
3. J. D. McGee and G. Felsenfeld, Nucleosome structure, *Annu. Rev. Biochem.*, 49:1115 (1980).
4. S. Weisbrod, Active chromatin, *Nature*, 297:289 (1982).
5. I. Isenberg, Histones, *Annu. Rev. Biochem.*, 48:159 (1979).
6. S. G. Franklin and A. Zweidler, Non-allelic variants of histones H2a, 2b and 3 in mammals, *Nature*, 266:273 (1977).
7. W. M. Bonner, M. H. West and J. D. Stedman, Two-dimensional gel analysis of histones in acid extracts of nuclei, cells and tissues, *Eur. J. Biochem.*, 109:17 (1980).
8. R. Kornberg, Structure of chromatin, *Annu. Rev. Biochem.*, 46:931 (1977).

9. C. M. Gorman, L. F. Moffat and B. H. Howard, Recombinant genomes which express chloramphenicol acetyltransferase in mammalian cells, Molec. Cell Biol., in press (1982).
10. R. Wu, Ed., "Recombinant DNA", Methods Enzymol., vol. 68, Academic Press, New York (1979).
11. R. Davis, D. Botstein and J. R. Roth, "Advanced Bacterial Genetics: A Manual for genetic Engineering," Cold Spring Harbor Laboratory, New York (1980).
12. R. Mulligan, B. H. Howard and P. Berg, Synthesis of rabbit β-globin in cultured monkey cells following infection with a SV40 β-globin recombinant genome, Nature, 277: 108 (1979).
13. M. L. Goldberg, "Sequence Analysis of Drosophila Histone Genes," Ph.D. Thesis, Stanford University (1979).
14. R. P. Lifton, M. L. Goldberg, R. W. Karp and D. S. Hogness, The organization of the histone genes in Drosophila melanogaster: Functional and evolutionary implications, Cold Spring Harbor Symp. Quant. Biol., 42:1047 (1977).
15. R. C. Mulligan, P. F. Southern, B. H. Howard, M. Yaniv, A. I. Geller and P. Berg, Construction and potential uses for a family of mammalian transducing vectors, J. Molec. Appl. Genet., in press (1982).
16. F. Graham and A. van der Eb, A new technique for the assay of infectivity of human adenovirus 5 DNA, Virology, 52: 456 (1978).
17. W. Schaffner, Direct transfer of cloned genes from bacteria to mammlaian cells, Proc. Natl. Acad. Sci. USA, 77:2163 (1980).
18. R. M. Sandri-Goldin, A. L. Goldin, M. Levine and J. C. Glorioso, High-frequency transfer of cloned Herpes simplex virus type 1 sequences to mammalian cells by protoplast fusion, Molec. Cell. Biol., 8:743 (1981).
19. S. Panyim and R. Chalkley, High resolution acrylamide gel electrophoresis of histones, Arch. Biochem. Biophys., 130:337 (1969).
20. A. Zweidler, Resolution of histones by polyacrylamide gel electrophoresis in the presence of nonionic detergents, Methods Cell. Biol., 17:223 (1978).
21. R. C. Mulligan and P. Berg, Expression of a bacterial gene in mammalian cells, Science, 209:1422 (1980).
22. R. C. Mulligan and P. Berg, Selection for animal cells that express the Escherichia coli gene coding for xanthine-guanine phosphoribosyltransferase, Proc. Natl. Acad. Sci USA, 78:2072 (1981).
23. P. Berg, Dissections and reconstructions of genes and chromosomes, Science, 213:296 (1981).
24. D. Schumperli, B. H. Howard and M. Rosenberg, Efficient expression of the E. coli galactokinase gene in mammalian cells, Proc. Natl. Acad. Sci. USA, 79:257 (1982).

25. P. J. Southern and P. Berg, Transformation of mammalian cells to antibiotic resistance with a bacterial gene under control of the SV40 early region promoter, J. Molec. Appl. Genet., in press (1982).
26. C. M. Gorman, G. T. Merlino, M. C. Willingham, I. Pastan and B. H. Howard, The Rouse sarcoma virus 3' long terminal repeat is a strong promoter when introduced into a variety of eucaryotic cells by DNA mediated transfection, manuscript submitted (1982).
27. C. R. Alfageme, A. Zweidler, A. Mahowald and L. H. Cohen, Histones of Drosophila embryos, J. Biol. Chem., 249:3729 (1974).
28. T. W. Borun, M. B. Scharff and E. Robbins, Rapidly labeled, polyribosome associated, RNA having the properties of histone messenger, Proc. Natl. Acad. Sci. USA 58:1977 (1967).

APPENDIX

Protoplast Fusion Transfer of Plasmid DNA to Animal Cells

I. Monolayer Cell Culture (e.g., CV-1 monkey cells)

1. Logarithmic phase bacterial cultures (A_{600} = 0.7-0.8; An A_{600} of 0.500 = approx. 2 x 10^8 bacteria) growing in LB are collected by centrifugation (10 min at 5,000 rpm at 4°C). About 2-3 x 10^9 bacteria are required per tissue culture flask (25 cm^2), thus set up appropriate volumes of starter bacteria cultures accordingly. Strain HB101 bacteria was used in these experiments.

   For 50 ml of log phase cells, take a 4 ml O/N culture of bacteria and inoculate into 50 ml of super broth. An A_{600} of 0.7-0.8 is reached in 2-3 hrs at 37°.

   (N.B. We have used bacteria from O/N stationary cultures in super broth, and have obtained good fusion results although it is more difficult to obtain good protoplasts from these cultures than it is from log phase cells. Also, O/N chloramphenicol amplified plasmid-containing bacteria are good for protoplasts.)

2. Resuspend bacteria in 20% sucrose (in 50 mM Tris, pH 8.0) at about 10^9 bacteria in 1.25 ml.

3. To each 1.25 ml of bacterial solution add 0.25 ml of fresh lysozyme solution (2 mg/ml in 0.25 M Tris, pH 8.0). If protoplasts rupture too easily at this lysozyme concentration, either decrease the lysozyme concentration or

decrease the time of incubation of the bacteria at 37° -see below.

4. Hold on ice for 5 min.

5. Add 0.5 ml of 0.25 M EDTA, pH 8, for each 1.25 ml of bacterial solution.

6. Hold on ice for 5 min.

7. Slowly (with very gently mixing) add 0.5 ml of 50 mM Tris, pH 8.0, for each 10^9 bacteria volume.

8. Incubate at 37° for 10-12 min (longer or shorter depending on the extent of wall digestion) until greater than 90-95% of the bacteria have lost their walls. The digestion is monitored every few minutes by observation with a phase microscope (40X) at each time point. The digestion culture is also gently mixed by swirling. It is very important not to overdigest the bacteria but still make sure most of them are indeed protoplasts--thus, a fine balance between the two extremes is needed.

9. SLOWLY (over a 5-7 min period) and very carefully dilute each 10^9 bacterial volume with 10 ml of serum-free DME medium containing 10% sucrose and 10 mM $MgCl_2$. This is the most difficult part of the procedure for it is at this stage that protoplast lysis usually occurs. The solution can be added dropwise with gentle swirling of the tube as the drops are added. However, we have found that if the drops are added via a 9-inch Pasteur pipet to the center of the bacterial solution as the test tube is held at a steep angle and as both the test tube and the pipet are slowly rotated to uniformly mix the solutions, lysis is minimized and, therefore, no DNase must be added to the solution to break up released DNA resulting from cell lysis.

   At the end of the mixing, check with the 40X phase microscope to see that the bacteria are now grayish spheres with scattered remains of cell walls attached as opposed to the original dark rods of about the same diameter.

10. Hold at room temp. for 10 min.

11. Remove medium from monolayer tissue culture cells and add about 10-12 ml of protoplast solution (containing about 10^9 bacteria) to the cells.

12. Centrifuge the tissue culture flask (Falcon #3031, 25 cm^2 with canted neck) at 1,500 xg (i.e., about 2500 rpm) for 8 min in a swinging bucket rotor head using a modified Cook "microtiter" plate holder (Cook #A109) adapted to hold the Falcon flask securely.

13. Remove supernatant by aspiration and drain flask by tilting for 30 sec and remove residual solution.

14. Add 2-3 ml of 47.5% polyethylene glycol-1000 (in PBS or Tris-saline). Add PEG along one side of the flask as it is held at an angle, then tilt the flask to cover the surface of the cells with the PEG. Hold for 90 seconds (no longer) at room temp. (N.B. Make sure the pH of the PEG is adjusted to pH 7.3-7.4 prior to use)

15. Aspirate off the PEG and rapidly rinse the flask three times with 5 ml of serum-free DME medium containing 200 μg/ml of gentamycin and 100 units per ml of penicillin and streptomycin.

16. To each flask add 5-10 ml of complete DME medium containing, in addition, 200 μg/ml of gentamycin.

17. After 48 hr of growth, the cells should be confluent and are ready for assay or for subculturing into selection medium.

II. Preparation of Monolayer Tissue Culture Cells for Protoplast Fusion:

The day before protoplast fusion, the tissue culture cells should be subcultured at a density that will grow to confluence in about 3 days. For CV-1 monkey cells this is about $4\text{-}5 \times 10^5$ cells per 25 cm^2 flask (Falcon #3031). The flask should be of the appropriate size to fit snugly into the microtiter plate centrifuge holder. On the day of fusion, three hours before the actual fusion, a complete medium change should be made on the cells. Since the PEG solution causes promiscuous membrane fusions, the monolayer tissue culture cells should not be touching each other too closely during the protoplast fusion step.

III. Protoplast Fusions to Cells Growing in Suspension (e.g., Friend erythroleukemia mouse cells).

Bacterial protoplasts are prepared as above. On the day before fusion the tissue culture suspension cells are subcultured at a density that will reach confluency or saturation in about 3 days (for Friend cells this is about 2.5×10^5 cells per 25 cm^2 flask). On the day of fusion, three hours before the experiment, the cells are pelleted by centrifugation (1,500 xg, 10 min) and resuspended in fresh medium.

Steps of Fusion

1. Add about $1-2 \times 10^9$ bacterial protoplasts per $1-1.5 \times 10^6$ suspension culture cells and pellet the two together in a 50 ml Corning Screw Cap centrifuge tube with a conical bottom (1,500 xg, 8 min). Carefully aspirate off the supernatant and resuspend cells and protoplasts in about 1 ml of serum-free DME containing 10% sucrose and 10 mM $MgCl_2$. Add 2-3 ml of 47.5% PEG with gentle agitation to evenly mix and leave at room temp. for 90 sec (no longer). Immediately add 40-45 ml of fresh, warm, complete DME medium containing 200 μg/ml of gentamycin. This rapid dilution is necessary to prevent the PEG from killing the cells. The actual concentration of PEG used and the length of exposure of cells may vary from cell type to type. After 1 hour incubation at 37°, the cells are gently pelleted at low speed (about 800 rpm, for 10-15 min) and the supernatant aspirated off. Fresh medium (about 10 ml) is added and the cells resuspended and put in a 25 cm^2 flask. After 48 hr the cells are ready for assay.

AN INSECT VIRUS FOR GENETIC ENGINEERING: DEVELOPING BACULOVIRUS POLYHEDRIN SUBSTITUTION VECTORS

Lois K. Miller, David W. Miller and Michael J. Adang

Department of Bacteriology and Biochemistry
The University of Idaho
Moscow, ID 83843

INTRODUCTION

Baculoviruses are exceptionally attractive candidates as vectors for propagating and expressing exogenous DNAs in a eukaryotic (invertebrate) environment (Miller, 1981a). Among the features which make baculoviruses highly advantageous as recombinant DNA vector systems are (1) a covalently-closed, circular, nuclear-replicating DNA genome, (2) an extendable rod-shaped capsid, (3) a group of genes, involved in occlusion, that are nonessential for infectious virus production and thus deletable, and (4) a strong promoter which is turned on after infectious virus production and controls the synthesis of the major occlusion body protein (polyhedrin), constituting approximately ten percent of the protein of infected cells. The replacement of the polyhedrin gene with passenger DNA was previously suggested as an approach to using baculoviruses as recombinant DNA vectors (Miller, 1981a). The initial experimental advances our laboratory has made in developing the baculovirus *Autographa californica* nuclear polyhedrosis virus (AcNPV) as a vector in insect cells are described herein.

IDENTIFICATION AND CHARACTERIZATION OF THE AcNPV POLYHEDRIN GENE

Location of the Polyhedrin Gene on the AcNPV Physical Map

The first step in utilizing the polyhedrin promoter to express

---

Published with the approval of the director of the Idaho Agricultural Experiment Station as Research Paper 82517.

exogenous DNA was to determine the location of the polyhedrin gene with respect to the physical map of AcNPV (see Fig. 1). Poly A-containing mRNA was isolated at 27 hours post-infection (a time of active polyhedrin synthesis) from AcNPV infected *Spodoptera frugiperda* (Lepidoptera:Noctuidae) cells. Complementary DNA (cDNA) was synthesized by reverse transcription using an oligo dT primer and duplex DNA was formed using *E. coli* DNA polymerase I. The ends of the cDNA were tailed by calf thymus terminal transferase, annealed to complementary tailed PstI-cut pBR322 plasmid vector DNA and the resulting DNA was used to transform *E. coli* (Adang and Miller, 1982). Of the 45 AcNPV-homologous clones isolated, 27% hybridized to the AcNPV HindIII-V region at 3.3 to 4.0 map units (Fig. 1). The largest of these clones, pMA-VI-1, was 0.74 Kb. The pMA-VI-1 DNA was used to hybrid select homologous mRNA. The pMA-VI-1-specific mRNA directed the *in vitro* synthesis of a 32K protein with a rabbit reticulocyte lysate system. This 32K protein was

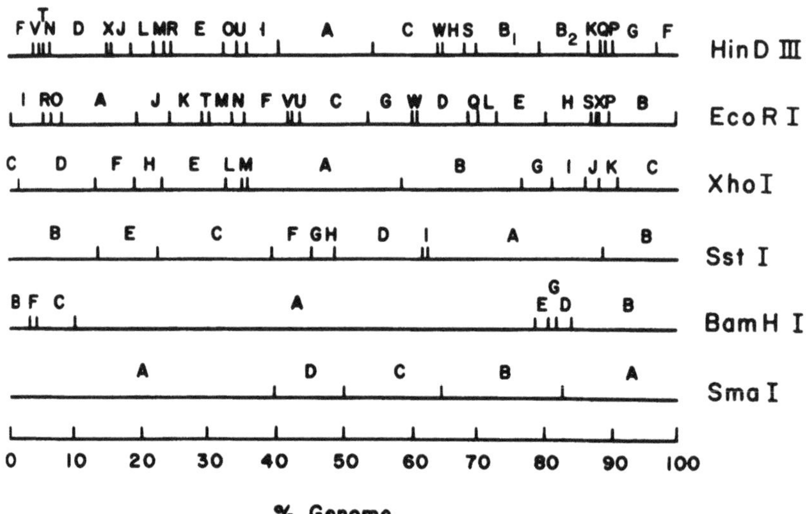

Fig. 1. A linear representation of the restriction endonuclease recognition sites in the circular DNA of the L-1 variant of AcNPV is shown. The fragment nomenclature and map orientation conforms with the recent proposal for uniform AcNPV nomenclature (Vlak and Smith, 1982). The L-1 variant has an additional HindIII site within HindIII-B and the two fragments are referred to as B_1 and B_2 (Miller and Adang, 1982). The total genome size is approximately 128 Kb.

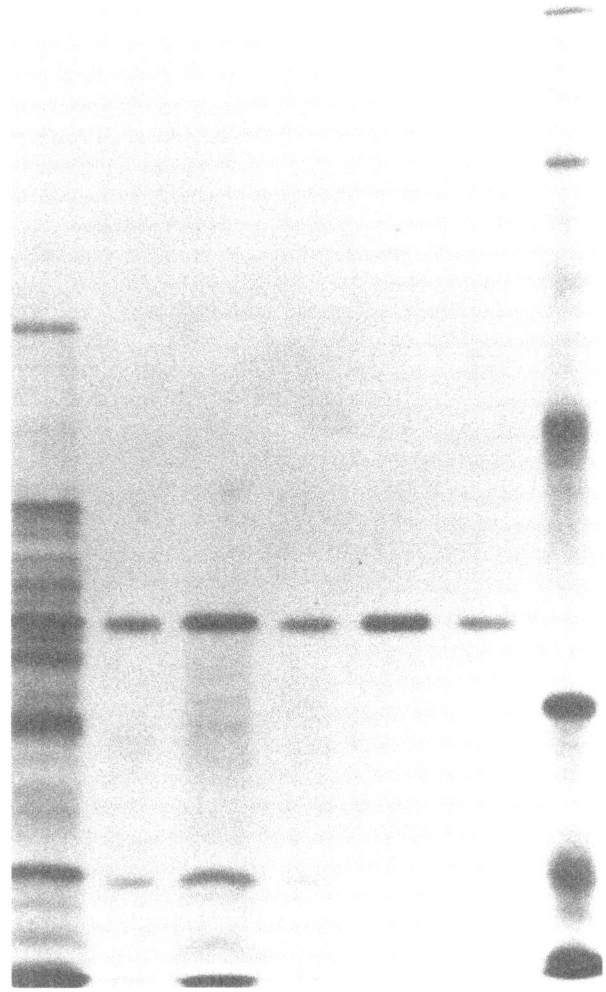

Fig. 2. In vitro translation of mRNA homologous to cDNA plasmid clone pMA-VI-1 results in the synthesis of polyhedrin as demonstrated by SDS-PAGE analysis of ^{3}H-leucine-labeled, in vitro synthesized proteins. Lanes from left to right are (1) proteins synthesized from poly A-containing mRNA isolated late in infection, (2) protein as in lane 1 immune precipitated with polyhedrin antisera, (3) proteins synthesized from pMA-VI-1 homologous poly A-containing mRNA, (4) proteins of lane 3 immune precipitated with polyhedrin antisera, (5) purified, in vivo synthesized polyhedrin, (6) lane 5 proteins immune precipitated by polyhedrin antisera, and (7) molecular weight standards of 200, 92.5, 68, 43, 25.7, 18.4 and 12.3 Kd.

immune precipitable with polyhedrin antibody and comigrated electrophoretically with in vivo synthesized polyhedrin (Adang and Miller, 1982; see Fig. 2). Since the method of cDNA cloning involved oligo dT priming, the 3' terminal portion of the polyhedrin mRNA, having a poly-A tail, is expected to be preferentially cloned. Thus, the 3' terminal portion of the polyhedrin gene is probably located between 3.3 and 4.0 map units of the AcNPV physical map.

The Nature of Polyhedrin Gene Transcription

The size of the polyhedrin gene transcript was determined by isolating total cellular RNA from AcNPV infected cells at various times post-infection, fractionating the RNA by size on an agarose gel, transferring the RNA to a nitrocellulose filter by a Northern blot procedure and locating the polyhedrin gene-homologous RNA(s) by hybridization with ^{32}P-labeled, nick-translated, pMA-VI-DNA. The results are shown in Fig. 3. Very little or no polyhedrin RNA was observed at 0 or 6 hours post-infection. At 12 hours post-infection, an RNA, approximately 1.2 Kb long, was observed and increased in quantity through 24 hours post-infection. Since RNAs from other regions of the viral genome are observed earlier in infection (Miller and Miller, unpublished results), the synthesis of polyhedrin mRNA is temporally controlled. The pMA-VI-1 cDNA, 0.74 Kb in length, thus represents approximately 62% of the total 1.2 Kb polyhedrin mRNA. Since pMA-VI-1 hybridizes only to the 0.87 Kb HindIII-V region of AcNPV, there are apparently few if any sequences within the HindIII-V region which are removed by splicing. From the experiments in Fig. 3, we cannot rule out the possibility of splicing within the polyhedrin gene; there is a trace of homologous RNA which hybridizes in the 5.0 Kb region of the Northern blot which may represent precursor RNA.

THE STRATEGY FOR DEVELOPING AN AcNPV POLYHEDRIN SUBSTITUTION VECTOR

General Considerations for the AcNPV Vector System

We now know the location of the 3'-terminal 62% of the 1.2 Kb polyhedrin gene of AcNPV. Our approach to replacing polyhedrin with a passenger DNA is to clone in *E. coli*, using a plasmid vector, a segment of AcNPV DNA from 0.0 to approximately 6.0 map units encompassing at least the 3' terminal segment of the polyhedrin gene from 3.3 to 4.0, if not the entire gene (the 5' terminus has not yet been identified). A restriction endonuclease, that recognizes a site or sites within the polyhedrin gene region, may then be used to open the recombinant plasmid DNA creating a site for the insertion of passenger DNA. BamHI has some potentially useful sites in this region and this possibility is currently being explored. Once the passenger DNA is inserted into the cloned plasmid, the plasmid can be used in a "marker rescue" fashion (Miller, 1981b). Using this

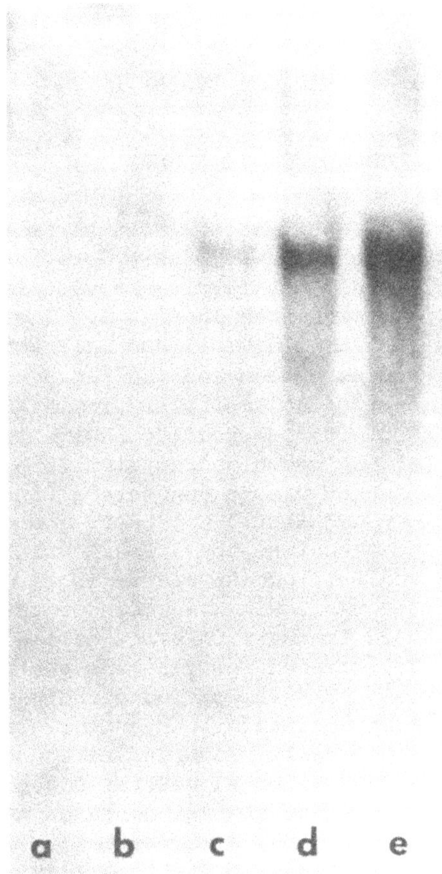

Fig. 3. Northern blot of 1.4% agarose gel containing mRNA isolated from AcNPV-infected cells at various times post-infection was hybridized to ^{32}P-labeled pMA-VI-1 DNA and the blot was autoradiographed. Lanes a-e represent 0, 6, 12, 18 and 24 hours post-infection respectively. The single major RNA transcript is approximately 1.2 Kb. A very weak region of homology was observed in the 5 Kb region of the blot.

technique, full length AcNPV DNA is cotransfected with a fragment of AcNPV DNA. Allelic replacement occurs either by gene conversion or a double recombination event resulting in the replacement of DNA in the full length viral DNA with DNA from the fragment. In the example above, it should be possible to replace the polyhedrin gene with a passenger DNA and select for passenger DNA-containing viruses by screening plaques for absence of occlusion bodies by visual observation of virus plaques under the light microscope. A total deletion of the polyhedrin gene is not necessary since the rod-shaped nucleocapsid of baculoviruses is extendable to greater lengths. The extendable nature of AcNPV has now been demonstrated by the characterization of a mutant of AcNPV carrying a 7.5 Kb copia-like transposable element (Miller and Miller, 1982).

Construction of a Plasmid Clone, pEXS942 Containing the Polyhedrin Gene

In order to pursue the possibility of inserting a passenger DNA into AcNPV L-1, we have cloned the 0.0 to 8.7 region of AcNPV L-1 DNA in *E. coli* using pBR325 (Bolivar, 1978) as a vector. The plasmid containing this region is presented in Fig. 4. The plasmid was constructed by digesting pBR325 with EcoRI and SalI which cleave within the chloramphenicol resistance gene and the tetracycline resistance genes, respectively, leaving the ampicillin resistance gene and replication origin intact with one EcoRI cohesive end and one SalI cohesive end. AcNPV L-1 DNA was digested simultaneously with EcoRI and XhoI; the original intent was to generate a viral DNA fragment containing an XhoI sticky end at 1.9 map units and an EcoRI sticky end at 5.9 map units and then fuse the 1.9-5.9 viral DNA fragment with the pBR325 EcoRI and SalI cohesive ends (SalI and XhoI generate identical cohesive ends). Following ligation of the EcoRI, XhoI or SalI digested viral/pBR325 fragment DNAs, *E. coli* RRl was transformed. $Ap^R Cm^S Tet^S$ colonies were screened for plasmids containing BamF. In the course of this screen, pEXS942 was found and has properties which in some respects were more desirable than the originally conceived plasmid type. pEXS942 apparently arose due to the cocloning of an AcNPV Xho-EcoRI fragment and an EcoRI partial digestion product containing EcoRI-I, R and O. Since pEXS942 contains the region from 0.0 to 8.7 rather than 1.9 to 5.9, a larger region of the AcNPV genome and more DNA on both sides of the HindIII-V region (3.3 to 4.0) has been obtained and this is expected to facilitate the double recombination (or gene conversion event) necessary for marker rescue between plasmid DNA and AcNPV L-1 DNA *in vivo*. Another advantage is the presence of the viral PstI site at 8.0 which will be useful in further constructions to insert passenger DNA into the polyhedrin region. Finally, the 0.0 to 8.7 region totally encompasses the HindIII-N region of AcNPV which rescues tsB113 (Miller, 1981b). Thus tsB113 and pEXS942 can be used together as an additional selection for allelic replacement.

Determining Essential Functions in the BamF Region of AcNPV L-1

It was of interest to determine whether the region of AcNPV L-1 encompassing BamF could be deleted in its entirety. To this end, pEXS942 DNA was digested with BamHI and religated so as to delete the BamF fragment. A plasmid lacking BamF was isolated and is heretofore referred to as pEXS942B3. During the course of isolating this deletion plasmid, we also isolated a plasmid pEXS942B6 which lacks the BamHI site at 4.5 (Fig. 1). Thus pEXS942B6 has only a

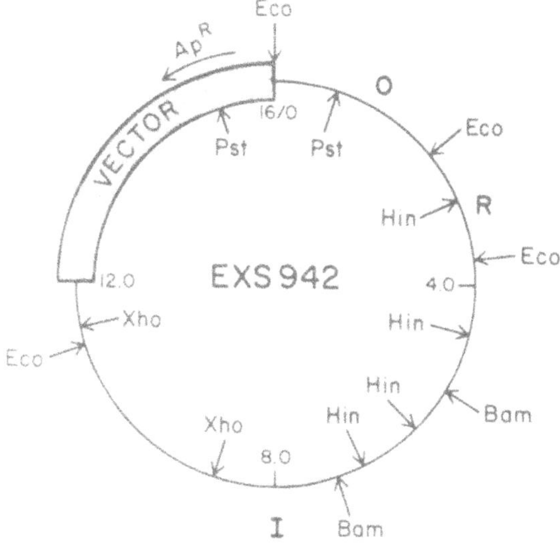

Fig. 4. A physical map of the pEXS942 plasmid DNA is presented. This plasmid contains the 0.0 to 8.7 region of AcNPV L-1 DNA (see Fig. 1) including EcoRI-I, R and O fragments (denoted in heavy letters. The vector segment was derived by EcoRI and SalI digestion of pBR325.

single BamHI site at 7.2 Kb map units (Fig. 4). The EXS942B3 and B6 plasmid DNAs were cotransfected with AcNPV tsB113 DNA into *Spodoptera frugiperda* cells using a slight modification of a previously described $CaCl_2$ transfection procedure (Potter and Miller, 1980). Plaques have been picked and are currently being analyzed to determine (1) if allelic replacement has occurred and (2) if pEXS942B3 and B6 allelic replacements result in viable viruses. These experiments should provide information on whether the Bam sites near the polyhedrin gene may be used as entry sites for passenger DNA insertion.

SUMMARY

Progress in developing the baculovirus AcNPV as a vector for propagating passenger DNA in insect cells has been rapid. The polyhedrin gene was previously recognized as a potentially valuable site for passenger DNA insertion since polyhedrin is synthesized in high quantity very late in infection (following extracellular progeny virus production). Thus passenger DNAs, including those with gene products causing cell death, may be propagated and possibly expressed at a high level in an invertebrate environment (Miller, 1981a). The location of the polyhedrin gene with respect to the physical map of AcNPV has now been determined. The 3' terminal 62% of the 1.2 Kb gene is located within AcNPV HindIII-V. Appropriate sites for inserting passenger DNA in the polyhedrin region have been identified.

Since there are no known unique restriction endonuclease sites in the virus genome, it will be necessary to employ a marker rescue technique to achieve allelic replacement of the polyhedrin gene with passenger DNA. In this procedure, the region of AcNPV surrounding the polyhedrin gene is cloned in E. coli; we have isolated a plasmid pEXS942 which includes the AcNPV region from 0.0 to 8.7 map units thus encompassing the polyhedrin 3' terminal 62% between 3.3 and 4.0. The polyhedrin region in pEXS942 or its derivatives can be replaced with an appropriate passenger DNA while in plasmid form. The resulting pEXS942-passenger plasmid DNA can then be cotransfected with wild-type AcNPV DNA. A double recombination or gene conversion event between the recombinant plasmid DNA and wild-type AcNPV should result in allelic replacement of the polyhedrin gene of AcNPV with passenger DNA. The basis for this allelic replacement step was previously developed for marker rescue of AcNPV ts mutations (Miller, 1981b). Successful allelic replacement of the polyhedrin gene with passenger DNA should result in viruses defective in occlusion body formation. This phenotype is visually selectable in plaque assays. In addition, a mutation in an AcNPV mutant, tsB113, maps adjacent to the polyhedrin gene so that successful allelic replacement within this region may also be selected by decreased temperature sensitivity.

Thus a potentially very valuable host/vector system is essentially ready to be employed for a variety of purposes (once an appropriate restriction site for passenger DNA insertion has been identified). We envision that this vector system may be of greatest value for those wishing to propagate and express large segments of eukaryotic passenger DNA in a eukaryotic environment. Initially we recommend the use of AcNPV in lepidopteran noctuid cell lines. We are aware of the interest in expressing the vector in other cell types and note that replication of AcNPV has been reported to occur in a mosquito (dipteran) cell line and in a mammalian cell line (Sherman and McIntosh, 1979; McIntosh and Sherry, 1980). Since the extracellular form of AcNPV is enveloped with a cell-derived unit membrane, fusion of the virus with a variety of cell types may be expected. Whether full expression of the viral genome can occur in the more diverse cell lines remains to be investigated. Since lepidopteran noctuid cell lines are easy to maintain and can be scaled up to commercial levels, the insect cell lines can currently be used advantageiously for a variety of applications.

ACKNOWLEDGMENTS

This research is supported in part by Public Health Service grant AI 17338 from the National Institute of Allergy and Infectious Diseases. The technical assistance of David Browne is greatly appreciated.

REFERENCES

Adang, M. J., and Miller, L. K., 1982, Molecular cloning of DNA complementary to mRNA of the baculovirus *Autographa californica* nuclear polyhedrosis virus: Location and gene products of RNA transcripts found late in infection, J. of Virol., in press.

Bolivar, F., 1978, Construction and characterization of new cloning vehicles. III. Derivatives of plasmid pBR322 carrying unique EcoRI sites for selection of EcoRI generated recombinant DNA molecules, *Gene*, 4:121.

McIntosh, A. H., and Shamy, R., 1980, Biological studies of a baculovirus in a mammalian cell line, *Intervirol.*, 13:331.

Miller, D. W., and Miller, L. K., 1982, A virus with an insertion of a copia-like transposable element. *Nature*, in press.

Miller, L. K., 1981a, A virus vector for genetic engineering in eukaryotes, *in*: "Genetic Engineering in the Plant Sciences," N. J. Panopoulos, ed., Praeger Publishers, New York.

Miller, L. K., 1981b, Construction of a genetic map of the baculovirus *Autographa californica* nuclear polyhedrosis virus by marker rescue of temperature-sensitive mutants, *J. of Virol.*, 39:973.

Potter, K. N., and Miller, L. K., 1980, Correlating genetic mutations of a baculovirus with the physical map of the DNA genome, *in*: "Animal Virus Genetics," B. N. Fields, R. Jaenisch, and C. F. Fox, eds., Academic Press, New York.

Sherman, K. E., and McIntosh, A. H., 1979, Baculovirus replication in a mosquito (dipteran) cell line, *Infect. and Immun.*, 26:232.

Vlak, J. M., and Smith, G. E., 1982, Orientation of the genome of *Autographa californica* nuclear polyhedrosis virus: A proposal, *J. of Virol.*, 41:1118.

GENETIC ENGINEERING OF PLANT CELLS: A RAPID OVERVIEW

Paul F. Lurquin

Program in Genetics and Cell Biology
Washington State University
Pullman, Washington 99164-4350 USA

The genetic manipulation of plant cells via DNA-mediated transformation has been a slow and frustrating enterprise.

Back in the pre-recombinant DNA days, at a time when neither E. coli nor mammalian cells had been conclusively shown to be transformable, it seemed as though plants were on the verge to destroy the old myth that DNA from a given species could never survive in the cells of another one[1,2].

Alas, repeated attempts to reproduce integration, replication and expression of prokaryotic DNA in plant cells consistently failed [3,4]. Later on, the discovery of the Agrobacterium tumefaciens pTi plasmid[5] and its involvement in crown gall definitely shattered the dogma. Quite certainly, DNA could be maintained in both a prokaryote and, ironically, plant cells[6,7]. Of course, in this latter case, it was not Man, but A. tumefaciens which was doing the job. Anyway, the Ti plasmid in its host are now being used as a means to introduce foreign DNA into plant cells. Difficulties to regenerate engineered real plants from crown gall tumors may be circumvented by using A. rhizogenes plasmids as vectors.

Nevertheless, and despite its enormous interest, the Agrobacterium system may not be the best nor the last one for use in plant genetic engineering. Indeed, the Ti plasmid technology is not very simple and Agrobacterium does not transform monocotyledonous plants, our major plant food source.

Therefore, the direct DNA-mediated transformation of plant cells retains all its importance. Since the early authoritative and unfortunately unsupported claims, ten years have elapsed. Where are we now? It seems that we may be able to see the light at the end of the tunnel. For one thing, it is generally accepted that plant protoplasts and not plant cells are suitable candidates for the transfer of DNA, thanks to the ability of the plasma membrane to fuse with other biological or synthetic membranes and thanks to its higher degree of permeability to macromolecules as compared to the plant cell wall.

Of course, this approach raises the question of the regeneration of plant protoplasts. This can be done in a number of plant species, most of them being totally devoid of economical interest. Again, one cannot refrain a feeling of discouragement when one notices that protoplasts isolated from monocotyledonous plants are the ones that are most refractory to regeneration.

Going back to DNA uptake and expression in plant protoplasts, it is interesting to note that the first demonstration of *Chlamydomonas* DNA transformation by a recombinant yeast plasmid[8] was made possible thanks to DNA uptake techniques established several years earlier[9,10,11] in the total absence of a biological assay system. Similarly, higher plant protoplasts seems to have been transformed using a closely related technique[12] or DNA encapsulated in liposomes[13] following reports that indeed liposomes loaded with nucleic acids could apparently deliver them into plant protoplasts without drastic damage[14,15].

In other words, DNA uptake experiments in plant cells do have a heuristic value, a question which I raised in a review article published in 1977[3]. Moreover, it has also been shown that protoplasts can be transformed when incubated with DNA in the presence of polyethylene glycol and Ca^{++} ions[16], an "old trick" used to "activate" the plasma membrane.

Are we being too shy? Do we know how to transform plant protoplasts and hesitate to do some crucial experiments? Or does Pasteur's statement hold true more than ever: "Quelle idée vous faites - vous donc du progrès dans la Science? La Science fait un pas, un autre, puis elle s'arrête et se recueille avant d'en faire un troisième."

References

1. Ledoux, L. and R. Huart. Fate of exogenous bacterial deoxyribonucleic acids in barley seedlings. *J. Molec. Biol.* 43:243 (1969).
2. Ledoux, L., R. Huart and M. Jacobs. DNA-mediated genetic correction of thiamineless *Arabidopsis thaliana*. *Nature* 249:17 (1974).

3. Lurquin, P. F. Integration versus degradation of exogenous DNA in plants: An open question. In: Progress in Nucleic Acids Research and Molecular Biology, W. E. Cohn, ed., Academic Press, New York, vol. 20, p. 161 (1977).
4. Kleinhofs, A. and R. M. Behki. Prospects for plant genome modification by nonconventioal methods. Ann. Rev. Genet. 11:79 (1977).
5. Zaenen, I., N. Van Larebeke, H. Teuchy, M. Van Montagu and J. Schell. Supercoiled circular DNA in crown gall inducing Agrobacterium strains. J. Molec. Biol. 86:109 (1974).
6. Chilton, M.-D., M. H. Drummond, D. J. Merlo, D. Sciaky, A. L. Montoya, M. P. Gordon and E. W. Nester. Stable incorporation of plasmid DNA into higher plant cells: The molecular basis of crown gall tumorigenesis. Cell 11:263 (1977).
7. Thomashow, M. F., R. Nutter, K. Postle, M.-D. Chilton, F. R. Blattner, A. Powell, M. P. Gordon and E. W. Nester. Recombination between higher plant DNA and the Ti plasmid of Agrobacterium tumefaciens. Proc. Natl. Acad. Sci. USA 77:6448 (1980).
8. Rochaix, J.-D. and J. van Dillewijn. Transformation of the green alga Chlamydomonas reinhardii with yeast DNA. Nature 296: 70 (1982).
9. Lurquin, P. F. and R. M. Behki. Use of molecular sieving on agarose gels to study DNA uptake by Chlamydomonas reinhardii. In: Genetic Manipuation with Plant Materials, L. Ledous, ed., Plenum Press, New York, p. 429 (1975).
10. Suzuki, M. and I. Takebe. Uptake of single-strand bacteriophage DNA by isolated tobacco protoplasts. Z. Pflanzenphysiol. 78:421 (1976).
11. Lurquin, P. F. and C. I. Kado. Escherichia coli plasmid pBR313 insertion into plant protoplasts and into their nuclei. Molec. Gen. Genet. 154:113 (1977)
12. Davey, M. R., E. C. Cocking, J. Freeman, N. Pearce and I. Tudor. Transformation of Petunia protoplasts by isolated Agrobacterium plasmids. Plant Sci. Lett. 18:307 (1980).
13. Dellaporta, S. L. and R. T. Fraley. Delivery of liposome-encapsulated nucleic acids into plant protoplasts. Plant Molec. Biol. Newslett. 2:59 (1981).
14. Lurquin, P. F. Entrapment of plasmid DNA by liposomes and their interactions with plant protoplasts. Nucl. Acids Res. 6:3773 (1979).
15. Matthews, B. F., S. Dray, J. Widholm and M. Ostro. Liposome-mediated transfer of bacterial RNA into carrot protoplasts. Planta 145:37 (1979).
16. Krens, F. A., L. Molendijk, G. J. Wullems and R. A. Schilperoort. In vitro transformation of plant protoplasts with Ti-plasmid DNA. Nature 296:72 (1982).

Bacterial-Plant Gene Cloning Shuttle Vectors for Genetic Modification of Plants

C. I. Kado and R. C. Tait

Department of Plant Pathology
University of California
Davis, California 95616 U.S.A.

Directed genetic transformation of plant cells is one of the fundamental requirements for tailoring plants' cells to harbor desirable characteristics. This requirement can be achieved by the development of systems for the delivery and integration of foreign genes into the plant genome. Two potential gene delivery systems have been the focus of considerable attention: the Ti plasmid of *Agrobacterium tumefaciens* and the DNA plant virion cauliflower mosaic virus (CaMV)[1-8]. Although these are the most thoroughly characterized systems, reports on the successful application of these vectors in the manipulation of the plant genome have been premature. The inherent limitations of these vectors have been previously pointed out [3,4,6,7], yet the design of a cloning vector capable of replication in bacteria and plants continues to center around the Ti plasmid and DNA plant viruses.

We have chosen to construct alternative cloning vectors that can potentially shuttle genes between *Escherichia coli* and plants. The design of these vectors attempts to take advantage of the known properties of existing vectors such as CaMV and the Ti plasmid while at the same time minimizing the deleterious aspects of these vectors. Our vector construction has been based on the criteria listed in Table 1.

We are currently investigating the function of three types of vector to determine their potential as plant cloning vectors.

Table 1. Desirable Properties of Gene Shuttle Vectors

1. The vector must replicate in diverse organisms (i.e., bacteria, yease, and plants) to facilitate the isolation and characterization of genes.
2. The vector must be easily recognized by selectable markers.
3. The vector should be sufficiently small in size to accomodate DNA inserts.
4. Cloned genes should be easily detected.
5. Useful quantities of the vector must be easily obtained.
6. The vector must be stable, non-pathogenic, and non-stress-inducing.
7. Vectors must effectively deliver genetic information for stable maintenance in alternate desired recipients.
8. The introduced genetic information should be stably maintained as a new heritable determinant.

Derivatives of pTAR, a Naturally Occurring Plasmid of Agrobacterium

In addition to the pTi plasmids that are present in *A. tumefaciens*, there are coexisting plasmids of various sizes. We have recently identified a 44 kbp plasmid that carries genetic determinants for the stereospecific catabolism of L-tartaric acid in *Agrobacterium* spp.[9] (D. Zaitlin, J. C. Kao, C. I. Kado, submitted). The origin of replication and associated replication functions have been located within a 7.5 kb region flanked by XhoI and SalI sites (Fig. 1). This region was cloned into the SalI site of pCK1Z, a derivative of the plasmid pBR325 that contains a kanamycin resistance (Km^r) gene derived from Tn5 in the position originally occupied by the tetracycline resistance gene of pBR325[9] (D. Zaitlin, in preparation). The resulting plasmid, pCK2G, contains the origins of replication of pTAR and pBR322 and can be introduced into either *E. coli* or *A. tumefaciens* by transformation. Transformants can be selected on the basis of Km^r or resistance to ampicillin (Ap^r) or chloramphenicol (Cm^r). DNA insertions in the PstI site in the Ap^r gene, the XmaI (SmaI) site in the Km^r gene, or the EcoRI site in the Cm^r gene will result in the loss of the appropriate antibiotic resistance, and recombinants at these sites can be detected by insertional inactivation of resistance phenotype. The StuI site and the XbaI sites are in an unessential region of the plasmid and are also available as cloning sites.

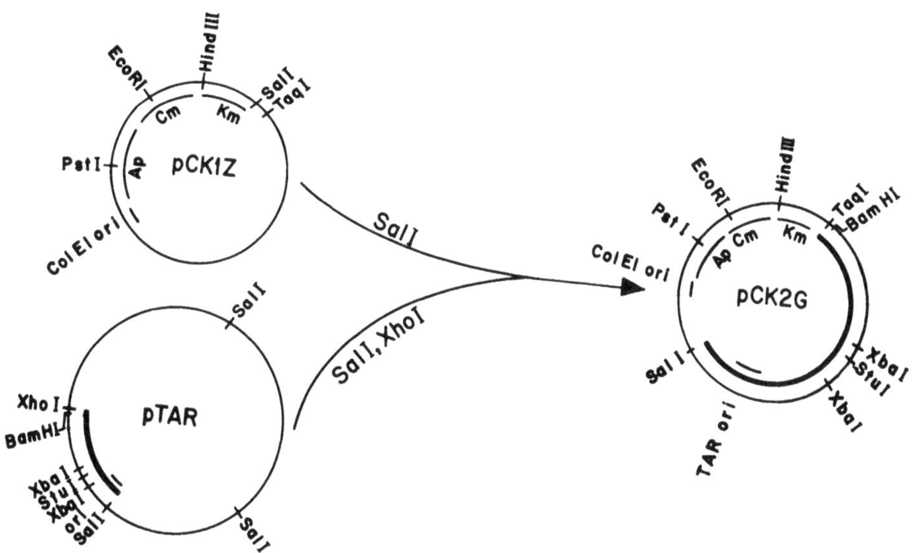

Figure 1. Construction of pCK2G

The plasmid pCK2G functions as a shuttle vector between E. coli and A. tumefaciens. We have cloned fragments of the plasmid pTiC58 in pCK2G and transferred the recombinants to A. tumefaciens containing mutant pTi plasmids in which the transposon Tn5 has been inserted into the virulence region or the T-DNA. Because pCK2G and the pTi plasmid are compatible, pCK2G recombinants can be used in a complementation analysis of the pTi plasmid. Furthermore, sequences present on both the recombinant plasmid and the pTi plasmid can be exchanged by homologous recombination. Thus, a pCK2G recombinant containing a fragment of the T-DNA might be used as a cloning vector for plant genes. A gene cloned in the T-DNA can then be introduced into the T-DNA of a pTi plasmid by homologous recombination, and the donor recombinant plasmid cured from the resulting recombinant by the introduction of the pTAR plasmid, which is incompatible with pCK2G in A. tumefaciens. Following transfer of the plant gene into the pTi plasmid, the gene can be transferred to plants through the normal infection process of A. tumefaciens. The transposition elements Tn5 and Tn7 were reported to be incorporated into the plant genome in such a manner[16,17].

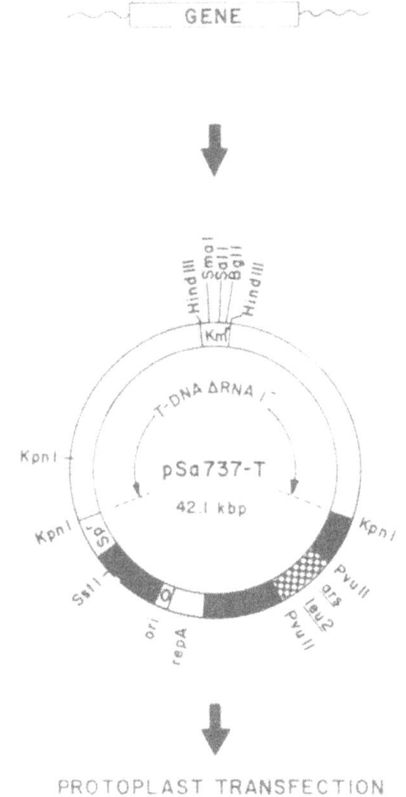

Figure 2. The potential vector pSa737-T

Construction of pSa737-T

We have recently reported the construction of pSa derivative plasmids that possess broad host range characteristics[9,10] (see Tait, R. C. et al. appearing elsewhere in this book). pSa737-T as shown in Fig. 2 is one of these derivatives that carries a partially deleted T-DNA of the Ti plasmid in the KpnI site just within the kanamycin resistance gene of plasmid vector pSa151[11]. The deletion of about 5 kb removes the gene encoding a product that limits the regulation of root and shoot development directed by the T-DNA in crown gall cells. Inserted in the PvuII site of pSa151 are the autonomously replicating sequence ars that was originally obtained from a chromosomal segment of the yeast *Saccharomyces cerevisiae*[19] and the leu2 gene also obtained from the yeast. Inserted in the T-DNA is a kanamycin (Km^r) resistance cartridge. This was accomplished initially by HindIII partial digestion of a T-DNA cloned in the KpnI site of pSa151. The Km^r cartridge, dissected from the transposon Tn5 by HindIII digestion, was then ligated to the T-DNA. The composite plasmid pSa737-T possesses cloning sites in the Km^r cartridge for SmaI (XmaI), SalI and BglI. None of these restriction recognition sequences are carried by pSa151[6] and DNA insertions can be detected by selecting for Km^s clones.

Based on the fact that _ars_ sequences have been obtained from plants[12], a plasmid such as pSa737-T should be suitable for replication in both in bacteria and in plants. As illustrated in Fig. 2, diverse types of DNA, cloned in either the SmaI, SalI or BglI site of the Km^r cartridge, may be delivered directly into plant protoplasts by transformation, which in turn can be made to regenerate into organized tissues and eventually into plants. Of course it should be emphasized here that almost any stably maintained plasmid of _E. coli_ could be harnessed in the same manner to shuttle genes into plants. For example, RSF1010 carrying yeast _ars_ sequences and T-DNA may be used as a similar cloning vector.

pSa737-T carrying a desirable gene that was cloned in the Km^r cartridge (selected on the basis of Km^s and Sp^r of the vector) can be inserted directly into protoplasts, which in turn can be regenerated to callus cultures that are able to regenerate into plants. Although further studies are required on the nature of T-DNA integration, the T-DNA with the help of adjoining left side sequences (KpnI, frag 9) nevertheless, may integrate into the plant genome. We had earlier established that _E. coli_ cloning vectors enter nuclei and are stably maintained although not as entirely complete circular molecules[13,14]. Since crown gall transformation, most likely involving T-DNA integration, occurs within a matter of a few minutes to a few hours[15], cloning vectors such as pBR313 and pBR322 that are stably incorporated for relatively long periods of time (48 hrs)[14] should provide sufficient time for the insertion of foreign DNA flanked by T-DNA integrative sequences.

Construction of pSa151-T

An alternative vector utilizes the origin of replication (ori) of the S strain of the cauliflower mosaic virus (CaMV-S) genome in the PvuII site of pSa151. Like pSa737-T, the "disarmed" T-DNA containing a Km^r cartridge and with the adjacent KpnI fragment 9 are inserted in KpnI site within the Km^R gene of pSa151. The resulting 42.7 kb vector, pSa151-T, replicates in _E. coli_ and carries clonable sites in the Km cartridge (Fig. 3). Genes cloned in the Km^r site of pSa151-T may be transferred to plants by transfecting plant protoplasts. It is assumed here that the CaMV-S _ori_ will function as effectively as the intact viral genome. Support of this contention is that CaMV DNA cloned in pBR322 retains infectivity but does not cause symptom expression in turnip plants because of the inability of the larger than CaMV genomic DNA to be packaged as an intact virion so that it can spread to adjacent leaf cells[6,7]. Nevertheless, CaMV DNA excised from its plasmid vector retains full infectivity by causing mosaic symptoms and generating progeny virions in the same host plant[6,7]. In our case, only the CaMV-S ori is considered and essentially CaMV-S is "disarmed" and unable to sustain viral infection. Thus, pSal51-T, capable of replication in the plant host, should induce no disease symptom expression, but will allow increased time for integration of the cloned genes to occur.

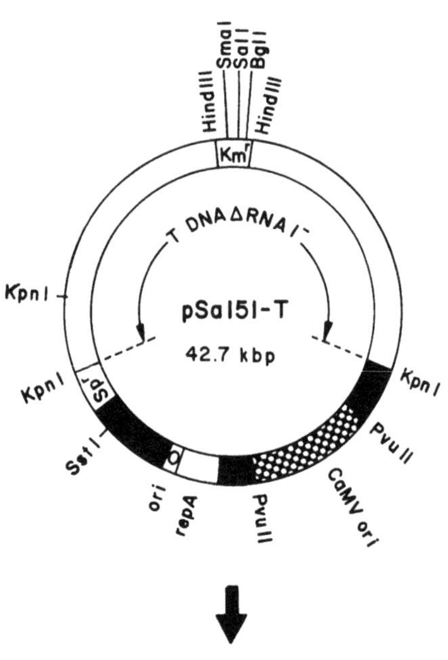

Figure 3. The potential vector pSal51-T

It should be stressed here that self replication of either pSa737-T or pSa151-T in plant cells does not ensure vector stability in the recipient cell. The addition of the disarmed T-DNA with essential sequences left of the T-DNA provide the means for stabilizing the cloned gene through its integration in the plant genomic DNA. Concerns of an effective promoter ahead of the gene have been purposely left unaddressed owing to the fact that T-DNA insertions now seem to be random and internal promoters seem to operate in the expression of foreign genes introduced in plants via Ti-plasmid vectors[18].

ACKNOWLEDGEMENTS

This work was supported, in part, by NIH grant CA-11526 from the National Cancer Institute, grant MV-102 from the American Cancer Society, and grants from the Competitive Grants Office, Science and Education Administration, United States Department of Agriculture. The authors gratefully acknowledge members of the Davis Crown Gall Research Group, in particular Ronald Lundquist, Michio Hagiya, David Zaitlin, Daniel Gallie, Christopher Schardl, Hans Rempel, Tom Quayle, Tim Close, Ray Rodriguez and Jeff Hall for useful discussions, use of facilities and expert assistance.

REFERENCES

1. P. J. J. Hooykaas, R. A. Schilperoort, and A. Rorsch, Genetic Engineering Vol. 1, p. 151-179, J. K. Setlow and A. Hollaender eds., Plenum Press, New York-London (1973).
2. C. I. Kado, Genetic Engineering Vol. 1, p. 223-239 (1979).
3. C. I. Kado, and A. Kleinhofs, Intl. Rev. Cytology, Suppl. 11B, 47-80, I. K. Vasil, ed., Academic Press, New York (1980).
4. M.-D. Chilton, Genetic Engineering of Osmoregulation p. 23-31, D. W. Rains, R. C. Valentine and A. Hollaender, eds., Plenum Press, New York-London (1980).
5. R. B. Meagher, and T. D. McKnight, Genome Organization and Expression in Plants, C. J. Leaver, ed., p. 63-75. Plenum Press, New York-London (1980).
6. S. H. Howell, Ann. Rev. Plant Physiol. 33:609-650 (1982).
7. T. Holn, K. Richards, and G. Lebeurier, Curr. Topics Microbiol. Immunol. 96:193-236 (1982).
8. J. Schell, and M. Van Montagu, Transfer of cell constituents into Eukaryotic cells, J. E. Celis, ed., p. 325-346. Plenum Press, New York-London (1980).
9. C. I. Kado, R. C. Tait, R. C. Lundquist, M. Hagiya, D. Zaitlin, and D. Gallie, Proc. Fourth Intl. Symp. Genetics Indust. Microorg., Kyoto, Japan (In Press) (1982).

10. R. C. Tait, T. J. Close, R. C. Lundquist, M. Hagiya, R. L. Rodriguez, and C. I. Kado, Proc. Natl. Acad. Sci. USA (submitted) (1982).
11. R. C. Tait, R. C. Lundquist, and C. I. Kado, Molec. Gen. Genet. 186:10-15 (1982).
12. D. T. Stinchcomb, M. Thomas, J. Kelley, E. Selker, and R. W. Davis, Proc. Natl. Acad. Sci. USA 77:4559-4563 (1980).
13. P. F. Lurquin, and C. I. Kado, Molec. Gen. Genet. 154:113-121 (1977).
14. S. M. Fernandez, P. F. Lurquin, and C. I. Kado, FEBS Letters 87:277-282 (1978).
15. J. A. Lippincott, and B. B. Lippincott, Ann. Rev. Microbiol. 29:377-405 (1975).
16. J.-P. Hernalsteens, F. Van Vliet, M. DeBeuckeleer, A. Depicker, G. Engler, M. Lemmers, M. Holsters, M. VanMontagu, and J. Schell, Nature 287:654-656 (1980).
17. D. J. Garfinkel, R. B. Simpson, L. W. Ream, F. F. White, M. P. Gordon, and E. W. Nester, Cell 27:143-153 (1981).
18. J. Schell, M. Van Montagu, M. Holsters, J. P. Hernalsteens, H. DeGreve, J. Leemans, L. Willmitzer, L. Otten, J. Schroder, and G. Schroder, Fourth Int. Symp. Genetic Industr. Microorg. Kyoto, Japan (Abstract) (1982).
19. K. Strahl, D. T. Stinchcomb, S. Scherer, and R. W. Davis. Proc. Natl. Acad. Sci. USA 76:1035-1039 (1979).

CONSTRUCTION OF CLONING VECTORS FROM THE *IncW* PLASMID pSa AND THEIR USE IN ANALYSIS OF CROWN GALL TUMOR FORMATION

R. C. Tait, T. J. Close[1], M. Hagiya,
R. C. Lundquist, and C. I. Kado*

Davis Crown Gall Group
Departments of Plant Pathology and Genetics[1]
University of California
Davis, California 95616 U.S.A.

ABSTRACT

A set of four cloning vectors has been constructed from the wide host range *IncW* plasmid pSa. Although the vectors are transfer defective, three of them can be efficiently transferred into a wide variety of Gram-negative bacteria by a separate mobilizing plasmid. One of the vectors is a cosmid and can be used for cloning large DNA fragments. The vectors, which can be selected on the basis of kanamycin, spectinomycin, or chloramphenicol resistance, contain cloning sites for seven different restriction endonucleases. DNA fragments from the *A. tumefaciens* plasmid TiC58 have been cloned into these vectors, and used to complement avirulent TiC58::Tn5 mutants.

INTRODUCTION

The analysis of gene structure and function has been facilitated in recent years by the construction of specialized cloning vectors that allow the isolation and characterization of both prokaryotic and eukaryotic genes[1-6]. Unfortunately, the vectors that have been most thoroughly characterized and are subsequently most easily applied to analysis of gene structure have a narrow host range. Their use in the *in vivo* complementation analysis of cloned genes is thus limited to the enteric bacteria. To perform such complementation analyses in Gram-negative bacteria like *Agrobacterium tumefaciens*,

*To whom correspondence should be addressed.

vectors that are functional in these bacteria must be used. The cloning vector pRK290 was constructed from the IncP group R factor RK2 and can be used in a wide variety of Gram-negative bacteria, but contains only tetracycline resistance (Tc^R) as a selectable marker[7].

We have constructed new cloning vectors from the IncW group plasmid pSa, a 29.6 kbp plasmid with broad host range properties[8, 9]. Two of these vectors encode resistance to kanamycin-gentamycin (Km^r) and spectinomycin-streptomycin (Sp^r), and two in addition encode resistance to chloramphenicol (Cm^r). The presence of cloning sites in the Km^r gene and the Sp^r gene allows the identification of recombinant plasmids by insertional inactivation of drug resistance phenotype. One of the vectors is a cosmid and can be used with *in vivo* λ bacteriophage packaging systems[5, 6] in the efficient construction of recombinant plasmids containing large DNA insertions. The replication of the vectors has been characterized, as have their host range properties. Although the vectors are all transfer defective by virtue of the deletion of a region involved in both conjugal transfer and in the inhibition of oncogenesis in *A. tumefaciens*[9], three of the vectors can be efficiently mobilized in the presence of a recombinant pBR322 plasmid containing the transfer genes of pSa. The vectors are functional in a variety of *Enterobacteriaceae*, *Rhizobiaceae*, and *Pseudomonadaceae* species. We describe here the construction of these vectors and their use in the analysis of the structure and function of various regions of the plasmid pTiC58, a large plasmid known to be involved in the formation of crown gall tumors by strains of *A. tumefaciens*[10].

RESULTS

Construction of Cloning Vectors

The regions of pSa that are required for DNA replication, the origin of conjugal transfer, Km^r, and Sp^r are all present on a 13.3 kbp DNA fragment obtained by digestion of pSa with *SstII* endonuclease[9]. This derivative, pSa151, served as the basis for the construction of three other vectors. A 1.36 kbp DNA fragment containing the Cm^r gene of Tn9 was used to introduce a third phenotypic marker into pSa151. This DNA fragment was generated by digestion of pBR325 with *HhaI* endonuclease[11] and purification by agarose gel electrophoresis. Plasmid pSa151 DNA was partially digested with *HhaI* and treated with alkaline phosphatase to prevent rearrangements of the plasmid during ligation. The purified Cm^r gene was then ligated to the partial digest of pSa151 and the ligated material used to transform *E. coli* RR1. Plasmid DNA was purified from Cm^r transformants and characterized by restriction endonuclease analysis. The second vector, pSa727, resulted from the ligation of the Cm^r gene to the linear pSa151 molecule, and the third vector, pSa4, resulted from the ligation of the Cm^r gene to an 8.0 kbp fragment of pSa151. The fourth vector, pSa747, is a cosmid that was constructed by purification of a 1.7 BglII kbp fragment of the cosmid pHC79. This fragment contains the intact λ cos sequence and can be inserted into a plasmid to convert it to a cosmid[6]. Although pSa151 contains a single BglII site, this site is adjacent to a region involved in plasmid mobilization and insertion of fragments at this site sometimes affects the efficiency of plasmid transfer. The cos fragment was therefore cloned into the single BamHI site of pSa151 to avoid interference with the transfer properties of the resulting vector. Restriction maps of these four vectors are shown in Figure 1.

Construction of the Mobilizing Plasmid pSa322

The deletion that resulted in the construction of pSa151 also removed from the plasmid two functions: conjugal transfer and inhibition of oncogenesis in *A. tumefaciens*[9]. The elimination of the interference with oncogenesis was important to the use of these vectors in the analysis of the Ti plasmids of *A. tumefaciens*, but conjugal transfer was desired to allow the use of these vectors with bacteria that are refractory to transformation. Using the pRK290:pRK2013 system as a model[7], a mobilizing plasmid was constructed by digesting pSa with BamHI and BglII to generate a 15 kbp DNA fragment containing the transfer genes of pSa. This was ligated into the single BamHI site of pBR322[1]. Ampicillin resistant (Ap^r) Tc^s transformants were screened for the presence of a single BamHI site in a 19 kbp plasmid; EcoRI and SstII were used to verify that the recombinant plasmid contained the expected pSa fragment. This plasmid was designated pSa322 and the transfer properties of the plasmid were determined.

As shown in Table 1, pSa322 is self-mobilizable at a frequency comparable to that of pSa, suggesting that pSa322 contains not only the transfer genes of pSa, but also an origin of transfer. The ability of pSa322 to mobilize each of the four vectors was determined by introducing pSa322 into a $recA^-$ strain containing each of the vectors. Transfer frequency was determined by measuring mobilization of the vectors to a Tc^r recipient strain containing Tn10. As shown in Table 1, pSa151, pSa727, and pSa747 were all mobilized by pSa322 at about 10% of the transfer frequency of pSa. However, pSa4 was not efficiently mobilized. In the absence of selective pressure for both pSa322 and pSa4, strains containing both plasmids rapidly lost pSa4 and maintained only pSa322. Apparently, the 5.3 kbp deletion involved in the construction of pSa4 removed a region of pSa151 required for efficient mobilization by pSa322.

Table 1. Mobilization of pSa derivatives by pSa322.

Plasmid present in donor HB101	Mobilization frequency transconjugants/donor*
pSa	1.6×10^{-1}
pSa322	7.7×10^{-2}
pSa151	1.5×10^{-6}
pSa727	1.5×10^{-6}
pSa4	4.2×10^{-6}
pSa151 + pSa322	8.4×10^{-2}
pSa727 + pSa322	8.0×10^{-2}
pSa4 + pSa322	5.2×10^{-6}

* pSa, pSa151, pSa727, and pSa4 donors were Sp^r Km^r, transconjugants were Sp^r Km^r Tc^r; pSa322 donors were Ap^r, transconjugants were Ap^r Tc^r. The recipient strain in the matings was *E. coli* E50 Tc^r (Tn10). The frequency of spontaneous Sp^rKm^r of E50 was $<10^{-8}$, as was the frequency of spontaneous Tc^R of *E. coli* HB101.

Table 2. Triparental conjugal transfer of pSa151 and pSa727 to various Gram negative bacteria

Family	Recipient	
Enterobacteriaceae		
	Escherichia coli K12	HB101, RR1
	Klebsiella pneumoniae	M5A1
	Providentia stuarti	164
	Serratia marcescens	ATCC 274
	Erwinia amylovora	1D39
Rhizobiaceae		
	Rhizobium leguminosarum	128C53
	Rhizobium trifolii	162P17
	Agrobacterium tumefaciens	1D135, 15955, C58, B6, 1D1, ACH-5, 1D1159
Pseudomonadaceae		
	Pseudomonas fluorescens	11D47
	Pseudomonas stutzeri	JM300
Uncertain affiliation		
	Alcaligenes eutrophus	ATCC 17707

Properties of the pSa Cloning Vectors

The cloning properties of these pSa vectors are summarized in Table 3. Together the vectors provide cloning sites for EcoRI, KpnI, HindIII, PvuII, BamHI, BglII, and SstII. Insertions in the BglII site can decrease the overall frequency of transfer by pSa322, and insertions at the KpnI site inactivate Km^r. Insertions in the EcoRI site of pSa151 inactivate Sp^r; the second EcoRI present in pSa727 and pSa4 is in the Cm^r gene and insertions in this site will inactivate Cm^r. Of the two PvuII sites in pSa727 and pSa4, one is in the Cm^r gene, and insertions will inactivate Cm^r. Cloning in the HindIII sites of these plasmids involves the deletion of two small HindIII fragments in the Sp^r gene and results in the inactivation of Sp^r in both recombinants and deletion derivatives.

Table 3. Properties of pSa cloning vectors

Vector	Phenotypic Markers	Mobilization by pSa322	Cloning Sites Available: Insertional Inactivation: KpnI[1]	EcoRI	PvuII[2]	HindIII[3]	Other: PvuII	BamHI	BglII	SstII
pSa151	Km^r Sp^r	+	–	Sp^s	–	Sp^s	+	+	+	+
pSa727	Km^r Sp^r Cm^r	+	Km^s	Sp^s, Cm^s	Cm^s	Sp^s	(2)	+	+	+
pSa747	Km^r Sp^r cos^+	+	–	Sp^s	–	Sp^s	(4)	–	+	+
pSa4	Km^r Sp^r Cm^r	–	Km^s	Sp^s, Cm^s	Cm^s	Sp^s	(2)	+	–	+

1. Insertion inactivates Km^r, 95% of insertions also inactivate Sp^r.
2. Two PvuII sites, one is in the Cm^r gene.
3. Three HindIII sites sithin 450 base pairs, two are in the Sp^r gene.
4. Two PvuII sites, one is adjacent to cos.

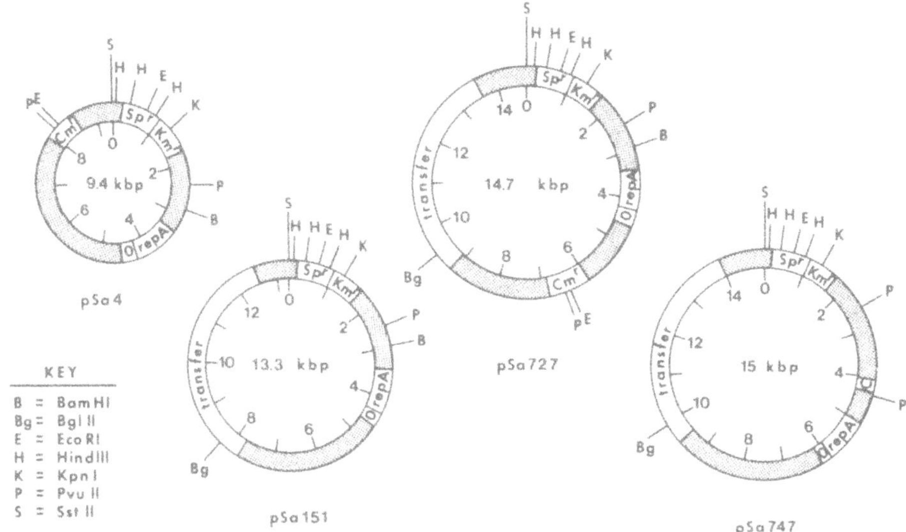

Figure 1: Restriction maps of pSa vectors. Restriction cleavage sites are indicated, as are the approximate locations of the Sp^r, Km^r, Cm^r, and repA genes. The location of the origin of replication is indicated by 0, and the location of the λ cos sequence by C.

Host Range of the Vectors

The host range of these vectors was determined by mobilizing pSa151 and pSa727 in the presence of pSa322 into a variety of Gram negative bacteria. The $recA^-$ *E. coli* strain HB101 was used as donor to minimize recombination between pSa322 and the vectors. Spot matings were allowed to proceed on non-selective medium for 24 hr, then the bacteria were diluted and plated on selective media to detect exconjugants. All the strains examined were found to support replication of pSa151 and pSa727 and are listed in Table 2. Sp^r and Km^r were detected at 50 μg/ml and 30 μg/ml, respectively, but a wide variation in Cm^r was observed. Although *E. coli* containing pSa727 was resistant to 200 μg/ml Cm, *A. tumefaciens* containing pSa727 was resistant to only 10-20 μg/ml Cm.

Polypeptides Encoded by the Vectors

The polypeptides encoded by the vectors were determined with the *E. coli* maxicell protein synthesis system. The polypeptides that have been assigned functions include a 35 kilodalton (kd) *repA* protein whose function is required at the origin of replication, the 28 kd Cm^r gene product, chloramphenicol acetyltransferase, a 31 kd Sp^r gene product, and a 26 kd Km^r gene product. The approximate size of these genes has been calculated from the polypeptide sizes and the location of the genes is indicated in Figure 1.

The mode of replication of the pSa origin has been characterized in detail[12]. Bidirectional replication initiates within a 400 bp region designated 0 in Figure 1. The gene for the 35 kd *repA* protein is located adjacent to the origin of replication and the function of the *repA* protein is required at the origin for efficient plasmid replication. Plasmids are maintained at a level of 2-3 copies per cell, and as a result of the requirement for the *repA* protein, the plasmid copy number cannot be amplified in the presence of inhibitors of protein synthesis. The genetic organization of the origin of replication is similar to that of the *IncX* group plasmid R6K[13], and nucleotide sequence analysis has revealed surprising homology between these two origins (R. Tait, manuscript in preparation).

Analysis of A. tumefaciens pTiC58

We have used the pSa vectors described above to perform complementation analyses of the *A. tumefaciens* plasmid pTiC58, which induces crown gall tumors in many plants and which may prove useful in genetic engineering of plants. For the initial phase of our analyses we have concentrated on a 25 kbp region of the plasmid which lies outside the T-DNA region, but is nevertheless essential for oncogenicity[10] (Fig. 3). Five different Tn5 insertion mutants across this region which are avirulent on all hosts were selected. Complementation of the mutants was attempted using wild type pTiC58 KpnI fragments cloned into pSa4. The clone bank of pTiC58 KpnI fragments was constructed by ligation of a complete KpnI digest of the plasmid to KpnI digested pSa4 DNA, and recombinant plasmids representing about 85% of the TiC58 genome were isolated and characterized.

The five avirulent C58 plasmids were introduced into LBA 4301, a recombination deficient *A. tumefaciens* strain[14], followed by transformation with the corresponding wild type KpnI fragment cloned on pSa4 (Fig. 2). After confirming that both the pTiC58 and recombinant pSa plasmids were present, the strains were assayed for virulence on tomato, and Kalanchoe. Three of the strains were in fact able to form tumors on all plants tested (Fig. 3). These results suggest that there are gene products in this region which are necessary for tumorigenesis, but which can be provided *in trans*. Tn5 insertion mutant 190 was not complemented under these conditions,

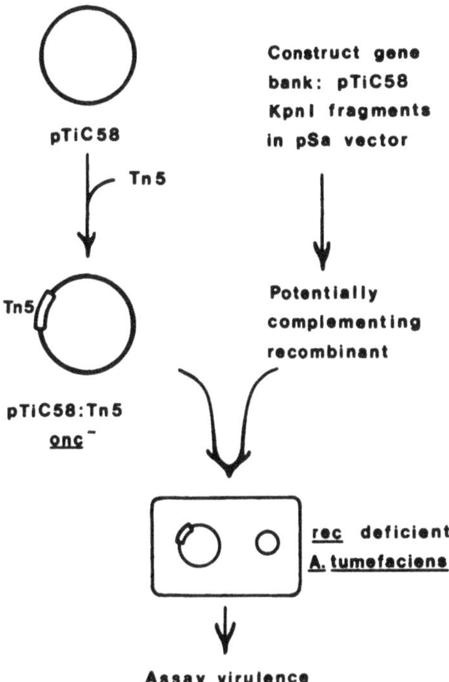

Figure 2: Illustration of the use of pSa vectors in the complementation analysis of pTiC58. A mutant pTiC58:Tn5 plasmid and a recombinant pSa plasmid containing pTiC58 DNA are introduced into a recombination deficient strain of *A. tumefaciens*. Plants are inoculated with this strain to assay complementation of the *onc*⁻ phenotype of the mutant pTi plasmid by the recombinant pSa plasmid.

possibly because the complete functional transcript for this mutation extends beyond the DNA contained in pSa4::Kpn5 (Fig. 3). Interestingly, mutant 104 was not complemented, although mutants on both sides were. A similar "cis-dominant" complementation effect has been observed with $pTiB_6806$[15]. A more detailed complementation analysis of TiC58 mutants should allow us to determine the number of gene products and eventually their mode of action during tumorigenesis.

Use of the pSa Vectors in Promoter Analysis

We have observed that the insertion of pTiC58 DNA fragments into the *KpnI* site of the pSa vectors results in the loss of Km^r and generally results in the loss of Sp^r. However, certain *KpnI* insertions maintain Sp^r. Km^r and Sp^r may be expressed from a common promoter, and insertions at the *KpnI* site may separate the promoter from the Sp^r structural gene. If the Sp^r gene retains a functional ribosomal

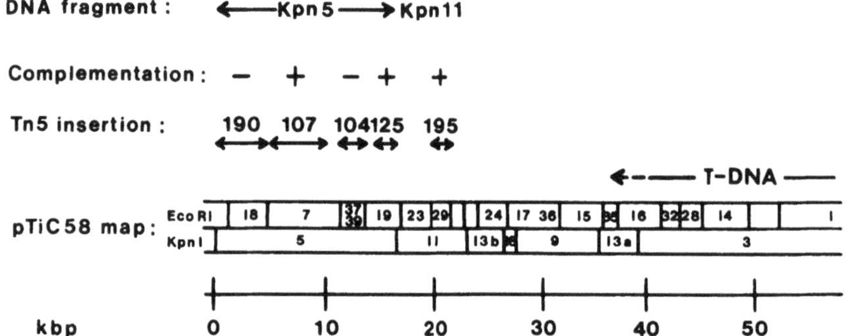

Figure 3: Complementation of avirulent pTiC58::Tn5 mutants. Rec$^-$ strains carrying mutant plasmids 190, 107, 104, and 125 were transformed with pSa4::Kpn5. The rec$^-$ strain containing mutant 195 was transformed with pSa4::Kpn11. Transformants were inoculated on sunflower, tomato, and Kalanchoe plants and scored for tumor formation after 4 and 6 weeks. + = virulence restored when recombinant pSa plasmid is present; - = remains avirulent when recombinan pSa is present.

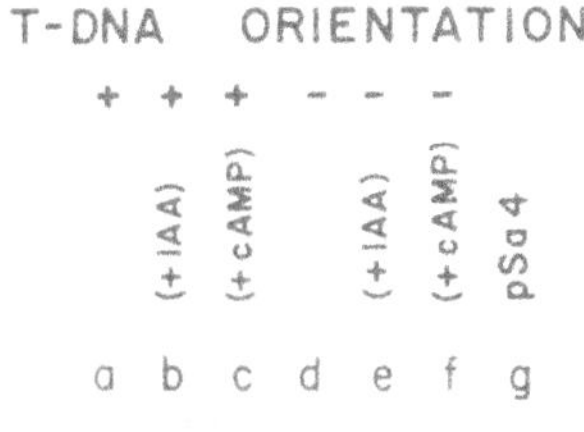

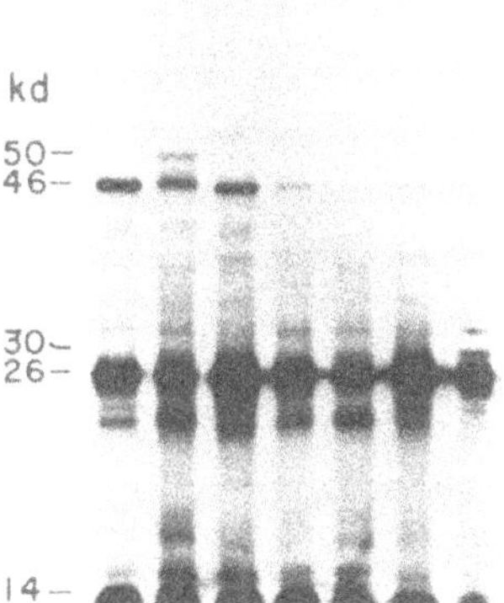

Figure 4: Synthesis of polypeptides in minicells. KpnI fragment 3 was cloned in pSa4 in the + Sp^r and $-Sp^r$ orientations and the recombinants examined in *E. coli* AS1522 minicells. Minicells were labeled in the presence of 5 mM IAA in lanes b and e, and in the presence of 5 mM cAMP in lanes c and f.

binding site, insertion of KpnI fragments that contain a functional promoter would restore Sp^r. If the Sp^r gene does not retain a ribosomal binding site, the restoration of Sp^r might be dependent on the production of a fusion protein consisting of a protein initiated within the inserted KpnI fragment and proceeding through the Sp^r gene in the correct translational frame to produce an active Sp^r fusion protein. We are currently determining the nucleotide sequence of the Sp^r gene to clarify the basis for Sp^r in these KpnI insertions.

KpnI fragment 3 contains about 90% of the T-DNA of pTiC58 (Fig. 3). When cloned in the KpnI site of pSa4 so that the left KpnI site is adjacent to the Sp^r gene (+ orientation), the recombinant plasmid will confer resistance to 30 μg/ml Sp, in contrast to a resistance of ≥100 μg/m Sp conferred by pSa4. Deletion analysis indicated that the region of KpnI fragment 3 that is responsible for this Sp^r is within 800 bp of the left KpnI site. When cloned in the opposite (-) orientation, no Sp^r was obtained. When these two recombinants were examined in *E. coli* minicells (Fig. 4), increased synthesis of a polypeptide of 46 kd was observed in the + orientation of KpnI fragment 3. In addition, the synthesis of a polypeptide of 50 kd was induced in the presence of indoleacetic acid (IAA) only in the + orientation of KpnI fragment 3. Deletion analysis indicates that the synthesis of these polypeptides is dependent on the presence of sequences at the right hand side of KpnI fragment 3, suggesting that these polypeptides are not the result of fusion with the Sp^r protein. One of these polypeptides may be a fusion involving the Km^r protein. The identity and potential function of these polypeptides in *Agrobacterium* remains under investigation.

Transfer of the Sp^r recombinant plasmids onto *A. tumefaciens* will determine whether the promoter responsible for the Sp^r is functional in both *E. coli* and *A. tumefaciens*. Preliminary results indicate that the + orientation of KpnI fragment 3 confers Sp^r in both bacteria. Further studies may allow a comparison of the structure of promoters in these bacteria.

SUMMARY

We have constructed and described a set of vectors designed for the cloning and analysis of *A. tumefaciens* plasmid DNA. These vectors allow the detection of recombinant plasmids by the insertional inactivation of antibiotic resistance phenotypes. The vectors can be transferred into a variety of Gram-negative bacteria by transformation or with a mobilizing plasmid by conjugation. These vectors are currently in use in the cloning and analysis of the plasmid pTiC58.

ACKNOWLEDGEMENTS

This work was supported in part by U.S. Public Health Service NIH grant CA-11526 from the National Cancer Institute, by NIH grant GM 29100-02, research grant MV-102 from the American Cancer Society and by grants from Competitive Grants Office, Science and Education Administration, United States Department of Agriculture. TJC was supported in part by NIH training grant GM-04767.

REFERENCES

1. F. Bolivar, R. L. Rodriguez, P. J. Greene, M. C. Betlach, H. U. Heyneker, H. W. Boyer, J. H. Crosa, and S. Falkow, Gene 2:95-113 (1977).
2. G. An, and J. D. Friesen, J. Bacteriol. 140:400-410 (1979).
3. R. W. West Jr., R. U. Neve, and R. L. Rodriguez, Gene 7:271-288 (1977).
4. U. Enquist, and N. Sternberg, Methods Enz. 68:281-298 (1979).
5. B. Hohn, Methods Enz. 68:299-309 (1979).
6. J. Collins, Methods Enz. 68:309-326 (1979).
7. G. Ditta, S. Stanfield, D. Corbin, and D. R. Helinski, Proc. Natl. Acad. Sci. (USA) 77:7347-7351 (1980).
8. A. P. Gorai, F. Heffron, S. Falkow, R. W. Hedges, and N. Datta, Plasmid 2:485-492 (1979).
9. R. C. Tait, R. C. Lundquist, and C. I. Kado, Mol. Gen. Genet. 186:10-15 (1982).
10. M. Holsters, B. Silva, F. Van Vliet, C. Genetello, M. DeBlock, P. Dhaese, A. DePicker, D. Inze, G. Engler, R. Villarroel, M. Van Montagu, and J. Schell, Plasmid 3:212-230 (1980).
11. X. Soberon, U. Covarrubias, and F. Bolivar, Gene 9:287-305 (1980).
12. R. C. Tait, T. J. Close, R. L. Rodriquez, and C. I. Kado, Gene, in press (1982).
13. R. Kolter, M. Inuzuka, D. Figurski, C. Thomas, D. Stalker, and D. R. Helinski, Cold Spring Harbor Symp. Quant. Biol. 43:91-97 (1979).
14. P. Klapwijk, P. van Beelen, and R. Schilperoort, Mol. Gen. Genet. 173:171-175 (1979).
15. H. J. Klee, M. P. Gordon, and E. W. Nester, J. Bact. 150: 327-331 (1982).

CONSTRUCTION OF RECOMBINANT Ti PLASMIDS CONTAINING THE *chlM* GENE FROM *E. COLI*

Thianda Manzara and Paul F. Lurquin

Program in Genetics and Cell Biology

Washington State University

Pullman, Washington 99164-4350

Introduction

The stable maintenance of foreign genes in plant cells is dependent upon the nature of the vector used in DNA transfer attempts. The potential vectors which presently exist can be divided into two categories: 1) vectors which integrate within the host genome and 2) vectors which can be established as independent replicons in plant cells. The first category includes the T-DNA from *Agrobacterium tumefaciens* and the T-DNA from *Agrobacterium rhizogenes*. The second class of vectors comprises the caulimovirus and germinivirus genomes, as well as cDNA copies of viroids. The pros and cons of each of those vectors have been recently reviewed by Howell[1].

We have chosen to use *A. tumefaciens* pTi as a vehicle to introduce foreign genes into plant cells since (a) its restriction endonuclease map is well known, (b) promoter sites in the T-DNA have been roughly located and (c) *A. tumefaciens* cells[2] or spheroplasts[3] are naturally able to introduce pTi into wounded whole plants, regenerating or freshly isolated plant protoplasts.

Even though it has proven difficult to regenerate plants from crown gall tumors, recent progress[4,5] has shown that proper engineering of the T-DNA might allow one to bypass these difficulties. It remains that *A. tumefaciens* is presently the best model system to study the expression of exogenous genes in plant cells.

The detection of such expression is itself dependent upon the ability to discriminate between transformed and untransformed plant cells. Aside from T-DNA markers (whose expression might be modified through pTi engineering), it is critical to use genetic markers which can be selected for at the level of the plant cells. One possibility is to use a donor gene which might possibly restore a wild-type-like phenotype in plant mutants and at the same time be easily distinguishable from its endogenous inactive counterpart. Such prerequisites seem to be offered by _Nicotiana tabacum_[6] and _N. plumbaginofolia_[7] nitrate reductase mutants unable to synthesize functional molybdenum cofactor (MoCo). On the other hand, the _chlM_ gene from _Escherichia coli_ has been cloned, and its product seems to be able to restore nitrate reductase activity in acellular extracts from corresponding plant mutants[8].

This paper describes the construction of recombinant DNA molecules which should make it possible to study the behavior of the _E. coli chlM_ gene in crown gall tumors generated from plant MoCo mutants

Construction of pTi Plasmids Containing a Potentially Selectable Marker

Three recombinant plasmids, pTM1, pTM2, and pTM3, have been constructed and partially characterized as shown in Figure 1. The construction of these recombinants involved insertion of a plasmid containing the _chlM_ gene (pFG1)[8] into the Bam H1 fragment 8 of pTiA6 cloned into the broad host range plasmid pRK248 (This vector, pMTB1, was kindly provided to us by Dr. Michael Thomashow). pMTB1 has 5 Hind III sites, all of which are located in the T-DNA fragment, while pFG1 has a unique Hind III site. Therefore, complete digestion of pFG1 and partial digestion of pMTB1 with Hind III followed by ligation allowed us to obtain recombinant plasmids with pFG1 inserted at different sites in the Bam 8 fragment. The desired recombinant plasmids carried ampicillin resistance from pFG1 and tetracycline resistance from pMTB1. In order to avoid selection of clones containing intact pFG1 and pMTB1, the pol A deficient strain, SF800 of _E. coli_ was used for transformation. Plasmids from three of the clones thus obtained were used for restriction mapping (Fig. 2). These intermediate vectors were then used to transfer pFG1 into the T-region of pTiA6.

Transfer of foreign DNA into the T-region using intermediate vectors has been described by others[9]. In this case, the recombinant plasmids were transformed into the octopine _Agrobacterium tumefaciens_ strain A136 carrying pTiA6, followed by conjugation with _E. coli_ carrying pPH1J1, a plasmid incompatible with pMTB1. Simultaneous selection for carbenicillin and gentamycin resitances (carried by pFG1 and pPH1J1, respectively) resulted in selection of clones in which marker exchange should have occurred. That is, crossing over between the engineered Bam H1 fragment 8 and the homologous region of pTiA6 should have occurred in such a way that there is insertion of pFG1 into the T-region of the pTi. Southern blotting will be performed to verify that pFG1 has been transferred to the T-region of pTiA6.

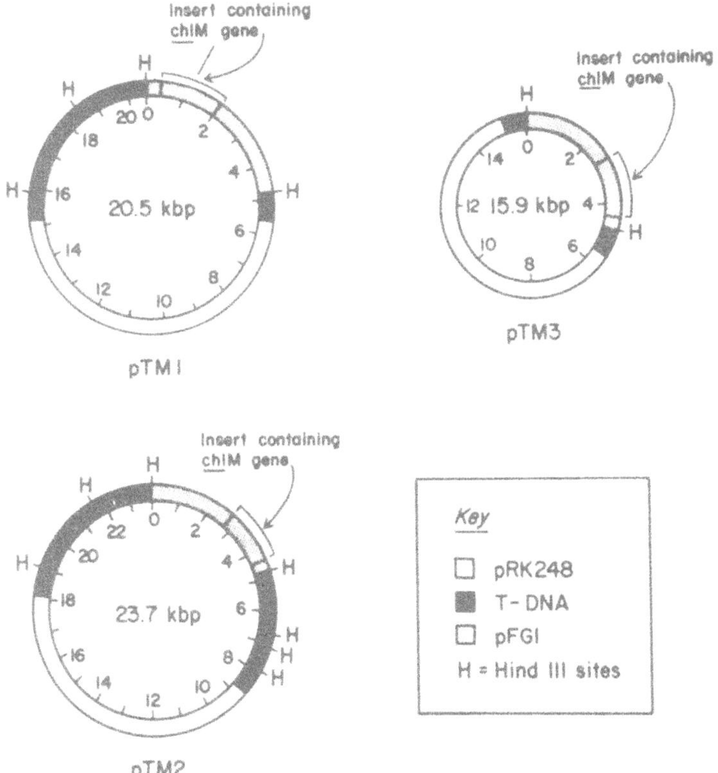

Figure 1. Hind III maps of the intermediate vectors pTM1, pTM2, and pTM3.

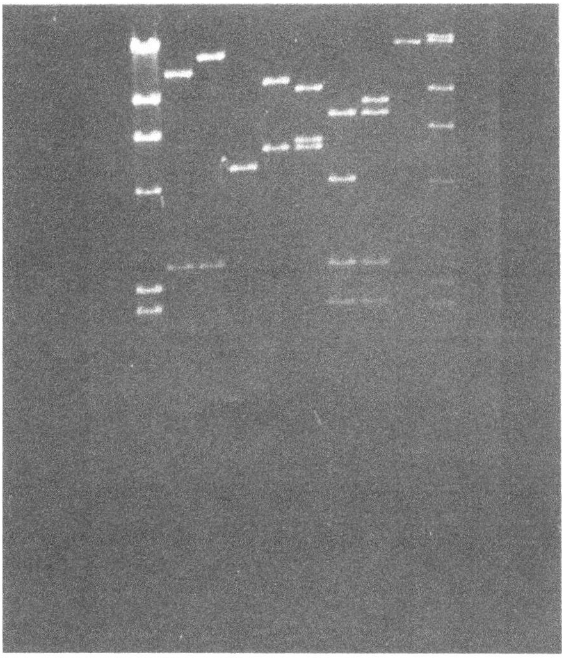

Figure 2. Mapping of pTM1. Lanes 1 and 10: Hind III digest of λ. Lane 2: pMTB1 digested with Bgl II. Lane 3: pTM1 digested with Bgl II. Lane 4: pFG1 digested with Eco R1. Lane 5: pMTB1 digested with Eco R1. Lane 6: pTM1 digested with Eco R1. Lane 7: pMTB1 digested with Sma I. Lane 8: pTM1 digested with Sma I. Lane 9: pTM1 digested with Pstl.

Transfer of Recombinant Plasmids to Plant Cells

Several methods will be used to transfer the engineered pTis to plant cells. The simplest and most obvious method is wounding and inoculation of intact plants with the engineered strains. For this purpose, mutant tobacco plants which are unable to synthesize functional molybdenum cofactor (MoCo) (courtesy of Dr. S. Evola) will be infected, and the resulting tumor tissue will be tested for its ability to grow on medium containing nitrate as the sole nitrogen source. The tumor tissue will be analyzed for the presence of pFG1 DNA by Southern blot hybridization and for the presence of mRNA complementary to pFG1 by Northern blot hybridization. Nitrate reductase activity in the tumor tissues will also be assayed.

Another approach will involve in vitro infection of protoplasts derived from suspension cultures of cnx68 tobacco cells, which are deficient in the ability to produce a functional molybdenum cofactor. Nitrate reductase activity has been shown to be restored to cell extracts of cnx68 by the chlM gene product[8]. Co-cultivation of these protoplasts with the engineered A. tumefaciens strains[2] and subsequent selection of transformants by their ability to grow on nitrate as the sole nitrogen source and to become sensitive to chlorate should provide the means of selecting and testing individual transformation events. A similar approach will involve fusion of cnx68 protoplasts with A. tumefaciens spheroplasts using polyethylene glycol, and subsequent elimination of spheroplasts using vancomycin[2].

The necessity of eliminating remaining A. tumefaciens cells can be avoided by introduction of the engineered pTis into cnx68 protoplasts via liposomes[14,15]. It has been demonstrated[10] that encapsulation of pTi in liposomes followed by fusion with protoplasts yields in vitro formation of crown gall tumors. Tumor tissues obtained from all three of the in vitro infection techniques will be analyzed as described for tumors resulting from infection of intact plants.

Discussion

In light of the recent findings by Leemans et al.[11] and of Willmitzer et al.[12], we can speculate as to the nature of the crown galls that will be obtained by infection with A. tumefaciens harboring the engineered pTis.

The pTi derived from marker exchange with pTM1 should be missing Hind III fragments 38c and 36b, and should have pFG1 inserted in this region. According to the above authors, this will most likely disrupt a message (transcript 1) which appears to suppress shoot induction. Therefore, one would expect to observe shoot induction on tobacco tumors obtained from infection with this strain. In order for the chlM gene to be expressed in the resulting tumor tissue, it would have to be under the control of the promoter of transcript 1. This promoter appears to be contained in the Eco R1 fragment 32[11] which lies directly outside of the pFG1 insertion in pTM1.

The situation in the case of the pTi derived from pTM2 is more difficult to predict, due to the fact that there are two Hind III fragments 22e, one on either side of the pFG1 insert. If the marker exchange between pTM2 and pTiA6 occurs in such a way that both of the Hind III fragments are retained, it is likely that looping out of the inserted DNA will occur, and that the insert will be lost.

Alternatively, the marker exchange may occur in such a way that pFG1 is simply inserted into the Hind III fragment 22e on the pTi. If this were to be the case, one, or possibly two, of the messages would be disrupted (transcript 2 and possibly transcript 1 as defined by Willmitzer et al.[12]), which are again transcripts that appear to be involved in suppression of shoot formation. In order for the chlM gene to be expressed in the resulting tumor tissue, it would be necessary for it to be under the control of the promoter for transcript 2.

The pTi derived from marker exchange with pTM3 should contain the corresponding deletion of Hind III fragments 18c, 22e, 38c and 36b, with pFG1 inserted at the site of deletion. According to Wilmitzer et al.[12], this will ablate transcripts 1, 2, 5, and 7. Tumors lacking the same transcripts were studied by Leemans et al.[11], who found that the resulting tissue grew as teratoma. Therefore, one would expect to see teratoma-like growth of tumors incited by this pTi. Since there will be no T-DNA promoters remaining that would be in the proper orientation, one would not expect that there would be the possibility of expression of the chlM gene in the tumor tissue.

The deletions and insertions which are present in pTM1, 2, and 3 and which are expected to occur in the corresponding pTis will most likely have the effect of reducing virulence of the resulting A. tumefaciens strains. Two strains harboring pTiB6S3 with TN7 transposons in the regions corresponding to transcripts 1 and 2 were found to require a longer time than wild-type strains to form visible tumors[11,13].

Although the tumorous phenotype should be expressed in the above examples, it has been found that T-DNA transfer can take place in the absence of crown gall induction[11]. This opens up new possibilities in plant genetic engineering in that it may simplify the production of phenotypically normal plants containing foreign DNA. Other selectable markers will be required, however, in order to detect transformation. If the chlM gene is expessed in MoCo$^-$ plant cells, it will provide a good system for detecting plant cell transformation.

Acknowledgements

We gratefully thank Elizabeth La Crosse and Suzanne Oelke for capable technical assistance. We also thank F. Grant, A. Kleinhofs, J. Taylor and M. Thomashow for gifts of plasmids and bacterial strains and for useful discussion. This work was supported by Department of Energy grant No. DE-AT06-82 ER 1207 to A. Kleinhofs and P. F. Lurquin and by funds provided to Washington State University through the NIH Biomedical Research Support Grant (T. Manzara).

References

1. Howell, S. H. (1982) Ann. Rev. Plant Physiol. 33:609-650.
2. Marton, L., Wullems, G. J., Molendijk, L. and Schilperoort, R. A. (1979) Nature 277:129-131.
3. Hasezawa, S., Nagata, T. and Syono, K. (1981) Molec. Gen. Genet. 182:206-210.
4. Wostemeyer, A., Otten, L., De Greve, H., Hernalsteens, J. P., Leemans, J., Van Montagu, M. and Schell, J. (1982) This volume.
5. Gordon, M. P. (1982) This volume.
6. Muller, A. J. and Grafe, R. (1978) Molec. Gen. Genet. 161:67-76.
7. Marton, L., Dung, T. M., Mendel, R. R. and Maliga, P. (1982) Molec. Gen. Genet. (in press).
8. Taylor, J. L., Bedbrook, J. and Kleinhofs, A. Submitted for publication.
9. Matzke, A. J. M. and Chilton, M. D. (1981) J. Molec. Appl. Genet. 1:39-49.
10. Dellaporta, S. and Fraley, R. T. (1981) Plant Molec. Biol. Newslett. 2:59-66.
11. Leemans, J., Deblaere, R., Willmitzer, L., DeGreve, H., Hernalsteens, J. P., Van Montagu, M., and Schell, J. (1982) The EMBO J. 1:147-152.
12. Willmitzer, L., Simons, G. and Schell, J. (1982) The EMBO J. 1:139-146.
13. DeGreve, H., Decraemer, H., Seurinck, J., Van Montagu, M. and Schell, J. (1981) Plasmid 6:235-248.
14. Lurquin, P. F. (1979) Nucl. Acid Res. 6:3773-3784.
15. Lurquin, P. F. and Sheehy, R. E. (1982) Plant Sci. Lett. 25:133-146.

REVERSAL OF PLANT TUMOR FORMATION

Milton P. Gordon

Department of Biochemistry
University of Washington
Seattle, WA

The transformation of plant tissues by the soil bacteria *Agrobacterium tumefaciens* and *Agrobacterium rhizogenes* results in tumor formation or a callus with excessive root formation, respectively. These processes are associated with the incorporation of bacterial plasmid DNA (T-DNA), into the genome of the host plant. Much effort is underway to utilize these processes to incorporate useful genes into plants by using the bacterial plasmid as a transformation vector. In order for the processes to be useful, it is necessary to have a procedure whereby normal fertile plants can be generated from the tumor tissue with retention of the foreign genes.

The first report of the formation of plants from a cloned crown gall tumor was that of Lutz (1966). Lutz was working with a tissue that was designated as habituated but which in the light of later investigation (Yang et al., 1980a), appears to have been a crown gall tissue. Somewhat later, Sacristan and Melchers (1969, 1977), were able to regenerate plants from single cell clones of crown gall tumors. In these pioneering studies, the loss or rearrangement of the T-DNA was not investigated and the tissues, unfortunately, are not available.

Braun and co-workers (1959, 1976), were able to reverse crown gall teratomas by repeated grafting onto normal tobacco plants. Relatively normal-looking shoots were obtained which retained tumorous traits. The tissues continued to synthesize nopaline and explants grew *in vitro* in the absence of phytohormones. Tissues resulting from meiosis such as haploid anther tissue and fertile seed set by these shoots appeared to be normal. Yang and co-workers (1980 b), investigated the T-DNA of these tissues and found that the normal appearing shoots obtained by grafting appeared to have lost some of the T-DNA present in the parental tissues. Tissues obtained after meiosis had no detectable T-DNA.

When the parental teratoma used in Braun's studies was treated with kinetin, shoots were generated which could be rooted. These shoots (F_0 generations), and subsequent generations obtained by selfing retained small fragments of the T-DNA (Yang and Simpson, 1981; A. Powell, unpublished).

The group at the State University of Leiden, The Netherlands, has reported two instances where plants have been regenerated from tumor tissue with retention of some of the T-DNA (Wullems et al., 1981; Ooms et al., 1982). In the first of these experiments plant protoplasts with partially regenerated cell walls were transformed with A. tumefaciens cells. Some of the resulting callus formed shoots which flowered. Upon fertilization with fertile male pollen, a number of the F_1 plants were nopaline positive. A second procedure used by this group was the fusion of streptomycin-resistant normal protoplasts with tumor protoplasts. Some of these fusion products regenerated plants. It is striking that the arrangement of the T-DNA in the regenerated plants differed from that of the T-DNA in the parental tumor (Ooms et al., 1982).

Octopine positive plants have been obtained by using "shooter" mutants generated by the insertion of bacterial transposons into the appropriate region of the tumor inciting plasmid of A. tumefaciens (Otten et al., 1981). Plants were generated from shoots obtained from infecting tobacco plants with a Tn 7 transposon mutant. The resulting plants sythesize octopine, and this trait was inherited as a single dominant trait with Mendelian segregation ratios. The T-DNA in these plants had an internal deletion which had eliminated the Tn 7 insertion and adjacent DNA. When large deletions are generated in the T region of Ti-Plasmid, the resulting mutants are essentially avirulent; nevertheless, bacteria containing these mutants are able to transform plant tissue. Thus, octopine synthetase and agropine were detected in carrot slices infected with avirulent mutants (Leemans et al., 1982), and octopine was detected in tobacco tissue infected with a very weakly virulent strain of A. tumefaciens containing a Ti-plasmid with a large deletion in the T region (W. Ream, unpublished).

It thus appears that a general feature occuring during the generation of plants from crown gall tumors is the loss of part of the T-DNA from the tumor.

Recently, much interest has been focused on the transformation of plant tissues by A. rhizogenes to produce tumors that show a large amount of roots, "hairy root disease." These tissues can be propagated in vitro in the absence of phytohormones and have the distinct advantage in that the roots spontaneously form shoots from which plants can be generated. The callus tissues, roots, and regenerated plants all contain DNA derived from a large plasmid,

Ri plasmid, present in the inciting organism (Chilton et al., 1982; White et al., 1982).

The simplicity of obtaining plants from rhizogenes-transformed tissues indicates that this procedure may be the system of choice for genetic engineering of plants.

REFERENCES

1. Braun, A.C. (1959). A demonstration of the recovery of the crown-gall tumor cell with the use of complex tumors of single cell origin. Proc. Natl. Acad. Sci. U.S.A. 45:932-938.

2. Braun, A.C. and Wood, H.N. (1976). Suppression of the neoplastic state with the acquisition of specialized functions in cells, tissues, and organs of crown gall teratoma of tobacco. Proc. Natl. Acad. Sci. U.S.A. 73:496-500.

3. Chilton, M.D., Tepfer, D.A., Petit, A., David, C., Casse-Delbart, F., and Tempé, J. (1982). Agrobacterium rhizogenes inserts T-DNA into the genomes of the host plant root cells. Nature, 295:432-34.

4. Leemans, J. Deblaere, R. Willmitzer, L., De Greve, H., Hernalsteens, J.P., Van Montagu, M. and Schell, J. (1982). The Embo Journal. 1(1):147-152.

5. Lutz, A. (1966). Obtention de plantes de tabac a partir de cultures unicellulaires provenant d'une souche anergée. C.R. Acad. Sci. Paris. 262:1856-58.

6. Ooms, G., Bakker, A., Molendijk, L., Wullems, G., Gordon, M.P., Nester, E.W., and Schilperoort, R.A., (1982). T-DNA organization in homogeneous and heterogeneous octopine-type crown gall tissues of Nicotiana tabacum. Cell (in press).

7. Otten, L., De Greve, H., Hernalsteens, J.P., Van Montagu, M., Scheider, O., Straub, J., and Schell, J. (1981). Mol. Gen. Genet. 183:209-213.

8. Powell, Ann T., Unpublished.

9. Ream, W., Unpublished.

10. Sacristan, M.D., and Melchers, G. (1969). The caryological analysis of plant regeneration from tumorous and other callus cultures of tobacco. Mol. Gen. Genet. 105:317-333.

11. Sacristan, M.D. and Melchers, G. (1977). Regeneration of plants from habituated and agrobacterium-transformed single-cell clones of tobacco. Mol. Gen. Genet. 152:111-117.

12. White, F., Ghidossi, G., Gordon, M.P., and Nester, E.W. (1982). Tumor induction of Agrobacterium rhizogenes involves the transfer of plasmid DNA to the plant genome. Proc. Natl. Acad. Sci. U.S.A. 79:3193-97.

13. Wullems, G.J., Molendijk, L., Ooms, G., and Schilperoort, R.A. (1981). Retention of tumor markers in F1 progeny plants from in vitro induced octopine and nopaline tumor tissues. Cell. 24:719-727.

14. Yang, F.-M., and Simpson, R. (1981). Revertant seedlings from crown gall tumors retain a portion of the bacterial T-DNA sequences. Proc. Natl. Acad. Sci. U.S.A. 78:4151-4155.

15. Yang, F.-M., Merlo, D.J., Drummond, M.H., Chilton, M.-D., Nester, E.W., and Gordon, M.P. (1980a). Plasmid DNA of Agrobacterium tumefaciens detected in a presumed habituated tobacco cell line. Mol. Gen. Genet. 177:704-714.

16. Yang, F.-M.. Montoya, A., Merlo, D.J., Drummond, M.H., Chilton, M.-D., Nester, E.W., and Gordon, M.P. (1980b). Foreign DNA sequences in crown gall teratomas and their fate during the loss of the tumorous traits. Mol. Gen. Genet. 177:707-714.

REGENERATION OF PLANTS FROM CROWN GALL CELLS

A step in the T-DNA mediated genetic engineering of plants

A. Wöstemeyer[+], L. Otten[+], H. De Greve*, J.P. Hernalsteens°, J. Leemans°, M. Van Montagu° and J. Schell+*

[+]Max-Planck-Institut für Züchtungsforschung - Köln(BRD)
*Laboratory for Genetics,State-University-Gent(Belgium)
°Laboratory for Genetical Virology, Free University of Brussels (Belgium)

INTRODUCTION

The mechanism whereby the plant pathogenic soil bacterium *Agrobacterium tumefaciens* induces Crown Gall plant tumors is the result of a remarkable example of naturally occurring genetic engineering. A fragment of about 20 kb (called the T-region) of a 120 kb plasmid (called Ti plasmid for tumor-inducing plasmid) is transferred to the plant cell where it becomes covalently linked to the nuclear DNA (1-7). This integrated DNA has been named the T-DNA. Crown Gall cells have two distinctive properties: They grow without hormones (8,9) and they produce so-called opines: compounds not found in normal plant cells and used specifically by *Agrobacterium tumefaciens* as a carbon, nitrogen and energy source with the help of a Ti plasmid-encoded uptake and degradation system (10-13). Opines moreover have the capacity to induce a plasmid transfer system which can spread the opine degradation system through an *Agrobacterium* population (14,15). For recent reviews see 3, 16-20.

This process in which a specific bacterial DNA segment invades wounded plant cells and forces these cells to proliferate and produce energy-rich compounds for the benefit of the bacterium has been called genetic colonization (3). *Agrobacterium* strains can be divided in several classes, both according to the morphology of the tumors they induce and to the type of opines these tumors contain (21). Four major groups are:

1. The nopaline strains induce tumors in which nopaline, nopalinic acid and agrocinopine are found as opines.
2. The octopine strains, inducing tumors with octopine, lysopine, octopinic acid, histopine and agropine,

3. The so-called null-type strains, originally thought to produce tumors without opines, but later found to produce tumors with agropine,
4. The Agrobacterium rhizogenes strains, producing agropine.

The T-DNA of Crown Gall cells is transcribed into polyadenylated messengers (22-26), which have been mapped by Northern anaylsis (26) for both the octopine tumors and the nopaline tumors (27,28). Only two proteins coded for by the T-DNA have thus far been identified in vivo and purified: the opine synthesizing enzymes lysopine dehydrogenase of octopine synthase (29) and nopaline dehydrogenase synthase (30). However, in vitro translation studies with Crown Gall messengers (31) and translation of cloned T-DNA fragments in Escherichia coli (32) into distinct proteins indicate that other T-DNA encoded proteins are present in Crown Gall cells which must be responsible for hormone-independent growth and tumor-morphology (33). The strongest argument in favour of this conclusion comes from an analysis of the abnormal morphogenetic properties of Crown Gall cells induced by Ti plasmids harbouring specific mutations in the T-region (33,34,35,49) (H. Joos, in preparation).

By transposon insertion it has been demonstrated that large pieces of extra DNA inserted into the T-region of the Ti plasmid can be transferred to the plant cell along with the normal T-DNA (36). This result has opened up the possibility to use the Ti plasmid as a vector in the genetic engineering of plant cells. However, to obtain the full regeneration of plants from such engineered cells it remained to be established whether the growth controlling functions carried by the T-DNA could be eliminated without interfering with the Ti plasmid DNA transfer mechanism and whether such DNA, once integrated into the plant genome would be stable and sexually transmittable.

Regeneration of teratoma derived from Crown Galls induced with wild-type Agrobacteria

Tobacco Crown Gall tissues induced by the nopaline strains T37 can form teratoma-like shoots (shoots showing aberrant growth) which retain the opine marker (37,38). These teratomas can be grafted onto normal tobacco plants in which case they can develop into shoots which can flower and set seed. It has been reported that T-DNA was present in all tissues of a grafted T37 teratoma, but absent in anther cultures of such grafted plants and in F1 plants (39,40). These results could be explained either by loss of the T-DNA during meiosis or by selection in favour of cells without T-DNA. If the T-DNA was originally present in a hemizygous state, absence of T-DNA in anther cultures and F1 generation could also have been the consequence of selective growth of gametes without T-DNA.

Although this tobacco tumor line called BT37 was derived from a single cell it was found to harbour several left and right hand T-DNA border fragments (39,40) (composite fragments containing T-DNA and plant DNA). Whether these different T-DNAs were present in all cells or whether this tumor line consisted of cells with different T-DNAs is unclear.

Protoplast cloning experiments carried out in our laboratory with the BT37 line showed that this callus contained normal, $NpDH^-$ cells, giving rise to normal tobacco plantlets. When teratoma shoots resulting from this cloning experiment were cloned again, they did not yield normal plants anymore (O. Schieder, personal communication).

In a different type of experiment, Yang et al. (41) observed normal shoot induction after hormone treatment of BT37 with 1 mg/l of kinetin. These shoots had lost all the phenotypic markers of transformed tissues (nopaline synthesis, hormone independent growth of leaf fragments of the grafted shoots, immunity against a second Agrobacterium infection) but they had apparently retained small border fragments of the T-DNA. The region common to both octopine and nopaline T-DNA and known to be responsible for hormone autotrophy was absent. These border sequences could also be found in the progeny of these plants. From the data presented by Yang et al. (41) it appears (although the authors did not mention this) that the original BT37 tissue already contained the T-DNA border fragments found in the regenerants obtained by the kinetin treatment. This would mean that the hormonal treatment merely allowed the selective growth of cells having spontaneously lost most of their T-DNA.

Fusion of normal SR-1 tobacco cells (SR-1 is a tobacco line containing a cytoplasmatically located streptomycin resistance) with non-regenerating octopine producing cells has yielded $LpDH^+$ teratoma shoots (45).

After coculturing tobacco protoplasts with an octopine Agrobacterium strain (46) many $LpDH^+$ teratoma shoots could be found. Like T37 derived teratoma shoots, these shoots could also be grafted onto normal tobacco plants and subsequently flowered (47). In the experiments reported, the flowers were found to be male sterile and after pollination with normal tobacco pollen, only normal $LpDH^-$ plantlets could be found. The male sterility was attributed by the authors to T-DNA activity. This is most probably incorrect since we found that control SR1 tobacco plants also exhibit male sterility and that T-DNA containing grafted shoots can be male fertile (see EXPERIMENTAL RESULTS). In the same way, $NpDH^+$ teratoma shoots were obtained (47), which were mostly found to be unable to transmit the NpDH gene to their offspring. Only one $NpDH^+$ plant was obtained, able to form roots, but which grew very slowly. As will be described further, when these experiments were independently repeated, we got significantly different results.

Whereas Crown Gall cells obtained with wild-type bacteria apparently cannot produce fully normal plants with functional T-DNA genes, we have been able to obtain such plants after infection with bacteria containing Ti plasmids with specific mutations in the T-region (48).

One such mutant contained a bacterial transposon (Tn7) within the T-region of pTiB6S3. This mutant, GV 2100, induced tumors on tobacco with numerous shoots, most of which were $LpDH^-$ and therefore probably derived from normal cells. Some $LpDH^+$ shoots were found to be able to regenerate into a normal tobacco plant. They contained a short T-DNA fragment (49) earlier shown to code for LpDH (50). This regenerant might have originated from a cell which at the time of infection acquired a deleted T-DNA fragment or from a cell which lost part of an originally bigger T-DNA. Whatever the mechanism, it is likely that such a cell was only able to form a shoot because the mutation in the T-DNA (in Eco 32g) sufficiently changed the conditions in the Crown Gall cells surrounding the regenerating cell. Indeed, cells containing short T-DNA fragments might also be present in wild-type Crown Galls but their regeneration would be prevented by the presence of cells containing an intact T-DNA segment.

A precise comparison between the regenerant and the original tumor tissue from which it was derived could show whether the T-DNA of the regenerant originated as a deletion of a once bigger T-DNA, since one can expect that in this case at least the left hand border fragment would be identical in both tissues.

As the regenerant was fully fertile, selfing and crosses with normal tobacco plants showed that the T-DNA was present in a hemizygous state (51). It was stably maintained through meiosis and inherited in a strictly Mendelian fashion.

In a second experiment the same region Eco 32g was mutated by substitution with a 5.8 Md derivative of the w-type wide host range plasmid S-a, yielding the mutant Ti plasmid GV 2206 (52). After screening shoots originating from callus obtained by infection tobacco with GV 2206, $LpDH^+$ shoots were again found (33), and regenerated into normal fertile plants (49). The results of crosses between both types of regenerants (from GV 2100 and GV 2206) showed that the two LpDH genes segregated independently of each other and were thus integrated at different loci (49). This confirmed earlier evidence obtained from T-DNA analysis where it was shown that the sizes of T-DNA border fragments differ in independently derived Crown Gall lines (3,39) and recent work by Zambryski et al. (59) which showed that T-DNA fragments reisolated from transformed tobacco lines are covalently linked to different plant DNA sequences.

EXPERIMENTAL RESULTS

In a comparative study of induction and regeneration of opine-positive shoots from tobacco and potato (A. Wöstemeyer, unpublished) the following approaches were used:

1. Infection of sterile shoots with wild-type octopine and nopaline bacteria on the one hand and with mutant octopine strains with a high shoot-inducing capacity (GV 2100 and GV 2206, see above) on the other hand.
2. Infection of protoplasts with the same strains, according to the method of Márton et al. (46)

1. Shoot infection

a. Tobacco

Sterile shoots of the tobacco line SR-1 (53) were infected with wild-type strains B6S3 and C58. They yielded undifferentiated tumors. However, when the *Agrobacterium* mutants GV 2100 was used, tumors formed numerous shoots. These were tested for LpDH activity. From 30 GV 2100 induced calli, 146 shoots were tested. 8 LpDH$^+$ shoots (5%) were found on 7 different calli. When cultured on medium without hormones, only 2 shoots retained the LpDH activity. 6 of the now LpDH$^-$ shoots rooted. After 3 more months in culture the 2 lines which had retained their LpDH activity also were found to have lost it, and subsequently rooted.

Apparently, infection with this mutant strain allows the regeneration of many normal plant cells, which complicates the detection of LpDH$^+$ shoots. Why the LpDH activity is sometimes lost in shoot cultures remains to be investigated. From our earlier results (49,51) with tobacco, it is clear that the presence of an actively expressed LpDH gene does not interfere with normal plant development. Furthermore when LpDH$^+$ plantlets (i.e. LpDH$^+$ shoots that form LpDH$^+$ roots when separated from the tumor base) were screened for (49), these turned out to be stably LpDH$^+$ over many generations.

Possibly the unstable, non-rooting LpDH$^+$ shoots observed in these studies, consisted of cells still expressing at least some of the T-DNA linked tumor-controlling genes. This might provide a selection for the formation of side shoots by those cells which would have lost (e.g. by deletion) the whole of the T-DNA including the LpDH gene. Indeed, LpDH$^+$ plants, from which all tumor controlling genes have been removed (49,51) are very stable with regard to the vegetative as well as the sexual inheritance of the LpDH gene.

b. Potato

Shoots of a diploid potato variety (HH 258) (54) with a high regenerative capacity in tissue culture were infected with wild-type octopine strain B6S3 and yielded undifferentiated tumor callus. After infection with nopaline strains C58 and T37 however, $NpDH^+$ teratomas were easily found. These were repeatedly grafted on tomato plants and some eventually flowered. However, all these teratoma grafts, developped into shoots which did not carry the opine marker. Since on tobacco C58 forms mostly undifferentiated tumors, the induction of teratoma clearly also depends on the host, as observed by others (55).

After infection of potato shoots with the mutant GV 2100 (see above) 7 shoot-regenerating tumors were obtained. 15 out of 90 investigated shoots were $LpDH^+$, 6 of which formed roots and retained the LpDH marker. 32 tubers formed on 12 $LpDH^+$ plants did not have a measurable LpDH activity. However, shoots originating from these tubers were all $LpDH^+$, indicating that the LpDH gene is transmitted through the tubers. The absence of activity in the tubers probably reflects the general dormancy of these tissues.

After fertilization of one $LpDH^+$ potato plant with normal potato pollen (the diploid potato line used is self-sterile) 31 of 123 resulting seedlings were found to be $LpDH^+$. All these plants had a normal morphology. The segregation figures deviate from the expected 1:1 ratio (assuming that the LpDH gene was present in a hemizygous state). The original $LpDH^+$ plant may have been a chimaera of cells with different T-DNA complements.

After infection of potato shoots with the mutant strain GV 2206, tumors with numerous shoots were obtained. However, none of 120 shoots investigated was $LpDH^+$. The difference between the number of $LpDH^+$ shoots observed on GV 2100 induced tumors relative to GV 2206 induced tumors both on potato and tobacco might be the result of a deletion activity resulting from the Tn7 transposon insertion in pGV 2100. Indeed, in the strain GV 2100 the Tn7 might induce deletions in the T-DNA, some of which take away the T-DNA part which is responsible for suppression of shoot formation by transformed cells. Such deletion mutants, which retain a segment of the T-DNA around the LpDH gene, would be able to regenerate shoots or even plants. This could explain why tumors of the GV 2100 strain produce more LpDH containing shoots than tumors of the strain GV 2206.

2. Protoplast infection

In a second type of experiment tobacco and potato protoplasts were infected with different bacterial strains as described by Márton et al. (46).

a. Tobacco

Tobacco protoplasts were prepared from SR-1 plants and infected with the nopaline strains C58 and T37 and the octopine strains LBA 4013 and B6S3. As observed by Wullems et al. (56) several types of calli were found (see Table 1). Here we shall limit ourselves to a description of experiments with C58 and LBA 4013 derived calli which formed opine-positive teratoma shoots. In both cases, shoots remained small and did not form roots. They were repeatedly grafted onto normal tobacco stems which resulted in a slow normalization and finally in flowering of the grafts.

Table 1. Properties of hormone-independent calli from regenerating SR-1 tobacco protoplasts infected with Agrobacterium strain C58, T37, LBA 4013, B6S3 and GV 2100.

S^+ = shootforming; S^- = shootless

Strain	opine (pos) calli		Opine (neg) calli	
	S^+	S^-	S^+	S^-
C58	6	21	6	5
T37	2	21	4	106
LBA 4013	6	8	4	9
B6S3	1	10	4	35
GV 2100	8	57	5	40

In contrast to normal tobacco leaves, leaf fragments of these grafted plants were able to grow when placed on hormone-free medium. Also, different parts of the grafted teratomas (stem, leaf, flower) retained the opine marker. The observations by Wullems et al. (47) that flowers of the $LpDH^+$ grafts are often male sterile was wrongly considered to represent a T-DNA controlled property. It is more likely due to a property of the SR-1 line itself, since male sterility was also observed in control plants (our observations). Moreover, in our experiments one of the two $LpDH^+$ grafts investigated, was found to be male sterile, whereas the other one was completely fertile.

After selfing of this fertile graft, two types of germinating plantlets were found: normally rooting plants without LpDH activity and rootless plantlets each of which contained high levels of LpDh activity.

When these rootless plantlets were cultured in vitro on hormone-free medium they formed callus at their base and developed into the type of teratoma-like tissue that was originally obtained from the infected protoplasts. When the fertile $LpDH^+$ graft was crossed with normal SR-1 pollen, 170 seedlings were normal and $LpDH^-$, 191 were rootless and $LpDH^+$. After selfing, this ratio was 38:110. The results indicate that in the original graft the LpDH gene and the gene(s) preventing root formation were 100% linked and present in a hemizygous state. Analysis of the T-DNA by Southern blotting of the fertile grafted plant showed that a large segment of the T-DNA, normally found in octopine tumors, was absent. The extent of the remaining T-DNA, as based upon preliminary observations, is shown in Figure 1. RNA analysis by hybridization of polynucleotide kinase labeled poly-A containing RNA isolated from polysomes to Southern blots containing defined segments of the T-DNA schowed the presence of messengers 4,6 and 3 (messengers of the TL-DNA have been numbered from 1 to 7 according to decreasing size (27). Recently both on the basis of detailed messenger studies and on the basis of DNA sequencing data, a region was found between gene 4 and 6, coding for a messenger called 6a (Willmitzer, Lemmers and Schreier, personal communication).

The results of the RNA mapping are shown in Figure 2. The analysis shows that the concentrations of transcript 4 and 6 were very low in leaf tissue whereas they were clearly present in callus tissue, obtained when the leaf tissue of the grafted material was brought into tissue culture and forced to dedifferentiate into callus tissue by the addition of 2mg/ml NAA and 0.2 mg/ml kinetin, or when the callus which grew at the base of seedlings on medium without hormones was used for RNA analysis. Whether this correlation between the lack of tissue organization and the levels of messengers 4 and 6 is the result of transcription regulation, or reflects events taking place at the level of messenger stability, processing or transport into polysomes is not known.

The presence of auxin and cytokinin at the concentrations used apparently does not inhibit the expression of gene 4 and 6, nor does the absence of hormones. As far as the function of messengers 4,6 and 6a is concerned, the following can be said:

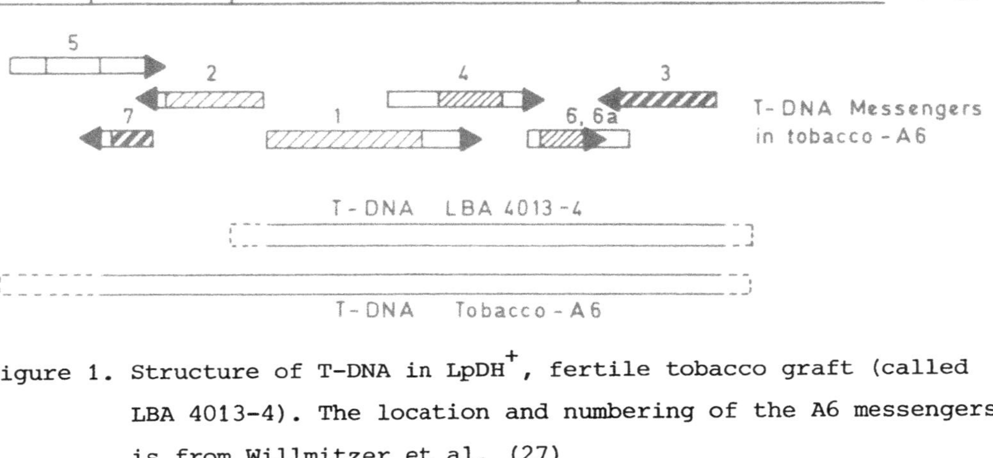

Figure 1. Structure of T-DNA in $LpDH^+$, fertile tobacco graft (called LBA 4013-4). The location and numbering of the A6 messengers is from Willmitzer et al. (27)

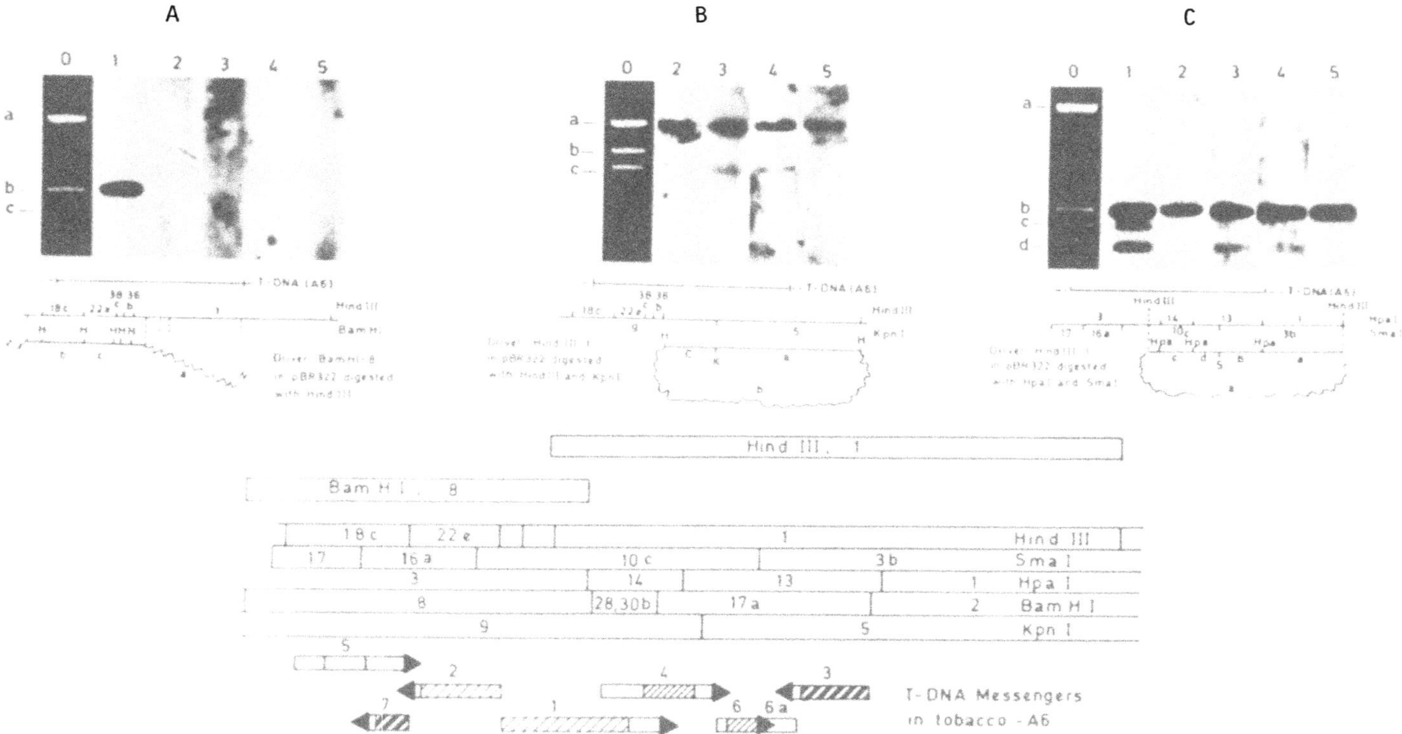

Figure 2. Mapping of RNA's from LBA 4013-4 (see text). Probe: polynulceotide kinase labeled poly-A^+ RNA from: 1. A6 tumor tissue; 2. leaf tissue from S1 seedlings of LBA 4013-4; 3. callus from the same; 4. callus tissue from leaf fragments of LBA 4013-4, grown on hormones. Drivers: pTi fragments cloned in pBR322, retricted as indicated. a,b,c and d correspond to the different restriction enzyme fragments indicated in the pTi map. For comparison, the map of the A6 messengers is included with numbering according to Willmitzer et al. (27).

Genes for messenger 4,6 and 6a are present in both octopine and nopaline T-DNA (27,28). As for the function of messenger 4, it has been observed both in octopine and nopaline T-regions that mutations in the gene coding for this messenger yield a new phenotype, i.e. tumors with protruding roots. On the basis of these results it could be postulated that the product of messenger 4 inhibits the formation of roots by both transformed and untransformed, T-DNA free cells (33). Thus the rootless character of the grafted plants in our experiments can be ascribed to the presence and expression of gene 4.

In parallel to our regeneration studies, T-DNA deletion mutants were contructed by in vitro mutagenesis (33,52). One of these mutants, GV 2219, contained only the genes for messengers 4,6,6a and3. This mutant was still virulent and produced tumors with numerous opine positive teratoma-shoots. It is expected that such teratoma-shoots will have properties identical to the grafted opine positive shoots described here.

In accordance with the model described above, which postulates that is is the activity of messengers 4, or 4,6 and 6a which prevents root formation, we predicted that $LpDH^+$ grafted shoots in which no or very low levels of these transcripts could be observed, would, when separated from their basis, be able to form roots. This was indeed observed to be the case. Such roots were also found to produce LpDH.

In regeneration experiments with the nopaline strain C58, $NpDH^+$, shoots were obtained. They behaved in the same way as the $LpDH^+$ shoots. A fully fertile shoot was obtained by grafting. Pollination of this shoot with SR-1 pollen yielded 214 normal plants and 95 rootless plants. Selfing yielded 58 normal plants and 111 rootless plants. Also, a 100% correlation was found in the seedlings between the presence of NpDH and the absence of roots. Although many $NpDH^+$ plantlets were found, the numbers of $NpDH^+$ plants deviate from what could have been expected on the basis of mendelian transmission of a hemizygous character. As we do not yet know the exact T-DNA structure in these plants, this result is difficult to interpret. Preliminary T-DNA mapping has shown that these grafted plants clearly have smaller T-DNAs. A more detailed analysis will be necessary to show whether the left borders of the T-DNA of the nopaline regenerants and the octopine regenerants correspond to identical positions within the T-region as in wild-type tumors or whether borders are derived from different plasmid sequences. These results are however in marked contrast to those obtained and described in previous publications where it was said that T-DNA containing plants could not or only very exceptionally transmit this T-DNA through meiosis (37,38,40,47). We had previously demonstrated (49,51) that these conclusions were not correct when most or all of the tumor-controlling genes were removed from the T-DNA without affecting the activity of the opine synthase gene. Most importantly the present experiments show that also tumor-controlling T-DNA genes (4,6,6a) can be readily transmitted through meiosis. It is unclear why Wullems et al. (47) in experiments essentially similar to those reported here, failed to observe this high rate of meiotic transmission of T-DNA linked tumor genes. Protoplasts of the potato lines HH 258 and HH 260 were grown in K8 medium (57). Infection with Agrobacterium however, was done in K3 medium (58) normally used for the infection and culturing of tobacco protoplasts (46), since in K8 the bacteria grew rapidly and killed the plant cells. After the removal of the bacteria the potato cells were again cultured in K8. In 3 out of 8 experiments with the wild-type strains C58, T37 and LBA 4013, calli and shoots could be regenerated on medium with hormones. All 38 calli investigated were opine negative. Upon transfer to hormone-free medium after 4 weeks, all calli died.

This last experiment shows that the successful bacterial infection of protoplasts of species other than tobacco will depend on efficient ways to control bacterial growth, on a better knowledge of the factors influencing the rate of transformation and/or those influencing the stability of the T-DNA in the absence of selection pressure through hormone-free conditions which in the case of protoplasts can only be applied at later stages of the cell culture.

GENERAL CONCLUSIONS

In the past, attempts to regenerate normal plants directly from Crown Gall tissues induced with wild-type bacteria have met with little success.

However, such regenerants have now been obtained by the use of Ti plasmids which were mutated in the T-DNA. Experiments with potato and tobacco have shown that T-DNA genes introduced into plant cells with the help of such mutants can be stably maintained both in mitosis and meiosis. In potato, such genes are also retained in vegetative propagation through tubers. These results demonstrate clearly that the T-region of *Agrobacterium tumefaciens* can be used as a vector to introduce foreign genes into plant cells without disturbing the normal regenerative capabilities of such cells.

To improve the frequency of occurrence of regenerants containing T-DNA, experiments are in progress to contruct *Agrobacterium* mutants which are deleted for most of the T-DNA.

REFERENCES

1. Chilton, M.-D., Drummond, H.J., Merlo, D.J., Sciaky, D., Montoya, A.L., Gordon, M.P., and Nester, E.W. (1977) Cell 11: 263
2. De Beuckeleer, M., De Block, M., De Greve, H., Depicker, A., De Vos, R., De Vos, G., De Wilde, M., Dhaese, P., Dobbelaere, M.R., Engler, G., Genetello, C., Hernalsteens, J. P., Holsters, M., Jacobs, A., Schell, J., Seurinck, J., Silva, B., Van Haute, E., Van Montagu, M., Van Vliet, F., Villarroel, R., and Zaenen, I. (1978) In: Proc. IV. Int. Conf. on Plant Pathogenic Bacteria, INRA, Angers, 115
3. Schell, J., Van Montagu, M., De Beuckeleer, M., De Block, M., Depicker, A., De Wilde, M., Engler, G., Genetello, C., Hernalsteens, J.P., Holsters, M., Seurinck, J., Silva, B., Van Vliet, F., and Villarroel, R. (1979) Proc. R. Soc. London B 204:251
4. Thomashow, M.F., Nutter, R., Montoya, A.L., Gordon, M.P., and Nester, E.W. (1980) Cell 19:729
5. Lemmers, M., De Beuckeleer, M., Holsters, M., Zambryski, P., Depicker, A., Hernalsteens, J.P., Van Montagu, M. and Schell, J. (1980) J. Mol. Biol. 144:355
6. Zambryski, P., Holsters, M., Krüger, K., Depicker, A., Schell, J., Van Montagu, M., and Goodman, H.M. (1980) Science 209:1385
7. De Beuckeleer, M., Lemmers, M., De Vos, G., Willmitzer, L., Van Montagu, M., and Schell, J. (1981) Mol. Gen. Genet. 183:283
8. Braun, A.C. and White, P.R. (1943) Phytopath. 33:85
9. Braun, A.C. (1956) Cancer Research 16:53
10. Petit, A., Delhaye, S., Tempé, J., and Morel, G. (1970) Physiol. Vég. 8:205
11. Bomhoff, G., Klapwijk, P.M., Kester, C.H.M., Schilperoort, R. A., Hernalsteens, J.P., and Schell, J. (1976) Mol. Gen. Genet. 145:177
12. Petit, A. and Tempé, J. (1978) Mol. Gen. Genet. 167:147
13. Klapwijk, P., Hooykaas, P., Kester, H., Schilperoort, R.A., and Rörsch, A. (1976) J. Gen. Microbiol. 96:155
14. Kerr, A., Manigault, P., and Tempé, J. (1977) Nature 265:560
15. Genetello, C., Van Larebeke, N., Holsters, M., Depicker, A., Van Montagu, M., and Schell, J. (1977) Nature 265:561
16. Gordon, M.P. (1979) In: "Proteins and Nucleic Acids, The Biochemistry of Plants", Vol. 6, A. Marcus ed. Acad. Press, New York, p. 531
17. Schilperoort, R.A., Klapwijk, P.M., Ooms, G., and Wullems, G.J. (1980) In: Genetic origins of tumor cells. F.J. Cleton and J.W. Simons eds. Martinus Nijhoff, The Hague, p. 87

18. Schell, J. and Van Montagu, M. (1980) In: "Genome Organization and Expression in Plants". C.J. Leaver ed. Plenum Press, New York, p. 453
19. Van Montagu, M. and Schell, J. (1979) In: Plasmids of medical, environmental and commercial importance". K. Timmis and A. Pühler eds. Elsevier, Amsterdam, p.71
20. Van Montagu, M., Holsters, M., Zambryski, P., Hernalsteens, J.P., Depicker, A., De Beuckeleer, M., Engler, G., Lemmers, M., Willmitzer, L., and Schell, J. (1980) Proc. R. Soc. London B 210:351
21. Guyon, P., Chilton, M.-D., Petit, A., and Tempé, J. (1980) Proc. Natl. Acad. Sci. USA 77:2693
22. Drummond, M.H., Gordon, M.P., Nester, E.W., and Chilton, M.-D. (1977) Nature 269:535
23. Gurley, W.B., Kemp, J.D., Albert, M.J., Sutton, D.W., and Callis, J. (1979) Proc. Natl. Acad. Sci. USA 76:2828
24. Willmitzer, L., Otten, L., Simons, G., Schmalenbach, W., Schröder, J., Schröder, G., Van Montagu, M., De Vos, G., and Schell, J. (1981) Mol. Gen. Genet. 182:255
25. Gelvin, S.B., Gordon, M.P., Nester, E.W., and Aronson, A.J. (1981) Plasmid 6:17
26. Alwine, J.C., Kemp, D.J., and Stark, G.R. (1977) Proc. Natl. Acad. Sci.USA 74:5350
27. Willmitzer, L., Simons, G., and Schell, J. (1982) EMBO J. 1: 139
28. Willmitzer, L., Dhaese, P., Schreier, P.H., Schmalenbach, W., Van Montagu, M., and Schell, J. (1982) submitted to Cell
29. Hack, E. and Kemp, J.D. (1980) Pl. Physiol. 65:949
30. Kemp, J.D., Sutton, D.W., and Hack, E. (1979) Biochemistry 18:3755
31. Schröder, J. and Schröder, G. (1982) Mol. Gen. Genet. 185:51
32. Schröder, J., Hillebrand, A., Klipp, W., and Pühler, A.(1981) Nucl. Acids Res. 9:5187
33. Leemans, J., Deblaere, R., Willmitzer, L., De Greve, H., Hernalsteens, J.P., Van Montagu, M., and Schell, J. (1982) EMBO J. 1:147
34. Garfinkel, D.J., Simpson, R.S., Ream, L.W., White, F.F., Gordon, M.P., and Nester, E.W. (1981) Cell 27:143
35. Ooms, G., Hooykaas, P., Molenaar, G., Schilperoort, R.A. (1981) Gene 14:33
36. Hernalsteens, J.P., Van Vliet, F., De Beuckeleer, M., Depicker, A., Engler, G., Lemmers, M., Holsters, M., Van Montagu, M., and Schell, J. (1980) Nature 187:654
37. Braun, A. and Wood, H.N. (1976) Proc. Natl. Acad. Sci.USA 73:496
38. Wood, H.N., Binns, A., and Braun, A.C. (1978) Differentiation 11:175

39. Lemmers, M., De Beuckeleer, M., Holsters, M., Zambryski, P., Depicker, A., Hernalsteens, J.P., Van Montagu, M., and Schell, J. (1980) J. Mol. Biol. 144:353
40. Yang, F., Montoya, A.L., Merlo, D.J., Drummond, M.H., Chilton, M.-D., Nester, E.W., and Gordon, M.P. (1980) Mol. Gen. Genet. 177:707
41. Yang, F. and Simpson, R.B. (1981) Proc. Natl. Acad. Sci. USA 78:4151
42. Scott, I.M. (1979) Pl. Sci. Lett. 16:239
43. Owens, L.D. (1982) Pl. Physiol. 69:37
44. Aerts, M., Jacobs, M., Hernalsteens, J.P., Van Montagu, M. and Schell, J. (1979) Pl. Sci. Lett. 17:43
45. Wullems, G.J., Molendijk, L. and Schilperoort, R.A. (1980) Theor. Appl. Genet. 56:203
46. Márton, L., Wullems, G.J., Molendijk, L. and Schilperoort, R. A. (1979) Nature 277:129
47. Wullems, G.J., Molendijk, L., Ooms, G., and Schilperoort, R. A. (1981) Cell 24:719
48. De Greve, H., Decraemer, H., Seurinck, J., Van Montagu, M., and Schell, J. (1981) Plasmid 6:235
49. De Greve, H., Leemans, J., Hernalsteens, J.P., Thia Thoong, L., De Beuckeleer, M., Willmitzer, L., Otten, L., Van Montagu, M., and Schell, J. (1982) submitted to Nature
50. Schröder, J., Schröder, G., Huisman, H., Schilperoort, R.A., and Schell, J. (1981) FEBS Lett. 129:166
51. Otten, L., De Greve, H., Hernalsteens, J.P., Van Montagu, M., Schieder, O., Straub, J., and Schell, J. (1981) Mol. Gen. Genet. 183:209
52. Leemans, J., Shaw, C., Deblaere, R., De Greve, H., Hernalsteens, J.P., Maes, M., Van Montagu, M., and Schell, J. (1981) J. Mol. Appl. Genet. 1:149
53. Maliga, P., Sz-Breznovits, A., Márton, L., and Joó, F. (1975) Nature 255:401
54. Binding, H., Nehls, R., Schieder, O., Sopory, S.K., and Wenzel, G. (1978) Physiol. Plant. 43:52
55. Gresshoff, P.M., Skotnicki, M.L., and Rolfe, B.G. (1979) J. Bacteriol. 137:1020
56. Wullems, G.J., Molendijk, L., Ooms, G., and Schilperoort, R. A. (1981) Proc. Natl. Acad. Sci. USA 78:4344
57. Kao, K.N. and Michayluk, M.R. (1975) Planta 126:105
58. Nagy, J.I. and Maliga, P. (1976) Z. Pflanzenphysiol. 78:453
59. Zambryski, P., Depicker, A., Kruger, K., and Goodman, H. (1982) J. Mol. Appl. Genet. 1:361

THE POTENTIAL USES OF *AGROBACTERIUM RHIZOGENES* IN THE GENETIC ENGINEERING OF HIGHER PLANTS: NATURE GOT THERE FIRST

David Tepfer

Laboratoire de Biologie cellulaire
I.N.R.A.
F 78000 Versailles, France

INTRODUCTION

The race has been on for some time to use genetic engineering, i.e. recombinant DNA technology, in a constructive, applied fashion. Although not a participant, I have enjoyed observing the original and often virtuostic exploits of the competitors. My own interest, in the meantime, has been to study with a minimum of manipulation, a natural parasexual genetic system, which I believe constitutes a precedent for the use of genetic engineering to introduce novel and potentially useful morphogenetic and physiological characters into plants.

Agrobacterium rhizogenes has been known for some time to cause the formation of adventitious roots on the stems of numerous plants (Hildebrand, 1934). Rhizogenicity was recently shown to be correlated with the presence of a large plasmid (Moore et al., 1979; White and Nester, 1980), subsequently named the Ri plasmid (Tepfer and Tempé, 1981) for "root-inducing" as a parallel to the Ti, or "tumor-inducing", plasmid of *Agrobacterium tumefaciens*. Roots induced on carrot discs by *A. rhizogenes* were cultured in the absence of contaminating micro-organisms and shown to synthesize agropine (Tepfer and Tempé, 1981), a marker for the presence of Ti plasmid DNA in plant tumors incited by *A. tumefaciens*. The hypothesis advanced by several authors, that *A. rhizogenes* engages in genetic transformation of higher plants in the same way as *A. tumefaciens*, that is by inserting a fragment of plasmid DNA, the transferred or "T-DNA", into the plant genome, was confirmed for carrot and *Nicotiana glauca* (Chilton et al., 1982; White et al., 1982). Thus it appears that the basic transformation phenomenon is similar in the *tumefaciens* and *rhizogenes* systems, and that at least one of the genes carried by the Ti T-DNA, agropine synthase, is also encoded in the Ri T-DNA.

Despite these molecular and genetic similarities the morphogenetic effects of the two T-DNAs in a plant cell are strikingly different: one causes tumors, the other roots. Tumors are clearly deleterious, while primary inoculations of *A. rhizogenes*, resulting in adventitious roots, were reported to confer drought tolerance on apple seedlings (Moore et al., 1979). In my experience, root-inducing primary inoculations are not harmful, and in some cases impart a certain vigor to the host plant. The results below indicate that the relatively benign, or perhaps even beneficial effects of Ri T-DNA insertion into adventitious roots can be generalized. Ri T-DNA presence in the whole plant and its progeny does not appear to be disadvantageous, and under some conditions might be of adaptive significance.

In this paper Ri T-DNA is traced from cultures of transformed roots, through regeneration of transformed plants, to their transformed progeny, using morphological markers and Southern hybridization. Possible applications in applied and basic research are proposed.

RESULTS

A. rhizogenes strains A4 and 8196 were maintained in log phase for several days, and then inoculated into wounded stems of tobacco (*Nicotiana tabacum* cv. Xanthi, diplohaploidized line XHFD8, Bourgin, 1978), *Convolvulus sepium*, *Convolvulus arvensis*, and onto the surface of carrot discs. All operations were performed under sterile conditions on surface sterilized material or *in vitro* germinated seedlings. Roots formed after several weeks in culture (fig. 1), while control tissue wounded in the same manner did not respond. These roots were used to establish continuous, axenic organ cultures. Control cultures were begun from primary roots excised from seeds germinated *in vitro*.

Morphological and physiological differences between the *A. rhizogenes* induced root cultures and the controls were immediately obvious in the four species. Roots originating from bacterial induction grow faster, are highly branched (apical dominance is reduced) and are plagiotropic, rather than positively geotropic, i.e. they grow horizontally, instead of downward.

The presence of Ri T-DNA has been reported in similar cultures of carrot and *N. glauca* (Chilton et al., 1982; White et al., 1982). Figure 2 shows that the roots of the same species, *C. sepium*, transformed by two different *A. rhizogenes* strains, A4 or 8196, contain T-DNA which hybridizes to plasmid DNA from 8196, but which is diffe-

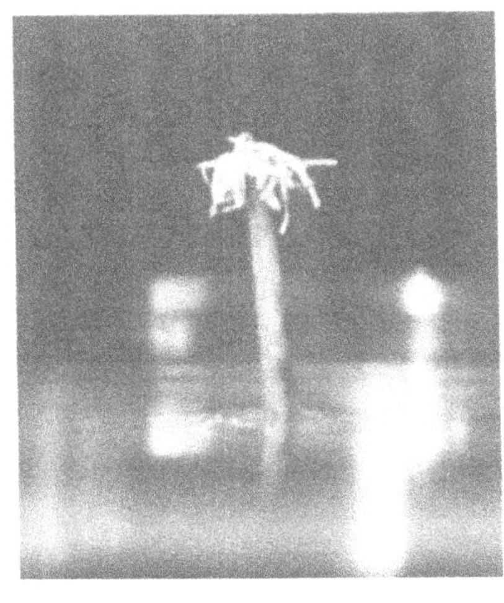

FIG. 1

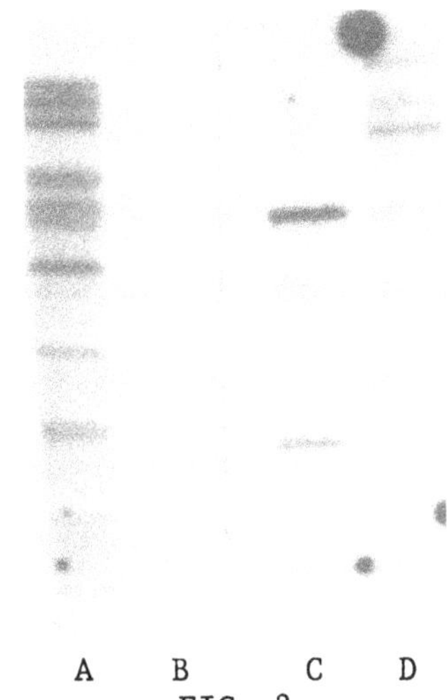

FIG. 2

Fig. 1. *Convolvulus arvensis* stem segment two weeks after *in vitro* inoculation with *A. rhizogenes* strain A4.

Fig. 2. T-DNA in axenic root cultures initiated by *A. rhizogenes*. Southern hybridization of *A. rhizogenes* strain 8196 plasmid DNA, labeled to 2×10^8 cpm/μg, against A) 8196 plasmid DNA, B) control *C. sepium* DNA, C) strain 8196 induced *C. sepium* root DNA, and D) strain A4 induced *C. sepium* root DNA.

rent in restriction pattern and hybridization intensity. Thus, A4 and 8196 contain Ri plasmids whose T-DNAs cross-hybridize, but have only partial sequence homology and differently arranged Bam H1 restriction sites. The pattern of opine synthesis is also different. *C. sepium* synthesizes agropine and mannopine, when transformed by strain A4, and synthesizes only mannopine, when transformed by 8196 (fig. 3). Although the molecular structures of these T-DNAs, as well as opinic type, are different, they have remarkably similar morphological and physiological effects in the host plant.

Transformed roots of tobacco and *C. arvensis* regenerated into whole plants spontaneously in culture (fig. 4). Carrot roots were regenerated by making cell suspensions and inducing somatic embryogenesis. In all three cases plants were obtained which are strikingly different from those regenerated from control root cultures. Their root systems are plagiotropic (fig. 5), with roots even growing along the surface of the soil; their roots are highly branched; and their leaves exhibit a marker first observed by Ackermann (1977) which I have named waffling (fig. 6). All regenerated plants exhibited the same morphological characteristics. Carrot plants, in addition, grew faster and produced more leaves than the controls (fig. 7). They were also annuals, rather than biennials, like the controls regenerated from normal roots. Plants regenerated from transformed roots contain T-DNA (fig. 8).

Transformed carrot plants were crossed with each other. *C. arvensis* was self-fertilized, and tobacco was crossed with non-transformed plants. The progeny of all three species included the transformed and non-transformed phenotypes. All markers for the presence of T-DNA segregate together, including the biennial-annual switch in carrot. The progeny from a transformed tobacco crossed by a normal plant were scored for root number when the seedlings were

Fig. 3. Opines in roots transformed by strains 8196 and A4. A) mannopine in *C. sepium* roots transformed by strain 8196. B) mannopine and agropine in *C. sepium* roots transformed by strain A4. C) mannopine, agropine and an apparently new opine in *C. arvensis* roots transformed by strain A4.

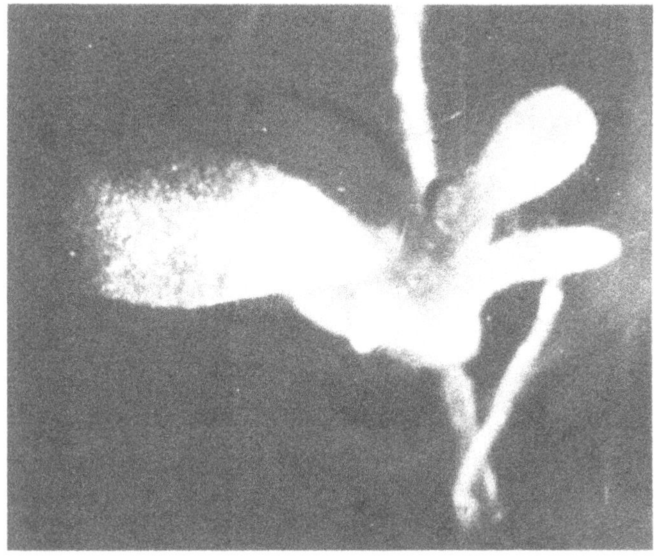

Fig. 4. Spontaneous regeneration of tobacco roots transformed by strain A4.

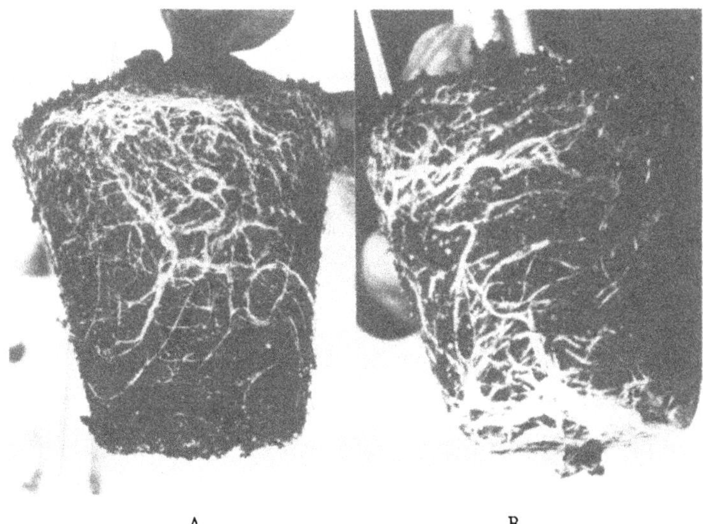

A B

Fig. 5. Differences in root geotropism associated with Ri T-DNA. A) Plagiotropic root system of a tobacco plant transformed by strain A4. B) Positively geotropic root system of control.

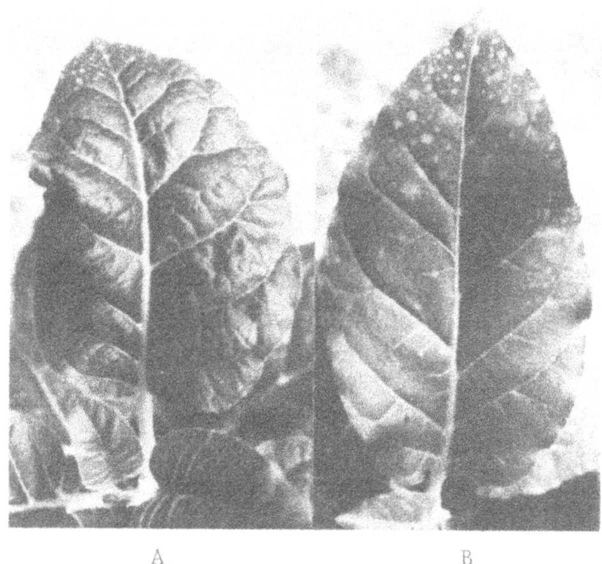

Fig. 6. Differences in leaf morphology associated with Ri T-DNA. A) Waffled leaf from transformed tobacco plant. B) leaf from control.

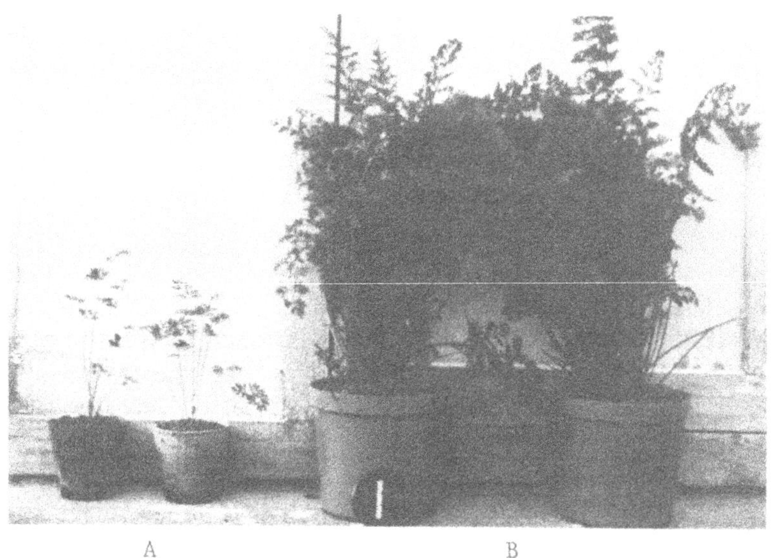

Fig. 7. Differences in leaf number and size in transformed carrot plants. A) Control regenerated from normal roots. B) carrot plants transformed by strain A4.

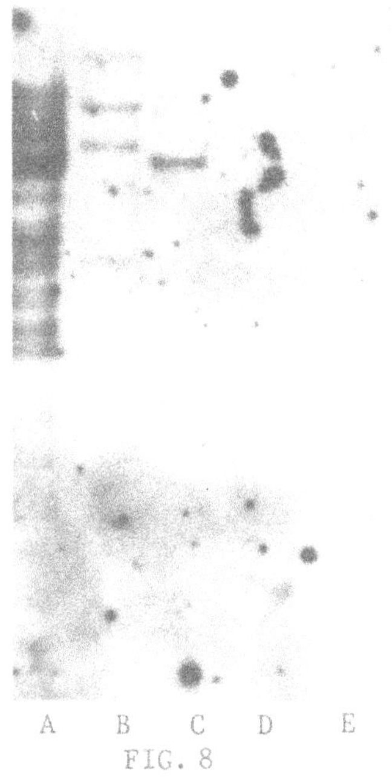

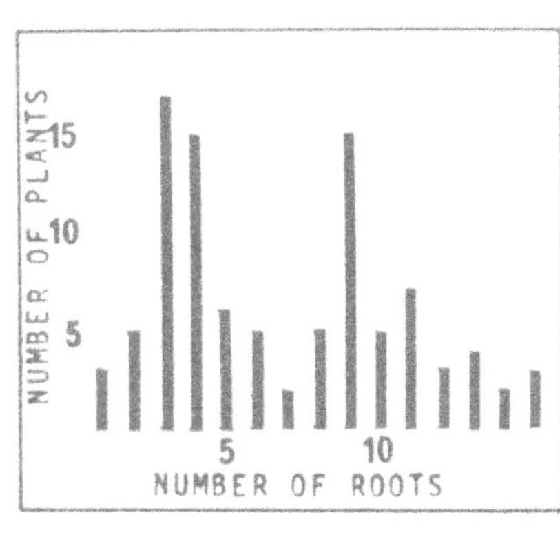

Fig. 8. T-DNA in plants regenerated from transformed roots. Southern hybridization of plasmid DNA from A4 against A) plasmid DNA from strain A4, B) DNA from regenerated tobacco transformed by A4, C) DNA from regenerated *C. arvensis*, transformed by A4, D) control tobacco DNA, E) control *C. arvensis* DNA.

Fig. 9. Histogram of roots per progeny arising from a tobacco plant carrying A4 T-DNA (female) crossed by a control plant (male).

three weeks old (fig. 9). There is an approximately 1:1 ratio between plants of low and high root number, suggesting that this T-DNA associated character is inherited as a dominant gene, present in a single copy in the transformed parent. The normal phenotype in the progeny of transformed tobacco and carrot (*C. arvensis* was not examined) is correlated with the absence of T-DNA, and the transformed phenotype in all three species is associated with the presence of T-DNA (fig. 10).

DISCUSSION

Although there are similarities between the *A. rhizogenes* and *A. tumefaciens* systems, i.e. they both depend on a transformation phenomenon, the two are fundamentally different from the point of view of the plant. *A. tumefaciens* is clearly a natural pathogen. In my hands *A. rhizogenes* strains A4 and 8196 are not, and I doubt that they are in nature. Whether or not *A. rhizogenes* is pathogenic, the argument for its apparent innocuousness, relative to the clear pathogenicity of *A. tumefaciens*, can be extended to the effects of their respective T-DNAs in cells and whole plants. In the species described above the presence of Ri T-DNA in adventitious roots or whole plants is compatible with regeneration and sexuality. In contrast, the T-DNA of *A. tumefaciens* disrupts these normal plant functions, making plant tumor cells transformed by the Ti T-DNA difficult to manipulate. Regeneration is problematical and T-DNA in whole plants goes through meiosis only rarely or when parts of the Ti T-DNA are deleted. These essential differences between *A. rhizogenes* and *A. tumefaciens* could be of importance to the bioengineer.

Despite the pathogenicity of the natural transformation systems previously proposed for the introduction of foreign genes into plants, numerous authors have imagined the imminent creation of new crops capable of synthesizing interferon or fixing nitrogen, through the

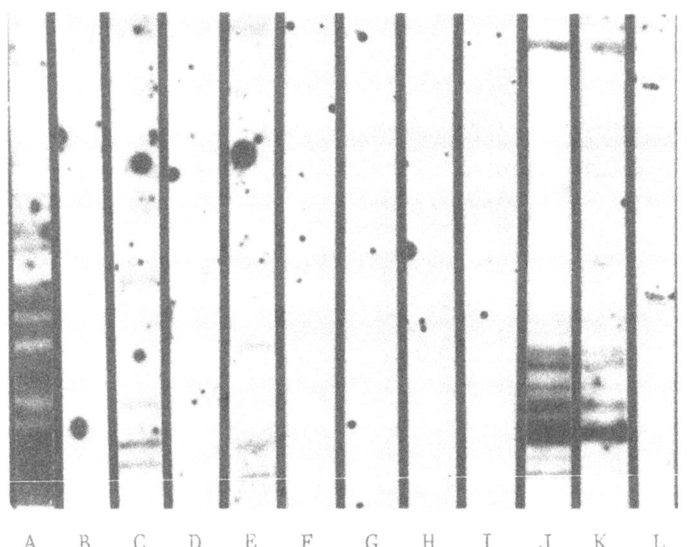

Fig. 10. T-DNA in the progeny of transformed carrot, tobacco and *C. arvensis*. Southern hybridization using A4 plasmid DNA as probe against A) DNA from a first sexual generation carrot plant with a normal phenotype, B) and C) DNA from plants with transformed phenotype, D) DNA from control, E), F) and G) DNA from first sexual generation tobacco plants with normal phenotype, H) with transformed phenotype, I) control, J) first sexual generation *C. arvensis* with transformed phenotype, K) control and L) A4 plasmid DNA.

parasexual introduction of the necessary gene(s) from another organism into an appropriate plant genome.

The assumptions inherent in many proposals to genetically "engineer" plants are, to name a few, 1) that foreign genes can be made to function at useful levels in plants, 2) that the products of these genes will be compatible with the normal physiology of the plant, 3) that transformed genotypes will be genetically stable, 4) that genes of agronomical interest, e.g. disease resistance, can be readily cloned, 5) that recombinant DNA technology and parasexual genetics are *a priori* a better way of modifying genotypes, 6) that parasexual genetic modification of plants is ecologically safe.

In the following discussion I suggest relatively modest uses of the *A. rhizogenes* system in applied and fundamental research, before addressing the possible advantages of *A. rhizogenes* over *A. tumefaciens* for the bioengineer. The applications are based on a biological interpretation of the transformation phenomenon I have described because I believe that understanding their overall biology is the key to using such systems in a constructive fashion.

The primary inoculation of *A. rhizogenes* into a wound on a root (carrot) or on a stem (*Convolvulus* and tobacco) results in the formation of roots that are morphologically, physiologically and genetically transformed. These roots synthesize agropine, a substance which nourishes the bacterium carrying the Ri plasmid (and some Ti plasmids). They grow rapidly, are highly branched, and are plagiotropic. All of these attributes are lacking in the normal root system. One can thus imagine that *A. rhizogenes* induces the formation of a secondary rhizosphere near the surface of the soil, composed of densely packed, horizontally radiating roots.

The possible advantage of this secondary root system might be better anckorage, ability to resist anoxia from flooding of the soil, increased drought resistance due to high root density, and greater chances of interactions with mycorhizal soil fungi, which establish exchange organs in the tissue produced by a growing root tip (Smith and Walker, 1981). In addition, in species where regeneration of plants occurs from roots, it would be advantageous to regenerate near the surface of the soil. One possible application of *A. rhizogenes* might be to inoculate certain plants, fruit trees for instance, in an attempt to establish such a secondary root system.

Another use of the root inducing properties of *A. rhizogenes* might be to stimulate root formation on cuttings. Many species are propagated vegetatively through cutting and rooting. In several cases, e.g. the root stock of some fruit trees, the rooting process is limiting. It remains to be shown that *A.rhizogenes* can accelerate this process without detracting from the agronomical interest of the plant.

Plants that regenerate from roots naturally, such as *C.arvensis* or those that can be induced to regenerate by tissue culture, such as tobacco and carrot, will tolerate the presence of Ri T-DNA in their cells and in the cases studied here, transmit this foreign DNA to their progeny. Thus novel genotypes can be created, which display the Ri T-DNA phenotype. This characters, waffled leaves, reduced apical dominance in roots and in shoots in the case of tobacco, plagiotropic roots, and increased leaf production and a switch from biennialism to annualism in carrot might be of use to the plant breeder. For instance increased leaf production could be advantagous in parsley, a close relative of carrot.

The synthesizing of agropine by certain clones of transformed roots, and the plants regenerated therefrom, may be of use in improving existing plant-microorganism symbioses, by the insertion of agropine catabolism genes from the Ri plasmid into *Rhizobium* by genetic means, and the agropine synthesis genes, carried by the Ri T-DNA, into a *Rhizobium* host in the manner described above.

The modification of plant genomes by transformation using a natural *A. tumefaciens* vector has been frequently proposed and attempted. To date foreign eukaryotic genes have been introduced into the Ti T-DNA, but their expression has not been achieved, at least to my knowledge, in plant cells, much less whole plants. The *A.rhizogenes* system might offer distinct advantages compared to that of *A. tumefaciens*. Briefly, 1) transformed roots are self-disinfecting. They outgrow contaminating bacteria. 2) Roots are semi, self-cloning, in that lateral roots probably originate from a small number of cells, if not a single cell. 3) Transformed roots are self-selecting due to their high growth rate compared to normal roots. 4) the transformed genome is maintained in differentiated (root) rather than undifferentiated (tumor) cells, which assures genetic stability. 5) Roots regenerate into plants and the Ri T-DNA does not impede this process. 6) Regenerated plants are vigorous. 7) The Ri T-DNA is readily transmitted sexually. 8) There exist morphological markers for the presence of T-DNA in the roots and leaves of transformed plants, which make them easily recognizable. After the initial parasexual process, the T-DNA can thus be traced through subsequent sexual manipulations, using the techniques of classical breeding, without constant dependence on complicated biochemistry. A geneticist could presumably screen, in the field, large quantities of plants for the presence of the Ri T-DNA vector, as well as other desirable traits, before the biochemist verifies the presence and expression of the foreign gene. These morphological markers should facilitate the integration of the expression of foreign genes into the endogenous physiology of the host plant.

Probably the most interesting application of the *rhizogenes* system is to the study of plant development. The Ri T-DNA is associated with the appearance of similar novel morphological and physiological characteristics in several different species, and thus must carry genes capable of functioning in different cellular environments, coding for, or controlling, the morphogenesis of particular structures, e.g. waffled leaves. By genetically modifying this T-DNA in the bacterium one might localize and study the gene(s) responsible for the Ri T-DNA associated phenotype. It is tempting to imagine that the metabolism of plant growth substances, e.g. cytokinins, is influenced by the Ri T-DNA, although such an oversimplification is certainly naive and premature. The possibility remains, however, that genes carried by the Ri T-DNA, governing morphological and physiological characters, can be studied, beginning with the DNA and ending with some understanding of how specific gene products influence phenotype.

A question raised by the results presented here is : to what extent do such non-pathogenic parasexual genetic systems operate in ecology and evolution ? Known natural transformation systems are pathogenic, e.g. viruses and *A. tumefaciens*. If the phenotype of the Ri T-DNA were of adaptive significance, it would be tempting to postulate a beneficial role for naturally occuring transformation in evolution. One would be led to question the origin of the Ri T-DNA, wondering if it encodes plant genes. The implication of such questioning is that micro-organisms might already serve in nature as intermediaries in parasexual genetic exchange among different species of higher plants.

ACKNOWLEDGEMENTS

I wish to acknowledge the assistance of my colleagues in the Laboratoire de Biologie Cellulaire, I.N.R.A. Versailles.

REFERENCES

Ackermann, C., 1977, Pflanzen aus *Agrobacterium rhizogenes*-Tumoren aus *Nicotiana tabacum*, Plant Sci. Lett., 8:23-30.

Bourgin, J.P., 1978, Valine-resistant plants from *in vitro* selected tobacco cells, Mol. Gen. Genet., 161:225-230.

Chilton, M., Tepfer, D., Petit, A., David, C., Casse-Delbart, F., and Tempé, J., 1982, *Agrobacterium rhizogenes* inserts T-DNA into the genomes of the host plant root cells. Nature, 295:432-434.

Hildebrand, E.M., 1934, Life history of the hairy-root organism in relation to its pathogenesis on nursery apple trees, Journal of Agricultural Research, 48:857-885.

Moore, L., Warren, G., and Strobel, G., 1979, Involvement of a plasmid in the hairy root disease of plants caused by *Agrobacterium rhizogenes*. Plasmid, 2:617-626.

Smith, S., and Walker, N., 1981, A quantitative study of mycorrhizal infection in *Trifolium* : separate determination of the rates of infection and mycellial growth. New Phytol., 89:225-240.

Tepfer, D., and Tempé, J., 1981, Production d'agropine par des racines formées sous l'action d'*Agrobacterium rhizogenes*, souche A4. C.R. Acad. Sc. Paris, 292:153-156.

White, F.F., and Nester, E.W., 1980, Hairy root : plasmid encodes virulence traits in *Agrobacterium rhizogenes*. J. Bacteriol., 141:1134-1141.

White, F., Ghidossi, G., Gordon, M., and Nester, E., 1982, Tumor induction by *Agrobacterium rhizogenes* involves the transfer of plasmid DNA to the plant genome. Proc. Natl. Acad. Sci. USA, 79:3193-3197.

Willmmitzer, L., Sanchez-Serrano, J., Buschfield, E., and Schell, J., 1982, DNA from *Agrobacterium rhizogenes* is transferred to and expressed in axenic hairy root plant tissues. Mol. Gen. Genet., 18:16-22.

VIROIDS AND GENETIC ENGINEERING

T. O. Diener*, R. A. Owens*, and D. E. Cress+

*Plant Virology Laboratory, Plant Protection Institute and +Cell Culture and Nitrogen Fixation Laboratory, Plant Physiology Institute, U.S. Department of Agriculture, Beltsville, Maryland 20705

INTRODUCTION

Viroids are low molecular weight RNAs that are present in certain species of higher plants afflicted with specific diseases. They are not detectable in healthy individuals of the same species, but, after introduction into such individuals, they are replicated autonomously and cause the appearance of the characteristic disease syndrome (Diener, 1979a). Unlike viral nucleic acids, viroids are not encapsidated.

Viroids constitute a novel class of subviral pathogens; they are the smallest known agents of infectious disease and represent minimal genetic and biological systems. To date, viroids are definitely known to exist only in higher plants; each consists of a unique covalently closed circular single-stranded (ss) RNA molecule. The five viroids whose nucleotide sequences have been determined contain 244-371 nucleotides. Although viroids have been discovered because they cause readily recognizable disease symptoms in certain hosts, viroids are often replicated in other hosts without causing obvious damage.

In recent years viroids have received increasing attention from molecular biologists with the result that our knowledge of their physical-chemical properties has increased dramatically (reviewed by Diener, 1979b and Gross and Riesner, 1980). Knowledge of viroid-host plant interactions has accumulated at a much slower rate. As the emphasis in viroid research begins to shift from physical-chemical studies of viroid structure to studies of mechanisms of viroid-host interaction, cloned viroid-complementary DNA (cDNA) will find many uses. Only three of the many potential applications of cloned potato spindle tuber viroid (PSTV) cDNA will be considered here -- (i) the development of a sensitive and reliable new method for detection of PSTV, (ii) identification of intermediates in viroid replication, and (iii) identification of regions of the viroid sequence involved in viroid-host interactions by directed *in vitro* mutagenesis of cloned viroid cDNA.

MOLECULAR CLONING OF PSTV cDNA

Determination of the 359 nucleotide sequence of PSTV established viroids as the first naturally occuring examples of covalently closed circular RNA (Gross et al., 1978). The molecular cloning and characterization of double-stranded (ds) PSTV cDNAs (Owens and Cress, 1980) has been facilitated by knowledge of the RNA sequence. In the latter work, ds PSTV cDNA was synthesized from a polyadenylated linear PSTV template and inserted in the *Pst*I endonuclease site of plasmid pBR322 using the oligo (dC)·oligo(dG) tailing procedure. Although one recombinant clone (pDC-29) contained a larger than expected 460 basepair (bp) insert, restriction endonuclease mapping and nucleotide sequence determinations demonstrated that all recombinants contained less than a complete copy of PSTV. Figure 1 shows the strategy used to construct clones containing full-length dsPSTV cDNA.

Restriction analysis of the PSTV-specific inserts from two of these clones, pDS-29 and pDC-22, suggested that these clones were partially overlapping and could be used to construct a full-length clone. The 285 bp *Ava*II-*Hae*III fragment from pDC-29 was ligated at the *Ava*II site to the contiguous 74 bp *Ava*II-*Hae*III fragment from pDC-22. *Hind*III oligodeoxynucleotide linkers were added to the *Hae*III blunt ends of this linear ligation product, and, following digestion with *Hind*III, this fragment was cloned in the *Hind*III site of pBR322. *Hind*III digestion of the resulting clones released the expected 365 bp PSTV-specific fragment.

Since use of this particular *Hind*III decanucleotide linker reconstructed the terminal *Hae*III sites of the PSTV insert, digestion of the recombinant DNA with *Hae*III relases a 359 bp fragment. This fragment is a full-length dsPSTV cDNA. Determination of the complete nucleotide sequence of this DNA by a combination of the Maxam-Gilbert chemical degradation and the M13 dideoxy chain termination methodologies has shown the cloned DNA sequence to be identical with that predicted by the RNA sequence published by Gross et al. (1978).

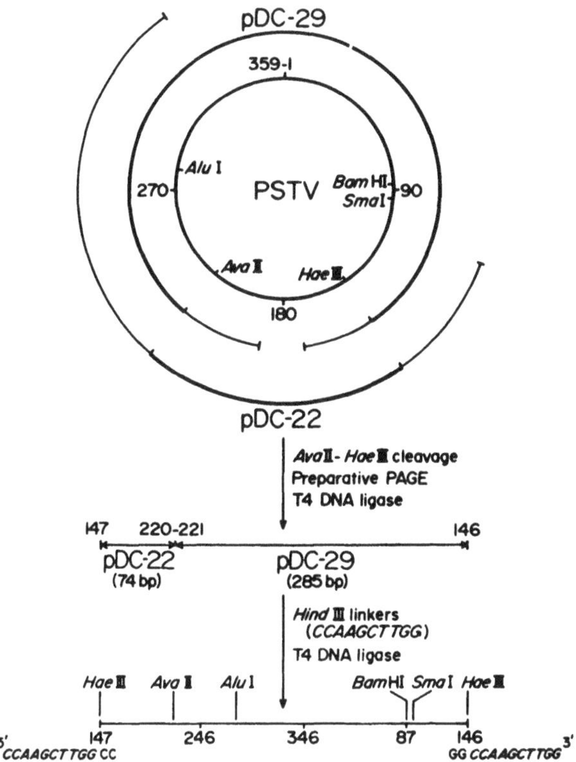

Fig. 1. Construction and molecular cloning of full-length dsPSTV cDNA.

SENSITIVE AND RAPID DIAGNOSIS OF PSTV

Practical Consequences of PSTV Infection

The potato spindle tuber disease poses a potentially serious threat in seed potato production, germ plasm collections, and potato breeding programs (reviewed by Diener, 1979a). PSTV is transmitted through vegetative propagation, foliar contact, and true seed and pollen.

A number of independently isolated PSTV strains have been described and can be classified as either severe or mild strains on the basis of the symptoms produced in Rutgers tomato. Tomato has been used as a diagnostic host for PSTV because symptoms in some potato cultivars are indistinct. Severe strains cause extreme shortening of the internodes, severe epinasty, shortening of petioles and midribs, and necrosis of stems, petioles and midribs in tomatoes. Symptoms of mild strains, on the other hand, are slow to develop and often so mild that they are easily overlooked (Fernow, 1967). The complete nucleotide sequences of a severe and a mild strain of PSTV differ in only 3 of the 359 nucleotides (Gross et al., 1981).

Depending on the potato cultivar, the strain of PSTV present, and environmental conditions, symptoms of PSTV infection in potato may vary considerably. Foliage symptoms are often obscure, and severity of the characteristic tuber symptoms --elongation with the appearance of prominent bud scales and growth cracks -- depend upon temperature and length of infection. While the disease causes neither total crop destruction nor storage losses, it can cause a serious reduction in total production. As long as control is effective in keeping the incidence of disease low, yield losses are of little consequence in temperate growing areas (1-2%). Inadequate control, however, can lead to catastrophic losses (~20% for mild strains or ~60% for severe strains) in a relatively short time (reviewed by Diener, 1979a).

In plants grown at high temperatures, however, PSTV may cause severe damage and total crop loss may ensue. Major efforts are underway to supplement the world's food supply by adapting the potato to growth in subtropical and tropical climates, and a lowland tropical potato cultivar has already been developed (Sawyer, 1978). Under these environmental conditions, PSTV poses a potentially serious threat and the importance of a sensitive, rapid, and reliable method for PSTV diagnosis is readily apparent.

Conventional Diagnostic Tests

Because PSTV lacks the antigenic protein coat characteristic of viruses, an assay based on the sensitive and widely used ELISA (enzyme-linked immunosorbent assay) technique has not been reported. Bioassay on suitable tomato cultivars (Raymer and O'Brien, 1962) and polyacrylamide gel electrophoresis (PAGE) of extracted nucleic acids (for example, Morris and Wright, 1975) have been used to detect PSTV. Although Fernow et al. (1969) have demonstrated that a double-inoculation technique can be used to detect and eliminate both mild and severe strains of PSTV from potato seed stocks before planting, bioassays on tomato are slow and often unreliable. Methods based on PAGE, on the other hand, are laborious and expensive. Neither method is suitable for the rapid screening of thousands of seed potato tubers. A third method, hybridization of highly radioactive PSTV cDNA with PSTV bound to a membrane filter and autoradiographic detection of the resulting DNA-RNA hybrids, is sensitive, rapid, and reliable (Owens and Diener, 1981). Automation of the testing procedure appears feasible.

PSTV diagnosis by nucleic acid hybridization

To simplify sample preparation when large numbers of samples must be processed, clarified plant sap rather than purified nucleic acid serves as the source of PSTV. A relatively high ionic strength and diethyldithiocarbamate concentration of the extraction buffer serve to release PSTV from nuclei and inhibit enzymatic polyphenol oxidation. After any PSTV present in the sap samples is bound to nitrocellulose membranes, the immobilized PSTV is hybridized with ^{32}P-labeled recombinant DNA; and the resulting ^{32}P-labeled PSTV cDNA-PSTV hybrids are detected by autoradiography.

Even though the presence of sap constitutents (presumably proteins) reduces the binding of PSTV to the membrane approximately tenfold as compared to purified nucleic acid samples, 100 pg of PSTV can still be detected when the specific activity of the ^{32}P PSTV cDNA probe is 2×10^8 cpm/mg (Owens and Diener, 1981). The entire procedure requires four days for completion and is approximately tenfold more sensitive than PAGE. A significant improvement over the tomato bioassay method (Fernow et al., 1969) is the ability to detect both mild and severe strains directly.

The feasibility and reliability of this method for the rapid and sensitive detection of PSTV by nucleic acid hybridization was demonstrated with tubers harvested from commercially important U.S. potato varieties that had been intentionally infected with PSTV (Owens and Diener, 1981). Recently, we have extended our initial studies in collaboration with Dr. L. F. Salazar of the International Potato Center (CIP), Lima, Peru.

Tubers from 24 clones currently under investigation at CIP were selected essentially at random for testing at Beltsville. Most of the selections had been tested by PAGE at CIP, but the results of these analyses were not revealed to us until our tests had been completed. As expected, clones that had tested "PSTV +" by PAGE also tested "PSTV +" by nucleic acid hybridization. Surprisingly, however, of 9 clones that had tested "PSTV -" by PAGE, 8 tested "PSTV +" by nucleic acid hybridization.

Three different analyses were then performed to reevaluate these initial results: bioassay on tomato, PAGE of low molecular weight RNA extracted from foliage of the inoculated tomatoes, and in some cases, a second hybridization analysis of the potato clones. Except for one clone which had given an ambiguous result in the first hybridization analysis, our initial results were confirmed. Clearly, the nucleic acid spot hybridization test not only is more rapid and convenient than previously used procedures, but also is more sensitive and permits detection of the viroid in plants that harbor it at a concentration too low to be detectable by PAGE.

These results illustrate the potential usefulness of cloned PSTV cDNA for viroid detection; they represent one of the first practical applications of genetic engineering in agriculture.

INTERMEDIATES IN VIROID REPLICATION

Cloned viroid-specific recombinant DNA (pDC-29) has been used also to study the mechanism of viroid replication. Labeled hybridization probes specific for RNA molecules having the same polarity as PSTV or the opposite polarity were prepared by labeling the 5' termini of Bam HI-cleaved pDC-29 with ^{32}P and cleaving the labeled DNA with PstI. Purification of the resulting products yielded a 110-base pair fragment that specifically hybridizes with cPSTV (Owens and Cress, 1980).

Hybridization experiments with this probe demonstrated the presence in extracts from infected cells of RNA molecules of the same mobility (and presumably molecular weight) as linear PSTV but of opposite polarity. PSTV-complementary RNA molecules of this size were found after treatment of the nucleic acid extracts with RNase, denaturation of the RNAs by heating for 2 min at 100°C in 50% formamide, quenching, and analysis by gel electrophoresis at 55° in the presence of 8M urea. Complementary PSTV (cPSTV) was found almost exclusively in the LiCl-supernatant (low molecular weight and double-stranded) fraction. The results also demonstrated that most, if not all, of cPSTV was present in nucleic acid extracts in the form of RNase-resistant duplex molecules, that is, base-paired with PSTV. This is indicated by the observation that the yield of cPSTV was not significantly reduced if the RNA·RNA annealing prior to RNase treatment was omitted (Owens and Cress, 1980).

Recent evidence by several investigators indicates that viroid-infected cells contain, in addition to full-length viroid complements, viroid-specific molecules longer than unit length (Branch et al., 1981; Hadidi and Hashimoto, 1981; Rohde and Sänger, 1981).

In our investigations, hybridization probes specific for either PSTV or cPSTV were prepared as described above, except that in these newer studies, the cloned insert consisted (as shown by direct DNA sequencing) of ds DNA representing the complete 359 nucleotide sequence of PSTV (Cress and Owens, 1981).

RNAs from PSTV-infected plants were separated by PAGE, transferred, and hybridized with the specific molecular probes. In agreement with the results of other investigators, blot hybridization experiments using these recombinant DNA probes revealed the presence in RNA extracts from infected tissue of viroid-related mostly ds RNA species that migrate in gels more slowly than unit-length PSTV (Owens

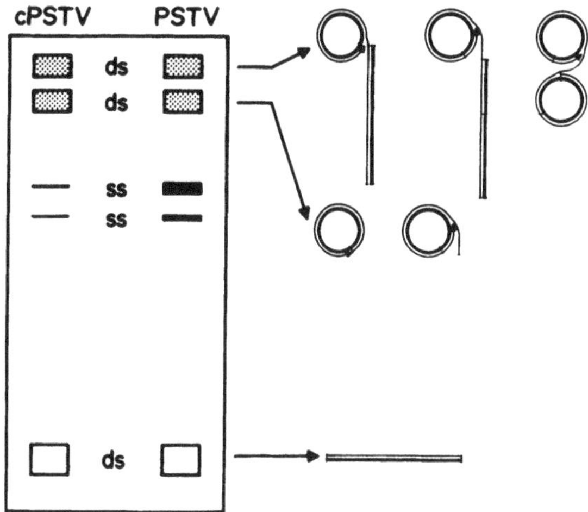

Fig. 2. Major viroid-related RNA species identified (left) and tentative structures for dsPSTV RNA (right). For explanation, see text. From Owens and Diener (1982).

and Diener, 1982). The two most prominent ones of these slowly migrating RNAs were separated from one another by cellulose chromatography and preparative gel electrophoresis and the composition, size, and configuration of the PSTV and cPSTV components of each were analyzed in a gel system that does not denature ds RNA, but prevents major reannealing of previously denatured RNAs. This gel system has the further advantage of separating circular from linear PSTV molecules (Owens and Cress, 1980). Untreated and RNase-treated separated ds components were analyzed in this system with or without prior denaturation (Owens and Diener, 1982).

The results of these analyses demonstrated that the two major, slowly migrating, viroid-specific ds RNAs are structurally related and that they are composed of unit-length circular and linear strands with the polarity of PSTV complexed with longer-than-unit-length RNA strands of opposite polarity. In Figure 2, a schematic summary of the results, as well as our interpretation of the molecular structures of the identified components is shown. At least five discrete zones of viroid-related RNAs are resolved (Fig. 2, left). Two zones contain ss RNAs, the circular and linear forms of PSTV and cPSTV. Only traces of the latter, however, could be detected. At least three zones contain ds RNA, as shown by RNase treatment. The most rapidly migrating ds RNA species, a linear duplex containing unit-length linear PSTV and linear cPSTV, was only detected if the RNA had been treated with RNase before analysis. It was not, therefore, considered a potential PSTV replication intermediate. The two more slowly migrating ds PSTV RNAs, however, were shown to possess several of the characteristics expected for such intermediates. The more rapidly migrating one of these two ds RNAs was shown to contain unit-length linear or circular PSTV, but complementary strands somewhat longer than unit-length. The more slowly migrating ds RNA was shown to also contain unit-length linear and circular PSTV and longer-than-unit-length cPSTV. In this component, however, the lengths of cPSTV ranged from unit length to at least twice that length. The formation of these structures can most readily be explained if one assumes that cPSTV is synthesized on a circular PSTV template and that this synthesis continues past the origin of replication, leading to the synthesis of linear dimers and higher multimers of cPSTV. Such a scheme resembles, in some respects, the "rolling circle" model previously advanced to explain replication of certain viral RNAs (Brown and Martin, 1965). Results further suggest that unit-length linear PSTV synthesized from the cPSTV template may be circularized while still complexed to the template.

In this view the more slowly migrating ds RNA zones would contain dimers and higher multimers of cPSTV, whereas the more rapidly migrating ds RNA zone would contain circular ds molecules of unit length with ss cPSTV tails of varying lengths (Fig. 2, right). That these structures probably are fragments of a larger PSTV replicative intermediate complex is indicated by the observation that synchronous synthesis of PSTV is accompanied by simultaneous synthesis of ds PSTV (Owens and Diener, 1982).

MECHANISMS OF VIROID-HOST INTERACTION

As mentioned earlier, viroids were the first naturally occuring examples of covalently closed circular RNA to be described (Gross et al., 1978). The origin of viroids is unknown, but with the discovery of split genes and RNA splicing in eukaryotic organisms it has been suggested that viroids may have originated by circularization of excised intervening sequences (Diener, 1979b; Crick, 1979). If such introns contained the appropriate recognition sequences, they might be transcribed (replicated) by a host enzyme able to function as an RNA-directed RNA polymerase and thus escape host cell control mechanisms. Such a hypothetical model for the origin of viroids has several interesting implications for the mechanisms of viroid-host interaction, because disease induction is most readily understood by postulating interference by the viroid with gene regulation (Diener, 1979b).

Comparisons of the nucleotide sequences of PSTV and cPSTV with the consensus sequence of eukaryotic intron-exon boundaries and the 5'-sequence of U1 RNA have been independently performed by three separate groups (Diener, 1981; Dickson, 1981; Gross et al., 1982). Both Diener (1981) and Gross et al. (1982) have noted the striking complementarity between the 5'-terminus of U1 RNA and nucleotides

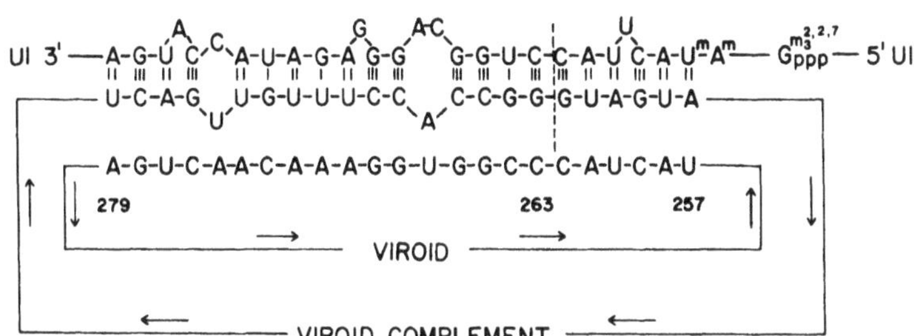

Fig. 3. Possible base-pairing interactions between the PSTV complement and the 5' end of U1 RNA. ---, Hypothetical splice junction. From Diener (1981).

257-279 of cPSTV (Fig. 3). Comparison of the corresponding regions from two other viroids, chrysanthemum stunt and citrus exocortis, have shown that this region is highly conserved (Gross et al., 1982). Dickson (1981) has proposed a different model for the involvement of viroids in RNA splicing -- one involving complementarity between plant intron sequences and 2 separate regions of PSTV itself, nucleotides 113-118 and 307-311. The minor sequence differences between a mild and a severe strain of PSTV fall within these regions (Gross et al., 1981), and a comparison of the sequences of PSTV and chrysanthemum stunt viroid showed that the degree of complementarity to plant splice junctions could be correlated with severity of disease induced in chrysanthemum. Although these hypotheses are intriguing and susceptible to experimental verification, as described below, the mechanism(s) of viroid pathogenesis must be more complex because neither avocado sunblotch viroid nor its complement contain these sequences (Symons, 1981).

Genetic analysis of viroid-host interaction depends on the isolation and characterization (sequencing) of mutants with defined phenotypic differences. Until now such analyses have depended upon sequence comparisons of known viroids or viroid strains. Lack of reliable local lesion hosts has hampered efforts to select desired viroid mutants following random mutagenesis. The development of methods for specific cleavage and enzymatic manipulation of DNA, cloning of DNA fragments, nucleotide sequence analysis, and rapid chemical synthesis of oligonucleotides of defined sequence allows mutations to be constructed at predetermined sites in a cloned DNA molecule (reviewed by Shortle et al., 1981). Racaniello and Baltimore (1981) have shown that transfection of cultured mammalian cells with pBR322 recombinant plasmids containing a complete cloned cDNA copy of the RNA genome of poliovirus leads to the synthesis of infectious poliovirions. If the same would be true for cloned PSTV cDNA, genetic analysis of viroid-host interaction would be greatly facilitated.

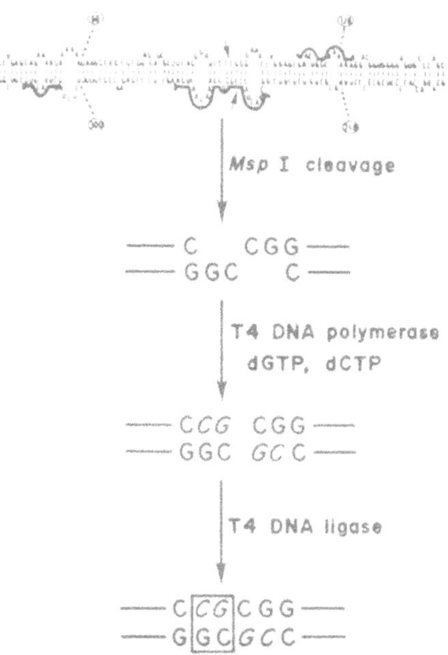

Fig. 4. Identification of viroid-host interactions by directed mutagenesis of cloned ds PSTV cDNA. Regions of the PSTV or complementary RNA sequence whose involvement in viroid-host interaction has been postulated are underlined. The sites of cleavage of the ds PSTV cDNA by MspI endonuclease are indicated by arrows. Sequential treatment of recombinant DNAs containing ds PSTV cDNA with MspI, T4 DNA polymerase, and T4 DNA ligase would allow isolation of derivatives containing a 361 bp ds PSTV cDNA. Half of these derivatives would contain a 2 bp insertion in the region (nucleotides 257-279) exhibiting a striking complementarity with the 5'-terminus of U1 RNA.

Figure 4 shows a specific example of the potential power of the directed mutagenesis technique as applied to viroids. The underlined regions of the sequence of the severe PSTV strain are those whose possible involvement in viroid-host interaction was discussed above. Cloned PSTV cDNA contains 2 recognition-cleavage sites for the restriction endonuclease MspI, and one of these sites falls within the region (nucleotides 257-279) identified by two groups (Diener, 1981; Gross et al., 1982) as possibly involved in PSTV pathogenesis. If the infectivity of cloned PSTV DNA can be demonstrated, it would be comparatively simple to introduce defined nucleotide insertions (shown in Figure 4) or deletions into this region and determine the biological effect of these changes. Introduction of defined mutations in this and other regions of the PSTV sequence will complement current attempts to correlate viroid structure and function by RNA sequence comparison.

CONCLUSIONS

Although cloned viroid cDNAs have only been availabe for approximately two years, they have already been applied to problems in both practical and basic agricultural research. Hybridization between highly radioactive recombinant PSTV cDNA and PSTV that has been attached to a solid support provides a sensitive and reliable method for the detection of PSTV (Owens and Diener, 1981). This technique will facilitate elimination of PSTV from potato varieties that are currently being developed for growth in tropical and subtropical climates. Using the appropriate homologous viroid cDNA clones, the same procedure could be used to detect other economically important viroids.

Cloned partial-length viroid cDNAs have also been important tools in basic studies of viroid replication and structure. Thus, Owens and Cress (1980) used strand-specific hybridization probes to demonstrate that PSTV-infected tomato tissue contains full-length RNA molecules complementary to PSTV, and Symons (1981) has used viroid cDNA fragments as primers for cDNA synthesis during the determination of the complete 247-nucleotide sequence of avocado sunblotch viroid. Full-length cloned viroid cDNAs have been used to demonstrate the presence in infected tissue of longer-than-unit-length viroid-complementary RNAs and to show that these structures probably are intermediates in the process of viroid replication (Owens and Diener, 1982).

We may anticipate even more results in the future, if the infectivity of newly available full-length PSTV cDNA clones can be demonstrated. Directed mutagenesis of infectious cloned PSTV cDNA will greatly facilitate genetic analysis of viroid-host interactions. Finally, the potential use of viroids as vectors in plant recombinant DNA technology should not be overlooked (Howell, 1982).

REFERENCES

Branch, A. D., Robertson, H. D., and Dickson, E., 1981, Longer-than-unit-length viroid minus strands are present in RNA from infected plants, _Proc. Natl. Acad. Sci. USA_, 78:6381.

Brown, F., and Martin, S. J., 1965, A new model for virus ribonucleic acid replication, _Nature (London)_, 208:861.

Cress, D. E., and Owens, R. A., 1981, Construction of a full-length double-stranded cDNA clone of potato spindle tuber viroid, Recombinant DNA, 1:90.

Crick, F., 1979, Split genes and RNA splicing. Science, 204:264.

Dickson, E., 1981, A model for the involvement of viroids in RNA splicing, Virology, 115:216.

Diener, T. O., 1979a, "Viroids and Viroid Diseases," John Wiley & Sons, New York.

Diener, T. O., 1979b, Viroids: structure and function, Science, 205:859.

Diener, T. O., 1981, Are viroids escaped introns?, Proc. Natl. Acad. Sci. USA, 78:5014.

Fernow, K. H., 1967, Tomato as a test plant for detecting mild strain of potato spindle tuber virus, Phytopathology, 57:1347.

Fernow, K. H., Peterson, L. C., and Plaisted, R. L., 1969, The tomato test for eliminating spindle tuber from potato planting stock, Am. Potato J., 46:424.

Gross, H. J., and Riesner, D., 1980, Viroids: a class of subviral pathogens, Angewandte Chemie, 19:231.

Gross, H. J., Domday, H., Lossow, C., Jank, P., Raba, M., Alberty, H. and Sänger, H. L., 1978, Nucleotide sequence and secondary structure of potato spindle tuber viroid, Nature (London), 278:203.

Gross, H. J, Liebl, U., Alberty, H., Krupp, G., Domdey, H., Ramm, K., and Sänger, H. L., 1981, A severe and a mild potato spindle tuber viroid isolate differ in three nucleotide exchanges only Biosc. Reports, 1:235.

Gross, H. J., Krupp, G., Domdey, H., Raba, M., Jank, P., Lossow, C., Alberty, H., Ramm, K., and Sänger, H. L., 1982, Nucleotide sequence and secondary structure of citrus exocortis and chrysanthemum stunt viroid, Eur. J. Biochem., 121:249.

Hadidi, A., and Hashimoto, J., 1981, Viroid-specific ribonucleic acid in cells infected with potato spindle tuber viroid: detection and characterization, Phytopathology, 71:222.

Howell, S. H., 1982, Plant molecular vehicles: potential vectors for introducing foreign DNA into plants, Ann. Rev. Plant Physiol., 33:609.

Morris, T. J., and Wright, N. S., 1975, Detection on polyacrylamide gel of a diagnostic nucleic acid from tissue infected with potato spindle tuber viroid, Am. Potato J., 52:57.

Owens, R. A., and Cress, D. E., 1980, Molecular cloning and characterization of potato spindle tuber viroid cDNA sequences, Proc. Natl. Acad. Sci. USA, 77:5302.

Owens, R. A., and Diener, T. O., 1981, Sensitive and rapid diagnosis of potato spindle tuber viroid disease by nucleic acid hybridization, Science, 213:670.

Owens, R. A., and Diener, T. O., 1982, RNA intermediates in potato spindle tuber viroid replication, Proc. Natl. Acad. Sci. USA, 79:113.

Racaniello, V. R., and Baltimore, D., 1981, Cloned poliovirus complementary DNA is infectious in mammalian cells, Science, 214:916.

Raymer, W. B., and O'Brien, M. J., 1962, Transmission of potato spindle tuber virus to tomato, Am. Potato J. 39:401.

Rohde, W., and Sänger, H. L., 1981, Detection of complementary RNA intermediates of viroid replication by Northern blot hybridization, Biosc. Reports, 1:327.

Sawyer, R. L., 1979, Annual Report, 1978, International Potato Center, Lima, Peru, p. iii.

Shortle, D., DiMaio, D., and Nathans, D., 1981, Directed mutagenesis, Ann. Rev. Genet., 15:265.

Symons, R. H., 1981, Avocado sunblotch viroid: primary sequence and proposed secondary structure, Nucl. Acids Res., 9:6527.

LIPOSOMES AS A TOOL FOR INTRODUCING BIOLOGICALLY ACTIVE VIRAL NUCLEIC ACIDS INTO PLANT PROTOPLASTS

Franco Rollo

Istituto di Microbiologia e Fisiologia Vegetale

Universita di Pavia, 27100 Pavia, Italy

Lipid vesicles (liposomes) have successfully been used to introduce a variety of biological macromolecules into mammalian cells. In particular large unilamellar vesicles prepared with the Ca^{++}-EDTA chelation technique (LUV) have been used for delivering infective poliovirus particles(1) and RNA(2) into permissive (HeLa) and non permissive (CHO,L) cells. More recently Fraley et al.(3) have reported the encapsulation of simian virus 40(SV40) DNA in large unilamellar vesicles prepared with the reverse-phase evaporation technique (4) and its delivery in an infectious form to monkey cells in culture.

In the last years the possibility of applying the technology of the recombinant DNA to the plant world has attracted the interest of an increasing number of workers and liposomes have been proposed as a means to protect DNA from degradation during incubation with plant protoplasts and to increase its efficiency of internalization. Several authors, Lurquin (5,6), Rollo et al. (7,8), Mathews and Cress (9), Lurquin and Sheehy (10), have shown that DNA-loaded liposomes are able to strongly interact with plant protoplasts under certain conditions. However, since convenient DNA-mediated transformation systems have not yet been established, these studies could not show whether the encapsulated nucleic acids are delivered into the cell in a manner in which they can function biologically. For this reason some researchers have been induced to use liposome-encapsulated plant virus or viral RNA as a model system for DNA transfer in an attempt to obtain conclusive evidences regarding the potential of liposome technology in plants. While only a few reports have so far appeared on this topic it is the opinion of the writer that they characterize with reasonable detail the liposome-mediated transfer technique in protoplasts as they have been obtained by using different virus, liposome and protoplast types.

Fukunaga et al. (11) have first used large unilamellar vesicles composed of phosphatidylserine (PS) and prepared by the Ca++-EDTA chelation method (12) for encapsulating tobacco mosaic virus (TMV) RNA and delivering it to plant protoplasts obtained from Vinca rosea suspension cultures. Infection of protoplasts was monitored by the immuno fluorescence technique (13). By this assay it was determined that infection at significant level does not result from the simple incubation of TMV RNA-loaded LUV with the protoplasts and no infection either was obtained after preincubation of the vesicles with either poly-L-ornithine or poly-L-lysine. On the other hand the addition of Polyethylene glycol (PEG) or polyvinyl alcohol (PVA) at relatively low concentration (10%) was shown to promote infection of up to 80% of the protoplasts.

Both the temperature during the inoculation and the duration of the incubation were shown to significantly influence the infection. Postinoculation washing with high pH-high Ca++ buffer was also shown to substantially enhance the percentage of infected protoplasts. On the other hand the infectivity of free TMV RNA was considerably lower than that of an equivalent amount of encapsulated RNA. In a similar study performed by the same group (Nagata et al.) (14) TMV RNA was entrapped into phosphatidylserine/cholesterol (PS/CHO) unilamellar vesicles prepared with the reverse-phase evaporation technique (REV) and delivered to tobacco protoplasts obtained from tobacco suspension cultures. Infectivity of encapsulated RNA was shown to be strictly dependent on the length of the sonication step during the preparation of REV liposomes. Under the same experimental conditions used in the previous work (Fukunaga et al. 11) TMV RNA-loaded REV were shown to mediate infection of tobacco protoplasts.

The above reported results have essentially been confirmed by Fraley et al. (15) and Fraley and Papahadjopoulos (16). Instead of immunofluorescence these authors used radio immuno assay (RIA) or enzyme-linked immuno assay (ELISA) to monitor the infection. In this case too, PVA and PEG were shown to be essential for the liposome-mediated infection. No significant infection could be observed after treatment with glycerol, dimethyl sulfoxide or ethylene glycol. Highest level of infection was observed when REV liposomes composed of PS/CHO were used while no infection was observed with REV liposomes composed of phosphatidylcholine and stearylamine (PC/SA). Interestingly similar results were obatined by the same authors by using RNA from cowpea mosaic virus (CPMV) and cowpea protoplasts.

As a model system for the liposome-mediated transfer of cauliflower mosaic virus (CaMV) DNA into plant protoplasts Rollo and Hull

(17) used turnip rosette virus (TRosV) particle and RNA and turnip protoplasts from leaf mesophyll. Initial experiments were performed with whole TRosV encapsulated in multilamellar liposomes (MLV) composed of phosphatidylcholine and β-sitosterol (PC/SS) or PC/SA. It was shown that PC/SS MLV-mediated infection takes place only in the presence of PEG and $CaCl_2$. A very low level of infection (0.4% of the protoplasts) was obtained by simply incubating TRosV-loaded PC/SA MLV with turnip protoplasts. Also in this case the infection was enhanced by PEG treatment. However no infection could be detected after incubation of turnip protoplasts with TRosV-RNA-loaded PC/SS MLV and PEG-$CaCl_2$ treatment. A possible cause of this failure can be the very low capture of MLV liposome. Another one can be the mechanism by which these vesicles interact with the protoplasts. In fact it has been very recently evidenced (Lurquin and Rollo, 18) that MLV-mediated transfer of radioactive DNA into carrot protoplasts seems not to be accompanied by the internalization of the liposomes. This fact suggests that a phenomenon of leakage of the liposome-content followed by its uptake by the protoplasts may occur. According to this model RNA in intact virions would maintain its biological activity during the transfer from the liposomes to the protoplasts while naked RNA would be inactivated by nucleuses. Additional experiments were performed by Rollo and Hull (17) using TRosV RNA encapsulated in REV liposomes composed of phosphatidylcholine, dicetyl phosphate and β-sitosterol (PC/DCP/SS). The sonication step during the preparation of the REV liposomes was avoided by modifying the solvent composition. Instead of diethyl ether alone a 1:1:1 mixture of chloroform, diethyl ether and methanol was used. In this way a one-phase system was obtained which does not need sonication. The encapsulated RNA incubated with turnip protoplasts in the presence of PEG and $CaCl_2$ turned out to be considerably (10^3 times) more infectious than the free RNA.

Very recently (Christen and Lurquin, personal communication) cowpea protoplasts from leaf mesophyll have been infected with cowpea chlorotic mottle virus (CCMV) RNA encapsulated in large unilamellar vesicles composed of PS/CHO and produced by the reverse-phase evaporation technique. Infection of the protoplasts (up to 50%) took place after PEG treatment followed by high pH-high Ca^{++} buffer washing. Under the same experimental conditions PC/SA MLV as well as PS/CHO large unilamellar liposomes generated by the freezing and thawing procedure (19) were shown not to produce infection in cowpea protoplasts.

A possible explanation for the failure of MLV liposomes has been given above. In the case of large unilamellar vesicles produced by freezing and thawing the failure seems to be attributable to their very low trapping capacity.

Conclusions and perspectives

The above reported data shed some optimism on the potential of the liposome technology in plant virus-plant protoplast systems as it appears that liposomes can indeed transfer biologically active RNA into plant protoplast with high efficiency. Unilamellar vesicles prepared with the reverse-phase evaporation technique (REV) emerge as the most suitable liposomes for efficient encapsulation and delivery of RNA. The drawback represented by the sonication step during the preparation of this type of liposome has been successfully resolved in two different ways i.e. short sonication time (Fraley et al. 3), (Nagata et al. 14) and one-phase system (Rollo and Hull 17). Also emerging from the papers reviewed here, is the strict necessity of fusogenic agents (PEG, PVA, Ca^{++}) shown by the different liposome-protoplast systems.

Concerning the mechanism of REV liposome-mediated transfer of viral RNA, the requirement for the above cited factors seems to suggest a mechanism of fusion of the liposome membrane with the protoplast plasmalemma. The lack of infectivity shown by viral particles and RNA (either free or encapsulated in liposomes) when they are simply incubated with the protoplasts without further additions indicate that plant protoplasts are not endowed with spontaneous endocytosis. However, a fusogen-mediated endocytosis cannot be excluded.

Owing to the encouraging results obtained with RNA viruses, it seems obvious to indicate cauliflower mosaic virus (CaMV) DNA (20,21) as the next candidate for experiments on liposome-mediated transfection of protoplasts. As reported above, a model system (TRosV RNA and turnip protoplasts) has been studied by Rollo and Hull (17). It has been shown by the same authors that CaMV DNA can be encapsulated without damage in REV liposomes composed of PC/DCP/SS. Another attractive candidate may be DNA from Geminivirus The fact that Geminivirus DNA seems to be bipartite (22) should not constitute an obstacle to its eventual use in liposome-mediated transfection experiments as it has been shown that liposomes can work efficiently with bipartite (CPMV) and even multipartite (CCMV) RNA genomes.

As a concluding remark it seems of interest to make a short comparison between liposome-mediated internalization and microinjection with glass needles. The latter technique has extensively been used to deliver foreign DNA into cultured mammalian cells (23).

This technique is still waiting for a systematic evaluation in plant cell systems. Halliwell and Gazaway (24) were able to infect cultured tobacco cells by microinjecting TMV particles into them. Of great interest in this work is the exceptionally low multiplicity needed for infecting 100% of the microinjected cells i.e. 620 viral particles. However, it must be stressed that a limiting factor in the use of microinjection is represented by the very small

Author/s	Virus	RNA size (MD)	Liposome composition	incubation conditions	protoplast type/source	% of infected protoplasts/ multiplicity
Fukunaga et al.	TMV	2.I	PS LUV	PEG,PVA/ high pH-ca^{++}	Vinca rosea /SC	$80/2x10^{6}$
Nagata et al.	TMV	-	PS/CHO (I/I) REV	PEG,PVA/ high pH-Ca^{++}	tobacco/SC	$59/2x10^{5}-4x10^{5}$*
Fraley et al.	TMVV	-	PS/CHO(I/I),PC, PC/SA(9/I),PS REV	PVA	tobacco/SC	$20/5x10^{5}$*
Fraley and Papahadjo-poulos	CPMV	2.4,I.4	-	PVA	cowpea/n.r.	n.r.
Rollo and Hull	TRosV	I.4	PC/DCP/SS(10/2 /10) REV	PEG-Ca^{++}	turnip/LR	$12/1.5x10^{5}$
Christen and Lurquin	CCMV	I.I,I.0,0.8	PS/CHO (I/I)	PEG/high	cowpea/LM	$50/1x10^{4}$*

SC, suspension culture; LM, leaf mesophyll; n.r. not reported; *data calculated from the quoted reports. All other abbreviations as in text.

number of cells (a few tenths) that can be treated in one experiment. On the other hand, according to the data reported in this review, several millions of protoplasts can be synchronously infected in a single experiment of liposome-mediated transfection.

Acknowledgement. The author wishes to thank Dr. P. F. Lurquin for helpful criticism and comments.

References

1. T. Wilson, D. Papahadjopoulos, and R. Taber, Proc. Natl. Acad. Sci., 74:3471-3475 (1977).

2. T. Wilson, D. Papahadjopoulos, and R. Taber, Cell, 17:77-84 (1979).

3. R. Fraley, S. Subramani, P. Berg, D. Papahadjopoulos, J. Biol. Chem., 255:10431-10435 (1980).

4. F. Szoka and D. Papahadjopoulos, Proc. Natl. Acad. Sci., 75:4194-4198 (1978).

5. P. F. Lurquin, Nucleic Acids Res., 6:3773-3784 (1979).

6. P. F. Lurquin, Plant Sci. Lett., 21:31-40 (1981).

7. F. Rollo, F. Sala, and R. Cella, and B. Parisi, Plant Cell Cultures: Results and Perspectives, pp. 237-246, Sala et al eds, Elsevier/North Holland Biomedical Press (1980).

8. F. Rollo, M.G. Galli, and B. Parasi, Plant Sci. Lett., 20:347-354 (1981).

9. B. F. Matthews and D. E. Cress, Planta, 153:90-94 (1981).

10. P. F. Lurquin and R. E. Sheehy, Plant Sci. Lett., 25:133-147 (1982).

11. Y. Fukunaga, T. Nagata, and I. Takebe, Virology, 113:752-760 (1981).

12. D. Papahadjopoulos, W. Vail, K. Jacobson, and G. Poste, Biochim Biophys Acta, 394:483-491 (1975).

13. Y. Otsuki and I. Takebe, Virology, 38:497-499 (1969).

14. T. Nagata, K. Okada, I. Takebe, and C. Matsui, Mol. Gen. Genet. 184:161-165 (1981).

15. R. Fraley, S. L. Dellaporta, and D. Papahadjopoulos, Proc. Natl. Acad. Sci., 79:1859-1863 (1982).

16. R. Fraley, D. Papahadjopoulos, Current Topics in Microbiology and Immunology, 96:171-191 P.H. Hofschneider and W. Goebel, eds. (1981).

17. F. Rollo and R. Hull, J. Gen. Virol., 60:359-363 (1982).

18. P. F. Lurquin and F. Rollo, Biology of the Cell (in press).

19. U. Pick, Arch. Biochem. Biophys., 212:186-363 (1981).

20. R. Hull, TIBS, 3:254-256 (1978).

21. T. Hon, K. Richards, G. Lebeurier, Current Topics in Microbiology and Immunology, 96:193-236, P. H. Hofschneider and W. Goebel, eds. (1981).

22. S. Haber, M. Ikegami, N. B. Bajet, and R. M. Goodman, Nature 289:324-326 (1981).

23. M. Capecchi, Cell, 22:479-488 (1980).

24. R. S. Halliwell and W. S. Gazaway, Virology, 65:583-587 (1975).

PLANT GENETIC MANIPULATIONS: APPLICATIONS FROM PLANT SOMATIC CELL GENETICS

E. C. Cocking

Plant Genetic Manipulation Group
Department of Botany
University of Nottingham
University Park
Nottingham NG7 2RD
UK

INTRODUCTION

Currently there is much interest in the extent to which studies in plant somatic cell genetics will contribute to plant genetic manipulations and thereby to crop improvement in general. Aspects of plant genetic manipulations have recently been reviewed[1], and the special role of protoplasts in this respect have been highlighted[2]. In this survey some of these aspects will be further discussed in the light of more recent work mainly from our Genetic Manipulation Group here at Nottingham, but other work will be discussed where relevant.

SOMATIC HYBRIDISATION BY PROTOPLAST FUSION

In higher plants, just as in the fungi, the first essential step in any parasexual cycle will be heterokaryosis as a result of fusion of somatic protoplasts. If this is followed by the fusion of nuclei and the development of hybrid cells after mitosis, then this somatic hybridization component of the parasexual cycle will be complete. Moreover, if diploidization associated with the fusion process results in the formation of amphiploid hybrid plants, then protoplast fusions will be providing an alternative to gametic fusions for plant hybridization[3].

The ready availability of enzymatically isolated protoplasts opened up the possibility of inducing such protoplasts to fuse and to produce heterokaryons[4], and during the past decade there has been extensive work with the objective of producing somatic hybrid plants from these heterokaryons. From the earliest of these experiments it was clear that adequate procedures for the selection of heterokaryons would be required if these somatic fusions were to be successfully utilized for various programmes of plant improvement. Several procedures, often based on principles of microbiological complementation selection[5], have been employed for selection; and studies within the *Petunia* genus produced amphidiploid somatic hybrid plants by using a complementation selection procedure which involved fusing wild-type leaf protoplasts of one species with albino protoplasts from cell suspension cultures of the other species. From these protoplast fusions flowering plants with 28 chromosomes of the somatic hybrid *Petunia parodii* (2n=14) ⓧ *Petunia hybrida* (2n=14), and of *Petunia parodii* (2n=14) ⓧ *Petunia inflata* (2n=14) were produced between these sexually compatible species. The consequences of fusion of sexually incompatible *Petunia parodii* leaf protoplasts with albino protoplasts from cell suspensions of *Petunia parviflora*[6] enabled the production of amphidiploid somatic hybrid plants with 32 chromosomes, *P. parodii* (2n=14) ⓧ *P. parviflora* (2n=18)[7]. Horticulturally this novel hybrid could be of considerable interest, particularly if further hybridizations either sexually or somatically could extend the range of floral types of this 'hanging basket' type *Petunia*. Indeed there are many possible applications of somatic hybridization to the improvement of horticultural species.

Whilst, as we have seen, significant advances have been made in our ability to produce somatic hybrids by protoplast fusions, one of the limitations in further advancement has been our lack of knowledge of the details of many of the stages involved in this multi-stage process. The successful outcome of somatic hybridization, whether it is to produce nuclear hybrids, limited gene transfer or cybrids will depend on a basic knowledge of the many steps in this procedure. These steps involve isolation of protoplasts, division of cells regenerated from protoplasts, controlled fusion of protoplasts, and the identification and selection of heterokaryons, hybrid and cybrid cells and the regeneration of plants. This further development of the subject is from a base line of experience mainly with tobaccos and *Petunias*, and often some of the difficulties encountered are related to special cultural features of crop species.

The use of protoplasts isolated from seedling roots[8,9] and from seedling cotyledons[10] could also be particularly advantageous when somatic hybridizations are being undertaken. The use of germinating seeds overcomes the difficulty encountered with the production of leaf material, and enables an adequate supply of experimental material to be produced rapidly with the minimum of resources. It has also been suggested for somatic hybridization assessments that protoplasts from roots and etiolated cotyledons could be used, instead of cell suspension protoplasts, for fusion with green cotyledon leaf material or leaf mesophyll protoplasts[10].

The regeneration of plants from protoplasts is central to the utilization of new developments in somatic cell genetics for plant breeding programmes, and the recent successes in regenerating from seedling root and cotyledon protoplasts is likely to enhance greatly the spectrum of species in which regeneration from protoplasts is possible. It is likely that during the next decade regeneration of plants from protoplasts of the major crops will have been accomplished. The regeneration of tomato plants from tomato leaf protoplasts is a step towards this goal. It should be mentioned that more than three years' work was required to perfect this regeneration procedure[11].

Recently we have developed a simple procedure for the aseptic manual isolation of individual heterokaryons. Heterokaryons were identified with bright field illumination using an inverted microscope, and isolated by means of a micromanipulator and capillary pipette coupled to a specially constructed syringe. When cell suspension protoplasts were labelled with fluorescein isothiocyanate and fused with mesophyll protoplasts, the heterokaryons exhibited an apple green cytoplasmic fluorescence (from cell suspension protoplasts) and a red chloroplast fluorescence (from mesophyll protoplasts). Using an inverted microscope with a suitable fluorescence attachment we have also observed that the differential fluorescence from chloroplasts and fluorescein isothiocyanate in individual heterokaryons persists in the cells of small colonies developed from such heterokaryons. Manual or fluorescence activated cell sorting procedures may not therefore be required, since selection of individual heterokaryons is not then required[12]. Such methods are also readily applicable to the selection of cybrids.

If fusion of protoplasts is also coupled with procedures for the inactivation of the nuclear genome of one of the species, and suitable selection procedures, a range of novel cybrids can theoretically be obtained. Rather than irradiating protoplasts to inactivate nuclei, fractionation of protoplasts into enucleate subprotoplasts or enucleate microplasts[13] may provide suitable enucleate units for fusions to produce this novel range of cybrids, thereby avoiding any irradiation effects on the cytoplasm.

Microcell-mediated chromosome transfer has proved to be a promising approach for chromosome assignment of genes for mammalian cells. Nuclear material of cultured mammalian cells is fragmented by treatment of the cells with colchicine. The fragments consist of a limited amount of genetic material encapsulated in a cell membrane. Microcells are fused with recipient cells using routine somatic hybridization methods. Until recently there seemed little possibility that any comparable system could be developed for cultured plant cells apart from the production of nucleate subprotoplasts (mini-protoplasts) and cytoplasts[14]. However, the discovery of the plant microplast system[13] could lead to the development of such a microcell system if fragmentation of the nuclear material can be induced with colchicine. Microplasts surrounded by an inner membrane of the cell, most probably derived from the tonoplast, can be readily isolated by rupturing auxin-induced highly vacuolated thin-walled callus cells of several plant species[13]. Even if fragmentation of nuclear material cannot readily be achieved, such enucleate sub-protoplasts and microplasts could be used for the transfer of a range of cytoplasmic factors by fusion with nucleated protoplasts. Transfer of cytoplasmic based male sterility, and herbicide resistance, could readily be achieved between sexually incompatible species[15]. The opportunity now exists to re-assemble cells by the fusion of microplasts and sub-protoplasts Electric field-induced fusion[16] could help greatly in this respect since fusion can be readily observed microscopically. If this is coupled with the isolation of fusion products using a simple micromanipulator system and an inverted microscope[12] hybrid and cybri cells of various types could be readily produced.

THE USE OF NITRATE REDUCTASE DEFICIENT MUTANTS FOR TRANSFORMATION ASSESSMENTS

There is a paucity of stable auxotrophs in higher plants, and one of the few such auxotrophs are nitrate reductase deficient lines of tobacco. These *nia* mutant lines, selected for chlorate resistance, lack nitrate reductase apoenzyme activity and cannot grow with nitrate as the sole source of nitrogen. Protoplasts can be readily isolated from the leaf mesophyll cells of *nia*-130 auxotrophs and show high plating efficiency, and cell colonies derived from the protoplasts can be regenerated into complete plants. No nitrate utilising revertants were observed when 1.8×10^7 *nia*-130 colonies were transferred from amino acid medium to selection medium containing nitrate as the sole source of nitrogen. Pental et al.[17] have suggested that this *nia* mutant protoplast system could be used to isolate genomic sequences of nitrate reductase of *Nicotiana*, or other higher plants, by functional complementation of mutant protoplasts by recombinant plasmids from a random genomic library of wild type plant DNA. This nitrate reductase deficient mutant should also be capable of detecting any nitrate reductase gene transfer by fusion. The nitrate reductase deficient mutant would be corrected to nitrate reductase proficiency if transformation of protoplasts were possible by fusion with a donor wild type protoplast system.

TRANSFORMATION INVESTIGATIONS

The singular attraction of *Agrobacterium tumefaciens* is that when interacting with plants it naturally manages to transfer, maintain and express its prokaryotic DNA in plant cells. Numerous workers are now busy trying to exploit this natural capability of the Agrobacterium bacterium to use the Agrobacterium tumefaciens Ti plasmid as a host vector system for introducing foreign DNA in plant cells. In many of these experiments on plant transformation it is not necessary, at least initially, to use protoplasts.

Recently the presence has been demonstrated, by DNA-DNA hybridization, of DNA sequences homologous to the Ti plasmid in phytohormone-independent colonies derived from plasmid-treated Petunia protoplasts[18].

Suspension cell protoplasts of Petunia hybrida were incubated with pTiACH5 using either glycine-NaOH buffer (pH 10.1) containing 20 mM $CaCl_2$ and 9% (w/v) mannitol, followed by mixing with 47% (w/v) polyethylene glycol 6000, or poly-L-ornithine (Mol. wt. 166,000) in 45 mM Na citrate buffer (pH 9.4) and 12% (w/v) mannitol. After nine months of subculturing, callus from eighteen hormone-independent clones from such plasmid-treated protoplasts was harvested, and the DNA analysed for the presence of Ti plasmid (pTiACH5) homologous sequences by DNA-DNA hybridization.

The transformants, analysed by DNA-DNA hybridization, each contained pTiACH5 homologous sequences, but their hybridization patterns were not typical of that of authentic Petunia crown gall tissue induced by strain ACH5 of Agrobacterium. The results showed that a small fragment of pTiACH5, of approximately 2Md, is stably maintained in each of the eighteen clones from plasmid treated protoplasts. It was suggested[18] that this DNA fragment could represent the smallest part of pTiACH5 necessary for protoplast transformation and the maintenance of phytohormone independent growth in derived colonies. There are, however, indications[19] from analysis of two calluses ensuing from Nicotiana tabacum leaf protoplasts incubated with octopine Ti-plasmid from the wild-type strain ACH5, in the presence of 40% w/v polyethylene glycol 6000 followed by a post-incubation with high Ca^{2+} concentration, that a larger part of the Ti-plasmid is integrated into the host genome than on infection with the whole bacterium. Whether these differences represent differing responses of different plant species must await further analysis, since only two calluses were analysed in the tobacco protoplast experiments for the presence of Ti-plasmid DNA sequences[19].

Positive selective markers which can be added to a normal prototrophic genetic background are highly desirable, and these studies utilising protoplasts with Ti-plasmid and also those utilising agrobacteria[1] and Agrobacterium spheroplasts[20] have already established a firm foundation for transformation. Additionally the transformation of yeast spheroplasts and animal cells to a state of resistance to the antibiotic G418 has re-stimulated the setting up of experiments in which plant protoplasts are similarly assessed for antibiotic resistance. The first detailed assessment utilised protoplasts prepared from cultured tobacco cells treated with ColE1-kan plasmid DNA, a hybrid of ColE1 and pSC105 plasmids bearing a gene for kanamycin resistance. Upon commencement of division, the treated cells were plated in medium containing kanamycin. No evidence was obtained for expression of the kanamycin resistance gene of ColE1-kan in tobacco tissue. G418 is considerably more toxic to plant cells than kanamycin[21], and in collaborative work with the Molecular Genetics Group at the Plant Breeding Institute, Cambridge, we have begun an assessment of the use of this antibiotic as a dominant selectable marker. *Salpiglossis sinuata* protoplasts were incubated with vectors containing the transposons Tn5 and Tn601 transposed into ColE1 derivative plasmids. 36×10^6 protoplasts were utilised per experiment with uptake stimulated by either poly-L-ornithine or polyethylene glycol. Selection for any induced resistance to G418 which the plasmid might confer on the protoplasts, and any cell colonies derived from them, was stepwise. Initial plating was without G418 and then on media containing 20, 50, 100, 200 and 500 µg G418/ml. Controls (no plasmid) were similarly treated. Spontaneously resistant lines have been found in control experiments, but presumptive transformants after the G418 vector treatment have appeared more frequently. DNA-DNA hybridization analysis of presumptive colonies has not as yet however proved positive Moreover, cloning of cells from several presumptive transformants by isolation of protoplasts has provided no evidence for any inherited enhanced resistance to G418 greater than from non-plasmid treated controls. Whilst there is a possibility that further analysis will reveal presumptive colonies which are truly transformed, these preliminary results are illustrative of the type of problems arising in such assessments when using positive drug selective markers with plant protoplasts. The exact nature of the plasmid in determining the efficiency with which the host plant cell can express the bacterial gene conferring resistance will clearly influence whether or not transformation is achieved in some of the protoplasts; but ability to detect readily such transformants will be markedly influenced by such leaky controls. Explanations for such leakiness may involve a general induced detoxification of deleterious substances within plant cells; and there remains the possibility that the required stepwise selection leads to gene amplification resulting in enhanced antibiotic resistance in some colonies in the control. Such gene amplification is already well established for murine cells incubated with methotrexate[22].

ACKNOWLEDGMENT

Original work described in this review was supported by a grant from the Agricultural Research Council.

REFERENCES

1. E. C. Cocking, M. R. Davey, D. Pental, and J. B. Power, Aspects of plant genetic manipulation, Nature 293:265 (1981).
2. E. C. Cocking, Somatic hybridization by the fusion of isolated protoplasts - an alternative to sex, in: "Plant Cell and Tissue Culture Principles and Applications", W. R. Sharp et al., ed., Ohio State University Press, Columbus (1979).
3. E. C. Cocking, Parasexual reproduction in flowering plants, N.Z. Jl. Bot. 17:665 (1979).
4. J. B. Power, S. E. Cummins, and E. C. Cocking, Fusion of isolated plant protoplasts, Nature 225:1016 (1970).
5. E. C. Cocking, Selection and somatic hybridisation, in: "Frontiers of Plant Tissue Culture", T. A. Thorpe, ed., Int. Assoc. Plant Tissue Culture (1978).
6. J. B. Power, S. F. Berry, J. V. Chapman, and E. C. Cocking, Somatic hybridisation of sexually incompatible Petunias: Petunia parodii, Petunia parviflora, Theor. Appl. Genet. 57:1 (1980).
7. E. C. Cocking, Plant cell hybrids and somatic hybrid plants, in: "Chromosomes Today, Vol.7", George Allen and Unwin (1981).
8. Z-H. Xu, M. R. Davey, and E. C. Cocking, Isolation and sustained division of Phaseolus aureus (Mung Bean) root protoplasts, Z. für Pflanzenphysiol. 104:289 (1981).
9. Z-H. Xu, M. R. Davey, and E. C. Cocking, Plant regeneration from root protoplasts of Brassica, Plant Sci. Letts. 24:117 (1982).
10. D. Y. Lu, D. Pental, and E. C. Cocking, Plant regeneration from seedling cotyledon protoplasts, Z. für Pflanzenphysiol. 107:59 (1982).
11. A. Morgan and E. C. Cocking, Plant regeneration from protoplasts of Lycopersicon esculentum Mill., Z. für Pflanzenphysiol. 106:97 (1982).
12. G. Patnaik, E. C. Cocking, J. Hamill, and D. Pental, A simple procedure for the manual isolation and identification of plant heterokaryons, Plant Sci. Letts. 24:105 (1982).
13. P. C. Bilkey and E. C. Cocking, Isolation and properties of plant microplasts: newly identified subcellular units capable of wall synthesis and division into separate micro cells, Eur. J. Cell Biol. 22:502 (1980).
14. H. Lörz, J. Paszhowski, C. Dierks-Ventling, and I. Potrykus, Isolation and characterisation of cytoplasts and miniprotoplasts derived from protoplasts of cultured cells, Physiol. Plant. 53:386 (1981).
15. E. C. Cocking, Opportunities from the use of protoplasts, Phil. Trans. R. Soc. Lond. B, 292:557 (1981).

16. U. Zimmermann and P. Scheurich, High frequency fusion of plant protoplasts by electric fields, Planta 156:26 (1981).
17. D. Pental, S. Cooper-Bland, K. Harding, E. C. Cocking, and A. J. Müller, Cultural studies on nitrate reductase deficient Nicotiana tabacum mutant protoplasts, Z. für Pflanzenphysiol. 105:219 (1982).
18. J. Draper, M. R. Davey, J. P. Freeman, E. C. Cocking, and B. J. Cox, Ti-plasmid homologous sequences present in tissues from Agrobacterium plasmid-transformed Petunia protoplasts, Plant Cell Physiol. 23:92 (1982).
19. F. A. Krens, L. Molendijk, G. J. Wullems, and R. A. Schilperoort, In vitro transformation of plant protoplasts with Ti-plasmid DNA, Nature 298:72 (1982)
20. S. Hasezawa, T. Nagata, and K. Syono, Transformation of Vinca protoplasts mediated by Agrobacterium spheroplasts, Mol. Gen. Genet. 182:206 (1981).
21. D. Ursic, J. D. Kemp, and J. P. Helgeson, A new antibiotic with known resistance factors, G418, inhibits plant cells, Biochem. Biophys. Res. Comm. 101:1031 (1981).
22. R. T. Schimke, R. J. Kaufman, F. W. Alt, and R. F. Kellems, Gene amplification and drug resistance in cultured murine cells, Science 202: 1051 (1978).

SELECTION OF TOBACCO PROTOPLAST-DERIVED CELLS FOR RESISTANCE TO AMINO ACIDS AND REGENERATION OF RESISTANT PLANTS

Jean-Pierre Bourgin

Laboratoire de Biologie Cellulaire
I.N.R.A.
F 78000 Versailles, France

ABSTRACT

Cell colonies derived from UV-mutagenized mesophyll protoplasts of haploid tobacco (*Nicotiana tabacum* L.) were submitted to selection in a medium containing toxic concentrations of either L-valine or L-lysine plus L-threonine. Among the plants regenerated from colonies thus recovered in various experiments seven were resistant to valine (Val^r mutants) and two to lysine plus threonine (LT^r mutants). These markers were transmitted to progeny as mendelian characters, either single dominant (LT^r mutants and Val^r mutants of the first type), or digenic recessive (Val^r mutants of the second type). The two types of valine resistance were further characterized by testing cells derived from mesophyll protoplasts from resistant plants for resistance to valine and to other amino acids. Cells of mutants of the first type had a low level of resistance to valine, whereas cells of mutants of the second type had a high level of resistance to valine and to other amino acids. According to the results of ^{14}C-labelled amino acid uptake experiments the amino acid resistance of mutants of the second type could be accounted for by a generally reduced uptake of amino acids. Possible uses of valine resistance as a marker in plant cell genetics are discussed.

INTRODUCTION

Protoplasts are the current target of many plant cell transformation experiments (e.g. Krens et al., 1982; Lurquin and Sheehy, 1982). The experience gained from establishing methods for biochemically selecting mutants from protoplast-derived cells might be helpful in devising selective procedures for the recovery of genetically transformed cells.

Cell suspension cultures have been the traditional source of plant material for biochemical selection of plant cell mutants, such as numerous cell lines resistant to various amino acid analogs (for review, see : Widholm, 1977a ; Widholm, 1977b ; Maliga, 1978 ; Maliga, 1980). Unfortunately, changes in chromosome number and karyotype accumulate during subculture (Sunderland, 1973 ; Bayliss, 1980). Possibly due to these karyotypic changes (Murashige and Nakano, 1967 ; Smith and Street, 1974), no or only abnormal plants can be regenerated from established cell cultures, a situation which precludes genetic analysis of characters selected at the cellular stage (e.g. Widholm, 1977a), unless parasexual techniques are used (Glimelius et al., 1978 ; White and Vasil, 1979 ; Harms et al., 1981 ; Lázár et al., 1981).

In contrast, protoplast suspensions, prepared directly from plant tissues such as leaf parenchyma (mesophyll) constitute instantaneous cell suspensions, the genome of which is that of the cells of the mother plant. If necessary, it can be haploid, whereas, with some exceptions (e.g. Evans and Gamborg, 1979 ; Vanzulli et al., 1980), stability of the haploid state in cell suspension cultures is difficult to attain (e.g. Rashid and Street, 1974 ; Furner et al., 1978 ; Bayliss, 1980). The mother plant, and thus the protoplast genome, can also display a mutant character, which can subsequently be used for cellular genetic manipulations. While suspensions of cultured cells are in fact essentially composed of cell aggregates of various sizes (Yeoman and Street, 1973), suspensions of protoplasts constitute homogeneous populations of independent cells, from which true cellular clones can be generated. At least 95% of the protoplasts prepared from mesophyll cells are at the G1 stage (Magnien and Devreux, 1980), a situation which may be used to obtain synchronization of the first divisions (Meyer and Cooke, 1979 ; Magnien et al., 1980 ; Zelcer and Galun, 1980). Finally, although variations in the procedures of preparation may lead to differences in physiological state, protoplasts constitute an identical plant material from one laboratory to the other. In a pioneering period, where difficulties are encountered in establishing standardized procedures for the isolation of defined plant cell mutants, this seemingly minor aspect should not be underestimated.

As early as 1973 Carlson obtained mutant tobacco plants resistant to methionine-sulfoximine from cell colonies derived from haploid protoplasts (Carlson, 1973). Nevertheless, while the number of mutant cell lines derived from cell suspension cultures increased regularly (Widholm, 1977b), experiments involving protoplasts were rare and not very encouraging (Aviv and Galun, 1977a; Aviv and Galun, 1977b). The aims of the experiments summarized in the present report were i) to verify the feasibility of isolating defined mutants from a population of mesophyll protoplasts, ii) to obtain biochemical markers for studying the efficiency of selection of mutant clones.

Tobacco (*Nicotiana tabacum* L.) was chosen for these experiments, because i) haploid plants were easily available through anther culture (Bourgin and Nitsch, 1967; Nitsch and Nitsch, 1969, ii) the regeneration of plants from cultured cells and in particular from protoplast-derived cell colonies, had been mastered (Nagata and Takebe, 1971; Nitsch and Ohyama, 1971) and iii) the plating efficiency of mesophyll protoplasts, in particular when prepared according to the procedure devised by our group (Chupeau et al., 1974), was reproducibly superior to 80%. The major disadvantage of tobacco is its amphidiploid structure (2n = 2n'+2n" = 48). Despite an apparent functional diploidization of genes governing certain characteristics (Smith, 1968), there are other characters which appear to be governed by duplicate factors belonging to the two parental genomes (Clausen and Cameron, 1950; Stines and Mann, 1960). Obviously this genetic situation might hamper the recovery of recessive mutants. For example, Carlson (1970) suggested that incomplete diploidization of certain essential genes could explain the leakiness of six different auxotrophic cell lines obtained from haploid tobacco cells.

One simple method to test the efficiency of mutagenic treatments on protoplasts is to calculate the frequency of chlorophyll deficient cell colonies induced by these treatments (Schieder, 1976; Krumbiegel, 1979; Sidorov and Maliga, 1982). However, this criterion cannot be used to test the efficiency of selection of mutant cells among a population of wild type cells. I have thus adapted to plant cells a system developed by Adelberg et al. (1965) for assessing the mutagenic efficiency of nitrosoguanidine treatments on *Escherichia coli* K-12 cells by calculating the frequency of colonies which have become resistant to toxic concentrations of L-valine. This method was then extended by screening for clones resistant to the toxic mixture of L-lysine plus L-threonine.

GROWTH INHIBITION OF TOBACCO CELLS BY VALINE AND LYSINE PLUS THREONINE

Colony formation from tobacco protoplasts or protoplast-derived cells is inhibited in media containing valine : for instance 100 µM L-valine greatly reduced the plating efficiency

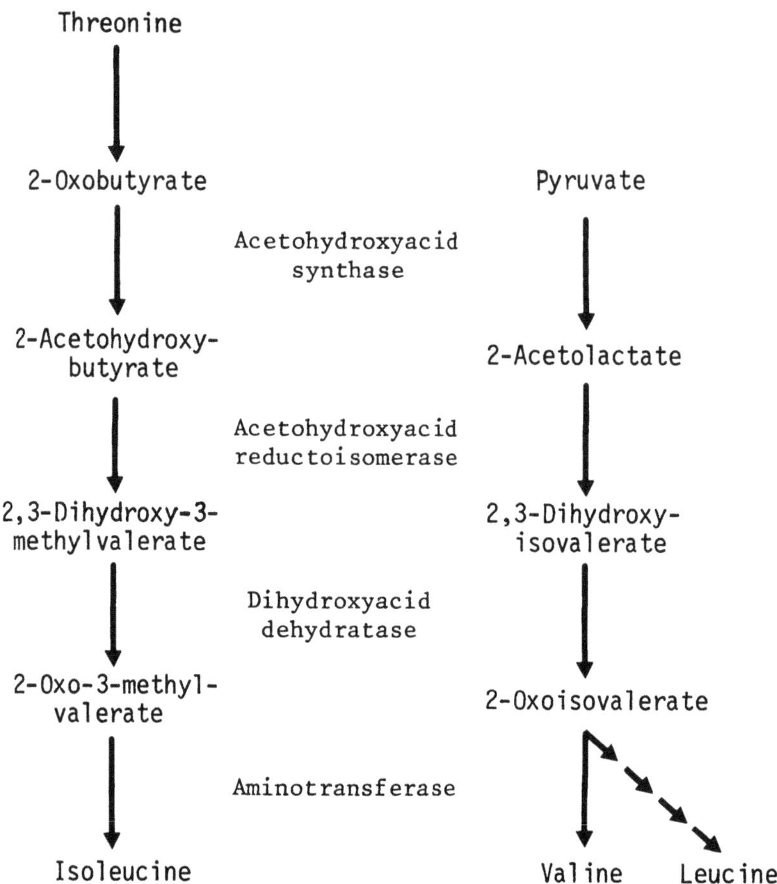

Fig. 1. Pathway for biosynthesis of isoleucine and valine.

of haploid protoplasts cultured at 65,000 ml^{-1}. This toxicity is specifically relieved by the simultaneous addition to the medium of isoleucine, but not by the addition of arginine, lysine or leucine (Bourgin, 1976; Bourgin, 1978; unpublished results).

An extensive biochemical and genetic analysis of the process of growth inhibition of microorganisms by valine has been performed by various laboratories, essentially on *E. coli* K-12 (Umbarger, 1969; De Felice et al., 1979). This phenomenon has also been studied in plant systems such as barley seedlings (Miflin, 1969; Miflin, 1973) and *Spirodela polyrhiza* fronds (Borstlap, 1972; Borstlap, 1981). One can infer from these studies that excess valine starves the cells for isoleucine. The last steps of the valine and isoleucine biosynthetic pathways are catalyzed by enzymes that are probably common to the two pathways (Bryan, 1980) (Figure 1.). Excess valine may inhibit the activity of the first of these common enzymes, acetohydroxyacid synthase, thus preventing valine, leucine, and isoleucine synthesis. Isoleucine is the only exogenous amino acid required for growth in these conditions, since valine is provided in the medium and leucine can probably be synthesized from valine (Borstlap, 1972). Similarly, exogenous isoleucine and leucine inhibit the growth of tobacco cells. In each case this toxicity is only relieved by a mixture of the two other branched-chain amino acids (unpublished results).

Another well-documented instance of antagonistic effects between related amino acids was also observed with tobacco protoplast-derived cells and plantlets : the combination of lysine plus threonine is toxic at concentrations at which the single amino acids are not or are only slightly inhibitory. Inhibition by lysine plus threonine is reversed by methionine or homoserine, but not by arginine and isoleucine (Bourgin et al., in preparation). The selection of resistants to lysine plus threonine was proposed as a means of isolating mutants with an altered level of the aspartate-derived amino acids, in particular methionine (Green and Phillips 1974, Chaleff and Carlson 1975). Indeed such mutants were obtained from mutagenized barley seeds (Bright et al., 1982) and from maize cultures initiated from scutellar tissue (Hibberd et al., 1980). Selected cell lines resistant to lysine analogs were also cross resistant to lysine plus threonine (Chaleff and Carlson, 1975; Widholm, 1976).

ISOLATION OF TOBACCO MUTANTS RESISTANT EITHER TO VALINE OR TO LYSINE PLUS THREONINE

Methods

Mesophyll protoplasts were prepared from plants of a haploid

Table 1. Number of clones manipulated at various steps in the isolation of amino acid resistant tobacco mutants.

Type of mutant	Val^r				LT^r
Experiment n°	1	2	3	4	1
Number of :					
- Selected colonies (clones)	15	72	149	228	119
- Clones from which plantlets were regenerated	6	19	67	174	59
- Presumed mutant clones after verification of resistance using shoot explants	1	5	2	2	4
- Confirmed mutant clones after testing progeny	1	4	1	1	2
Mutants isolated	Val^r-1	Val^r-2 Val^r-3 Val^r-4 Val^r-5	Val^r-6	Val^r-7	LT^r-1 LT^r-2
Frequency of mutant clones	7.7 10^{-7}	1.6 10^{-6}	1.7 10^{-6}	1.7 10^{-6}	2.5 10^{-6}

line obtained by anther culture and in vitro vegetative propagation. A portion of the protoplast population was submitted to UV-irradiation by a germicidal lamp at doses chosen to reduce the plating efficiency to values between 50 and 80% of that of the controls. Two or four weeks after irradiation, cultured suspensions of cell colonies derived from protoplasts were included in an agar-solidified medium containing the appropriate concentrations of L-valine (final conc.: 2.0, 3.0, 4.0, 4.3 or 8.6 mM) or of L-lysine plus L-threonine (final conc.: 2.0, 3.0 or 4.0 mM each). Between two and four months later the microcalli which had developed from cell colonies under the selective conditions were transferred to a regeneration medium.

After rooting of the shoots thus obtained, the plantlets were vegetatively propagated and their resistance to the appropriate amino acid(s) was assessed by culturing shoot explants (1 cm long) possessing one axillary bud on a medium containing either 2 mM L-valine or 1 mM L-lysine plus 1 mM L-threonine. Progeny testing of the adult plants obtained from the plantlets was carried out by germinating seeds on similar selective media.

Results

Four experiments produced valine resistant clones and one produced lysine plus threonine resistant clones. (Table 1) Details of the conditions of mutagenesis and selection are given elsewhere (Bourgin, 1982). Diploid or quasi-diploid plants were obtained from seven valine resistant clones and from two lysine plus threonine resistant clones, all originating from the UV-irradiated protoplast population. Four plants out of nine were male sterile, but female fertile, permitting successful crossing by wild type plants. Resistance was transmitted to the progeny of all nine plants.

Discussion

Most selected clones were lost, because colonies did not survive a possibly premature transplantation. A few others were not studied due to lack of shoot regeneration or, exceptionally, to lack of rooting of the shoots. This apparent loss of regenerative capacity might have been due to prolonged culture in the selective medium, since this phenomenon, common in established cell cultures, was not observed in protoplast-derived colonies not submitted to selection (e.g. Schieder, 1976 ; Evans, 1979). Another explanation for loss of regenerative capacity could be the mutagenic treatment itself, since ultraviolet irradiation of tobacco cells was shown to reduce their regenerative capacity (Eapen, 1976).

Diploid plants may have originated from spontaneously fused haploid protoplasts (Withers and Cocking, 1972), but this hypothesis was not substantiated by subsequent progeny testing. Otherwise in vitro culture conditions, which commonly lead to endopolyploidization and aneuploidization (Ogura, 1976 ; Bayliss, 1980) could account for this diploidization, like that observed in plants regenerated from haploid *Datura* protoplasts (Schieder, 1976).

The fact that all the proven resistant clones arose from the UV-treated protoplasts and none from the control population is evidence in favor of the mutagenic efficiency of this irradiation. Indeed other morphological and physiological variants were observed among the plants regenerated from irradiated protoplasts such as i) plants with abnormal leaf or flower coloration or shape and ii) a plant that requires short days for flowering, whereas the original Xanthi cultivar used in this study is a day-neutral variety. This mutation, however, could have occured spontaneously in tissue culture, since it has also been observed among tobacco plants regenerated from non-mutagenized protoplasts (Melchers, 1975). The use of UV-irradiation is more convenient than other mutagenic treatments (Howland and Hart, 1977). Its mutagenic effect on pollen grains has been well documented (Stadler and Sprague, 1936) and attributed essentially to point mutations (e.g. Pfahler and Linskens, 1977). In contrast to other mutagenic treatments which produced a fraction of mixed clones composed of mutant and wild type cells,UV-mutagenesis was shown in yeast to produce 100 % pure mutant clones, a situation attributed to the fact that the DNA repair process responsible for the UV-mutagenesis is replication independent (Nasim et al., 1981). Limited evidence has been given for the mutagenic efficiency of UV-irradiation on cultured plant cells (Eriksson, 1967 ; Widholm, 1977c). The present results should thus give wider acceptance to this treatment for mutagenizing protoplasts.

As observed in other reports (e.g. Carlson, 1973 ; Sung, 1976 ; Horsch, 1979), a significant fraction (74-99%) of the selected clones appeared sensitive when retested for amino acid resistance. Verification thus appears essential when the frequency of resistant clones is used for estimating the efficiency of a mutagenic treatment, which can also increase the frequency of pseudo-resistant clones (Horsch, 1979). It is perhaps unavoidable that some non resistant colonies escape the selection procedure, possibly due to secondary physiological alterations subsequent to the mutagenic treatment, such as those produced by UV-irradiation (e.g. Wright and Murphy, 1978). However, it is advisable to reduce as much as possible this "background noise" by optimizing the selection.

TRANSMISSION OF RESISTANCE MARKERS TO PROGENY

Results

Tests of resistance of progeny seedlings showed that:

i) all resistance markers obtained are inherited like mendelian characters and not cytoplasmically.

ii) they can be classified into two types:

- dominant: clones designated Val^r-1, Val^r-6, Val^r=7, LR^r-1 and LR^r-2;
- recessive: clones designated Val^r-2, Val^r-3, Val^r-4, and Val^r-5. However, tests carried out on protoplast-derived cells from mutant plants cultured at low density indicated that cells heterozygous for the Val^r-2 marker were slightly more resistant to valine than wild type cells (Bourgin et al., 1982). It thus would seem more appropriate to call this marker (and those of the same type) partially dominant rather than strictly recessive.

iii) Val^r-2, Val^r-3, Val^r-4 are transmitted like digenic characters (Val^r-5 F2 seedlings were not tested): composition of the F2 progeny fitted as 1 resistant: 15 (sensitive plus partially resistant) segregation pattern. Distribution of the partially resistant seedlings into the expected intermediary classes was not possible, due to their low level of resistance.

Crosses between the various Val^r mutants were carried out. F1 hybrid seedlings from crosses between the pseudo-recessive types were resistant, which indicates that the corresponding markers are allelic. Study of the F2 generation obtained by self-fertilization of hybrid plants indicated that Val^r-2 segregates independently from Val^r-1, Val^r-6 and Val^r-7.

Discussion

The resistance characters obtained were transmitted as stable mendelian markers through several sexual generations (and through androgenesis in the case of Val^r-1 and Val^r-2, for which anther culture was carried out). This definitely establishes that they are due to mutations, and not to stable physiological adaptations, such as auxin independence, an epigenetic change which frequently arises in tissue culture and which has led to increased levels of resistance to amino acid analogs in several established cell lines studied by King and Strauss (cited by Thomas et al., 1979). Even an epigenetic change capable of passing through the sexual cycle, as the tricotyly studied by Chaleff and Keil (1981), would probably not obey such strict patterns of inheritance.

In retrospect the use of haploid cells does not appear necessary for the selection of the LT^r mutants and of the Val^r mutants of Val^r-1 type, which are transmitted as dominant markers. On the other hand, the use of haploid cells is essential for the isolation of the Val^r mutants of Val^r-2 type, which are transmitted as digenic recessive traits. Relationships between the two hypothetical genes involved have not been determined. One might suppose that they are located on homeologous chromosomes from the two parental genomes of tobacco. Müller et al. (cited by Pental et al., 1982) have also observed that nitrate reductase deficient plants regenerated from a chlorate resistant tobacco cell line (Müller and Grafe, 1978) were homozygous for two unliked recessive mutations.

Although tobacco (*Nicotiana tabacum*) is the species from which most plant cell mutants have been obtained so far (Maliga, 1980), these results confirm that amphiploidy might complicate both the isolation of recessive mutants and their genetic analysis. *Datura innoxia*, *Daucus carota*, *Hyoscyamus muticus*, *Petunia hybrida* are candidates for replacement of tobacco as model species (e.g. Maliga et al., 1982). Other candidates are diploid species of the genus *Nicotiana*. Our group has been particularly involved in research on the feasibility of using the protoplast system in diploid *Nicotiana* species (Chupeau et al., 1974 ; Bourgin et al., 1976 ; Bourgin and Missonier, 1978 ; Bourgin et al., 1979). We looked for a species in which the three following technical steps could be mastered : i) production of haploids through anther culture, ii) regeneration of cell colonies from mesophyll protoplasts with a satisfactory plating efficiency, iii) regeneration of plants from protoplast-derived cell colonies. Among the species which were shown to have these advantages and were proposed as possible model species in plant cell genetics (Bourgin et al., 1979) *Nicotiana plumbaginifolia* seems to have rapidly gained a wide acceptance. The first established haploid clones (Bourgin et al., Maliga et al., unpublished results) are available and the other favorable characteristics for protoplast culture have been confirmed by other groups (Magnien et al., 1980 ; Negrutiu, 1981 ; Maliga et al., 1982 ; Shields, pers. comm.). We have also easily obtained bud regeneration from roots cultured in vitro, a characteristic which might interest the researchers involved in the use of *Agrobacterium rhizogenes* as an agent of plant transformation (Tepfer, this volume). Finally an array of various auxotrophic and chlorophyll-deficient mutants has already been obtained (Sidorov et al., 1981 ; Maliga et al., 1982 ; Sidorov and Maliga, 1982 ; Negrutiu, pers. comm. ; Muller and Caboche, unpublished results). Genetic analysis of these mutants should benefit from the relatively short life cycle of *N. plumbaginifolia* (Steinberg, 1959).

SEARCH OF THE MECHANISM(S) RESPONSIBLE FOR VALINE RESISTANCE

Results

Protoplasts were prepared from plants of the mutant clones and the plating efficiency of protoplast-derived cells subcultured in media with various concentrations of valine was measured. According to their response to exogenous valine the Val^r mutant clones were classified in two groups (Bourgin et al., 1980).

i) Cells of mutants of the Val^r-2 type (Val^r-2, Val^r-3, Val^r-4, Val^r-5) displayed a high level of resistance : the LD 50 was between 20 and 40 times higher than for wild type cells.

ii) Cells of mutants of the Val^r-1 type (Val^r-1, Val^r-6, Val^r-7) displayed only a low level of resistance (LD 50 between 3 and 7 times higher than for wild type cells), which could only be detected when using a particularly sensitive test of culture at low cell density (100 - 300 cells. ml^{-1}) developed according to the method established by Caboche (1980).

I tried to extend to tobacco cells a test routinely used for distinguishing among Val^r mutants of *E. Coli* K-12 those which owe their resistance to an altered valine uptake from those which are resistant due to some other intracellular alteration. The first category is still sensitive to glycyl-valine, as this dipeptide is taken up by a transport system different from those involved in the transport of amino acids and liberates valine inside the cell under the action of a peptidase (Guardiola and Iaccarino, 1971). Conversely the latter mutants, which owe their valine resistance to an alteration of one of the acetohydroxyacid synthases involved in the biosynthesis of branched-chain amino acids, or to a modification of the regulation of the responsible operon, are also resistant to glycyl-valine (De Felice et al., 1979). Since the highest concentrations of glycyl-valine tested (10 mM) were not toxic to tobacco cells this approach was abandoned. However control experiments showed that cells of mutants of the Val^r-2 type were resistant to inhibitory levels of glycine. Further study showed that they were also resistant to isoleucine, leucine, serine and threonine.

Uptake experiments of ^{14}C-labelled amino acids were carried out. Val^r-2 cells displayed a reduced uptake not only for valine and leucine, but also for other neutral amino acids (glycine and threonine), for an acidic one (aspartic acid) and for a basic one (histidine). The uptake of valine, leucine, and glycine by Val^r-1 cells could not be distinguished from that of wild type cells (Bourgin et al., in prep.).

Discussion

The resistance of mutants of the Val^{r}-2 type to amino acids can be simply explained by a general reduction in amino acid uptake, the cause of which has not been determined. However it was observed that the uptake of a sugar, 3-o-methylglucose, by Val^{r}-2 cells was not affected. Alteration in the mechanism of amino acid uptake might be similar to that of a parafluorophenylalanine resistant tobacco cell line isolated by Berlin and Widholm (1978), which displayed a generally reduced uptake of amino acids. Further study of the Val^{r}-2 mutant could be helpful for the analysis of amino acid uptake by higher plant cells.

One would expect that this reduced amino acid uptake could affect their transport through tissues of whole plants and that this would alter the normal growth of mutant plants. Preliminary experiments in growth chambers showed indeed that i) whereas growth of Val^{r}-2 plants was comparable to that of wild type plants when cultured at 30°C, it was strikingly reduced at 20°C, ii) at 20°C leaves of Val^{r}-2 plants displayed numerous spots of necrosis, which might be due to locally toxic accumulations of amino acids.

As for the mechanism responsible for the valine-resistance of Val^{r}-1 cells, reduction in the uptake of amino acids has been ruled out. Since the inhibitory effect of valine might be due to an inhibition of acetohydroxyacid synthase, I suggest that this enzyme might have a reduced sensitivity to valine in the mutant clones of the Val^{r}-1 type. Altered feedback properties of control enzymes were demonstrated in various plant cell lines resistant to amino acid analogs (e.g. Widholm, 1977a). Similarly, in mutants of barley and maize resistant to lysine plus threonine aspartokinase had reduced sensitivity to these feedback inhibitors (Hibberd et al., 1980 ; Bright et al., 1982). The same mechanism might be involved in our tobacco LT^{r} mutants.

Few other plant cell lines have been selected for resistance to natural amino acids. The isolation of tobacco callus lines resistant to valine, methionine or threonine was recently reported (Maisuryan et al., 1982). Beside the growth inhibitions due to antagonisms between biosynthetically related amino acids, most amino acids were reported as inhibiting plant cell growth on nitrate as sole nitrogen source (Heimer and Filner, 1970 ; Behrend and Mateles, 1975). Heimer and Filner (1970) selected a tobacco cell line resistant to threonine-induced inhibition of growth on nitrate. Resistance was attributed to an altered regulation of nitrate uptake.

GENERAL CONCLUSIONS

Mesophyll protoplasts, a system for the isolation of plant cell mutants

Different types of tobacco mutant plants were obtained from protoplast-derived cells biochemically selected in vitro : at least i) one type which is resistant to lysine plus threonine, and ii) two types which are resistant to valine, one of which is also cross-resistant to other amino acids. For most putative mutant clones normal fertile plants were obtained, which allowed subsequent genetic analysis. This study thus amply confirms the usefulness of mesophyll protoplasts as a source of plant cells in the selection of biochemical mutants. Lately other types of mutants have been obtained from protoplast-derived cells : i) antibiotic resistants in *N. tabacum* (Maliga et al., 1980), ii) auxotrophs in *Hyoscyamus muticus* (Gebhart et al., 1981 ; Strauss et al., 1981) and in *N. plumbaginifolia* (Sidorov et al., 1981 ; Maliga et al., 1982 ; Márton et al., 1982 ; Sidorov and Maliga, 1982).

Valine resistance, a possible marker for estimating the efficiency of mutagenic treatments in plant cells

Selection for valine resistance has led to the isolation of two types of resistant mutants : cells of mutants of the Val^r-1 type display a low level of resistance, whereas cells of mutants of the Val^r-2 type display a high level of resistance. Availability of these markers allowed us to study the efficiency of selective procedures. Using the low cell density medium devised by Caboche (1980) we have carried out reconstruction experiments for determining the optimal conditions for recovery of rare Val^r cells among populations of wild type cells (Bourgin et al., 1980). Valine resistance of the Val^r-2 type is simple to select. Thus, even though it is a digenic character in tobacco, frequency of new valine resistant clones of the Val^r-2 type can be used as a criterion for estimating the efficiency of mutagenic procedures, and work has been engaged along this line in our group (Caboche and Muller, 1980 ; Grandbastien et al., unpublished results).

Possible uses of available Val^r markers for plant somatic cell genetics

The high level of resistance expressed by Val^r-2 cells appears to be very useful as an accessory marker, e.g. for recovering cells after their microinjection and co-culture with wild type, non-manipulated cells (Caboche, pers. comm.). Shillito et al. (1981) took a further advantage of the characteristics of Val^r-2 cells in the course of a study on the conditions for selection of auxotrophic plant cells. In the presence of valine, Val^r-2 cells continue to grow, whereas wild type cells become isoleucine requiring.

Val^r-2 seems inappropriate as a marker for somatic hybridization and transformation experiments since heterozygous (Val^r-2/+) cells were shown to display only slight resistance to valine (Bourgin et al., 1982). However, one might take advantage of this pseudo-recessiveness to recover homozygous Val^r-2 cells after manipulation of heterozygous cells. For instance, one can envisage employing such a selective scheme for estimating the efficiency of potentially haploidizing treatments (e.g. Katz and Sussman, 1972; Lo Schiavo et al., 1980). Otherwise, combined with the use of a cytoplasmic trait such as the streptomycin resistance selected by Maliga et al. (1973, 1975), one could adapt this selective scheme to the specific selection of a particular nucleo-cytoplasmic combination (Bourgin et al., in prep.).

Val^r-1, which is transmitted as a dominant trait, could theoretically be used to select somatic hybrid cells or cells modified through gene transfer mediated by protoplast fusion (Dudits et al., 1980) or transformation. However, due to the low level of expression of this trait by cultured cells, reconstruction experiments with Val^r-1 cells have shown that this recovery could only be obtained among cells cultured at a low density (between 500 and 1000 cells ml^{-1}). Obviously this would only be feasible if the efficiency of the genetic manipulation is high. Conversely, since valine resistance of Val^r-1 seedlings is quite high, it is tempting to use this marker for estimating the efficiency of the transformation procedure through X-irradiated pollen (Pandey, 1978; Pandey, 1980; Jinks et al., 1981).

ACKNOWLEDGEMENTS

I gratefully acknowledge the excellent assistance of M.C. Chupeau, C. Missonier, J. Goujaud and the helpful collaboration of J. Guern, C. Martin, and C. Pethe. I am also indebted to colleagues of the Laboratory for helpful discussions, in particular to D. Tepfer for critical reading of the English manuscript, and to the colleagues, who communicated pre-prints or other unpublished results. This work was supported in part by grants from the CNRS (ATP n° A 651-2610 and n° A 651-4109).

REFERENCES

Adelberg, E.A., Mandel, M., and Chen, C.C.G., 1965, Optimal conditions for mutagenesis by N-methyl-N'-nitro-N-nitrosoguanidine in *Escherichia coli* K-12, Biochim. Biophys. Res. Comm., 18: 788-795.

Aviv, D. and Galun, E., 1977a, Isolation of tobacco protoplasts in the presence of isopropyl N-phenylcarbamate and their culture and regeneration into plants, Z. Pflanzenphysiol., 83: 267-273

Aviv, D. and Galun, E., 1977b, An attempt at isolation of nutritional mutants from cultured tobacco protoplasts, Plant Sci. Lett. 8: 299-304.

Bayliss, M.W., 1980, Chromosomal variation in plant tissues in culture, in: "Perspectives in Plant Cell and Tissue Culture ", I.K. Vasil ed., Int. Rev. Cytol. suppl. 11, Academic Press, New York : pp 113-144.

Behrend, J. and Mateles, R.I., 1975, Nitrogen metabolism in plant cell suspension cultures. I. Effect of amino acids on growth, Plant Physiol., 56: 584-589.

Berlin, J. and Widholm, J.M., 1978, Amino acid uptake by amino acid analog resistant tobacco cell lines, Z. Naturforsch. 33c, 634-640

Borstlap, A.C., 1972, Changes in the free amino acids of *Spirodela polyrhiza* (L.) Schleiden during growth inhibition by L-valine, L-isoleucine, or L-leucine. A gas chromatographic study. Acta Bot. Neerl., 21: 404-416.

Borstlap, A.C., 1981, Interactions between the branched-chain amino acids in the growth of *Spirodela polyrhiza*, Planta, 151: 314-319

Bourgin, J.P., 1976, Valine-induced inhibition of growth of haploid tobacco protoplasts and its reversal by isoleucine, Z. Naturforsch., 31c: 337-338.

Bourgin, J.P., 1978, Valine-resistant plants from in vitro selected tobacco cells, Mol. Gen. Genet., 161: 225-230.

Bourgin, J.P., 1982, Isolement de mutants de tabac (*Nicotiana tabacum*) résistants à de fortes doses d'acides aminés à partir de cellules dérivées de protoplastes, Thèse, Université Pierre et Marie Curie, Paris: pp 1-122.

Bourgin, J.P. and Nitsch, J.P., 1967, Obtention de *Nicotiana* haploïdes à partir d'étamines cultivées in vitro, Ann. Physiol. vég., 9: 377-382.

Bourgin, J.P., Missonier, C., and Chupeau, Y., 1976, Culture de protoplastes de mésoplylle de *Nicotiana sylvestris* Spegazzini et Comes haploïde et diploïde, C.R. Acad. Sci. Paris, sér. D., 282: 1853-1856.

Bourgin, J.P. and Missonier, C., 1978, Culture de protoplastes de mésophylle de *Nicotiana alata* Link et Otto haploïde. Z. Pflanzenphysiol., 87: 55-64.

Bourgin, J.P., Chupeau, Y., and Missonier, C., 1979, Plant regeneration from mesophyll protoplasts of several *Nicotiana* species, Physiol. Plant., 45: 288-292.

Bourgin, J.P., Hommel, M.C., and Missonier, C., 1980, Expression of resistance to valine in protoplast-derived cells of tobacco mutants, in: "Plant Cell Cultures: Results and Perspectives", F. Sala, B. Parisi, R. Cella and O. Ciferri eds., Elsevier/North Holland Biomedical Press, Amsterdam: pp 167-177.

Bourgin, J.P., Chupeau M.C. and Missonier, C., 1982, Amino acid-resistant plants from tobacco cells cultured in vitro, in: "Regeneration of Plants from Cell and Tissue Culture and Genetic Variability", E.D. Earle and Y. Demarly eds., Proeger Publishers, New York, in press.

Bright, S.W.J., Miflin, B.J., and Rognes, S.E., 1982, Threonine accumulation in the seeds of a barley mutant with an altered aspartate kinase, Biochem. Genet., 20: 229-244.

Bryan, J.K., 1980, Synthesis of the aspartate family and branched-chain amino acids, in: "The Biochemistry of Plants, P.K. Stumpf and E.E. Conn eds., Vol. 5, Amino Acids and Derivatives, B.J. Miflin ed., Academic Press. New York: pp 403-452.
Caboche, M., 1980, Nutritional requirements of protoplast-derived, haploid tobacco cells grown at low cell densities in liquid medium, Planta, 149: 7-18.
Caboche, M. and Muller, J.F., 1980, Use of a medium allowing low cell density growth for in vitro selection experiments: isolation of valine-resistant clones from nitrosoguanidine-mutagenized cells and gamma-irradiated tobacco plants, in: "Plant Cell Cultures: Results and Perspectives", F. Sala, B. Parisi, R. Cella and O. Ciferri eds., Elsevier/North Holland Biomedical Press, Amsterdam: pp 133-138.
Carlson, P.S., 1970, Induction and isolation of auxotrophic mutants in somatic cell cultures of *Nicotiana tabacum*, Science, 168: 487-489.
Carlson, P.S., 1973, The use of protoplasts for genetic research, Proc. Nat. Acad. Sci. U.S., 70: 598-602.
Chaleff, R.S. and Carlson, P.S., 1975, In vitro selection for mutants of higher plants, in: "Genetic manipulations with plant material", L. Ledoux ed., Plenum Press, New York: pp 351-363.
Chaleff, R.S. and Keil, R.L., 1981, Genetic and physiological variability among cultured cells and regenerated plants of *Nicotiana tabacum*, Mol. Gen. Genet. 181: 254-258.
Chupeau, Y. Bourgin J.P., Missonier, C, Dorion, N., and Morel, G., 1974, Préparation et culture de protoplastes de divers *Nicotiana* C.R. Acad. Sc. Paris, Sér. D, 278: 1565-1568.
Clausen, R.E. and Cameron, D.R., 1950, Inheritance in *Nicotiana tabacum*. XXIII. Duplicate factors for chlorophyll production, Genetics 35: 4-10.
De Felice, M., Levinthal, M., Iaccarino, M., and Guardiola, J., 1979, Growth inhibition as a consequence of antagonism between related amino acids: effect of valine in *Escherichia coli* K-12, Microb. Rev., 43: 42-58.
Dudits, D., Fejér, O., Hadlaczky, G., Koncz, C., Lázár, G.B., and Horvath, G., 1980, Intergeneric gene transfer mediated by plant protoplast fusion, Mol. Gen. Genet., 179: 283-288
Eapen, S., 1976, Effect of gamma- and ultraviolet-irradiation on survival and totipotency of haploid tobacco cells in culture, Protoplasma, 89: 149-155.
Eriksson, T. 1967, Effects of ultraviolet and X-ray radiation on in vitro cultivated cells of *Haplopappus gracilis*, Physiol. Plant., 20: 507-518.
Evans, D.A., 1979, Chromosome stability of plants regenerated from mesophyll protoplasts of *Nicotiana* species, Z. Pflanzenphysiol., 95: 459-463.
Evans, D.A. and Gamborg, O.L., 1979, Effects of para-fluorophenylalanine on ploidy levels of cell suspension cultures of *Datura innoxia*, Environ. Exp. Bot., 19: 269-275.
Furner, I.J., King, J., and Gamborg, O.L., 1978, Plant regeneration from protoplasts isolated from a predominantly haploid suspension culture of *Datura innoxia* (Mil.), Plant Sci. Lett., 11: 169-176

Gebhardt, C., Schnebli, V., and King, P.J., 1981, Isolation of biochemical mutants using haploid mesophyll protoplasts of *Hyoscyamus muticus*. II. Auxotrophic and temperature-sensitive clones, Planta, 153: 81-89.

Glimelius, K., Eriksson, T., Grafe, R., and Müller, A.J., 1978, Somatic hybridization of nitrate-reductase-deficient mutants of *Nicotiana tabacum* by protoplast fusion, Physiol. Plant., 44: 273-277.

Green, C.E. and Phillips, R.L., 1976, Potential selection system for mutants with increased lysine, threonine, and methionine in cereal crops, Crop Sci., 14: 827-830.

Guardiola, J. and Iaccarino, M., 1971, *Escherichia coli* K-12 mutants altered in the transport of branched-chain amino acids, J. Bacteriol., 108., 1034-1044.

Harms, C.T., Potrykus, I., and Widholm, J., 1981, Complementation and dominant expression of amino acid analogue resistance markers in somatic hybrid clones from *Daucus carota* after protoplast fusion, Z. Pflanzenphysiol., 101: 377-390.

Heimer, Y.M. and Filner, P., 1970, Regulation of the nitrate assimilation pathway of cultured tobacco cells. II. Properties of a variant cell line, Biochim. Biophys. Acta, 215: 152-165

Hibberd, K.A., Walter, T., Green, C.E., and Gengenbach, B.G., 1980, Selection and characterization of a feedback-insensitive tissue culture of maize, Planta, 148 : 183-187.

Horsch, R.B., 1979, Somatic plant cell genetics: a model system using cultured plant cells of *Haplopappus gracilis*, Thesis, University of California, Riverside: pp 1-91.

Howland, G.P. and Hart, R.W., 1977, Radiation biology of cultured plant cells, in: "Applied and Fundamental Aspects of Plant Tissue Culture", J. Reinert and Y.P.S. Bajaj eds., Springer-Verlag, Berlin and New York: pp 731-735.

Jinks, J.L., Caligari, P.D.S., and Ingram, N.R., 1981, Gene transfer in *Nicotiana rustica* using irradiated pollen, Nature, 291: 586-588.

Katz, E.R. and Sussman, M., 1972, Parasexual recombination in *Dictyostelium discoideum*: selection of stable diploid heterozygotes and stable haploid segregants. Proc. Natl. Acad. Sci. US., 69: 495-498.

Krens, F.A., Molendijk, L., Wullems, G.J., and Schilperoort, R.A., 1982, In vitro transformation of plant protoplasts with Ti-plasmid DNA, Nature, 296: 72-74.

Krumbiegel, G., 1979. Response of haploid and diploid protoplasts from *Datura innoxia* Mill. and *Petunia hybrida* L. to treatment with X-rays and a chemical mutagen. Environ. Exp. Bot., 19: 99-103.

Lázár, G.B., Dudits, D., and Sung, Z.R., 1981, Expression of cycloheximide resistance in carrot somatic hybrids and their segregants, Genetics, 98: 347-356.

Lo Schiavo, F., Nuti Ronchi, V. and Terzi, M., 1980, Genetic effects of griseofulvin on plant cell cultures, Theor. Appl. Genet., 58: 43-47.

Lurquin, P.F. and Sheehy, R.E., 1982, Binding of large liposomes to plant protoplasts and delivery of encapsulated DNA, Plant Sci. Lett., 25: 133-146.

Magnien, E. and Devreux, M., 1980, A critical assessment of the protoplast system as a tool for radiosensitivity studies, in: "Plant Cell Cultures : Results and Perspectives", F. Sala,

B. Parisi, R. Cella, and O. Ciferri eds., Elsevier/North Holland Biomedical Press, Amsterdam: pp 121-126.

Magnien, E., Dalschaert, X., and Devreux, M., 1980, Different radiosensitivities of *Nicotiana plumbaginifolia* leaves and regenerating protoplasts, Plant Sci. lett., 19: 231-241.

Maisuryan, A.N., Khadeeva, N.V., and Pogosov, V.Z., 1982, Isolation of tobacco cell lines resistant to high concentrations of amino acids, Soviet Plant Physiol., 28: 561-564.

Maliga, P., 1978, Resistance mutants and their use in genetic manipulation. in: "Frontiers of Plant Tissue Culture", University of Calgary Press, Calgary, Alberta: pp 381-392.

Maliga, P., 1980, Isolation, characterization, and utilization of mutant cell lines in higher plants, in: "Perspectives in Plant Cell and Tissue Culture", I.K. Vasil ed., Int. Rev. Cytol. suppl. 11A, Academic Press, New York: pp 225-250.

Maliga, P., Sz-Breznovits, A., and Márton, L., 1973, Streptomycin-resistant plants from callus culture of haploid tobacco, Nature, New Biol., 244: 29-30.

Maliga, P., Sz-Breznovits, A., Márton, L., and Joó, F., 1975, Non-mendelian streptomycin-resistant tobacco mutant with altered chloroplasts and mitochondria, Nature, 225: 401-402.

Maliga, P., Xuan, L.T., Dix, P.J., and Cséplő, A., 1980, Antibiotic resistance in *Nicotiana* in: "Plant Cell Cultures : Results and Perspectives", F. Sala, B. Parisi, R. Cella and O. Ciferri eds., Elsevier/North-Holland Biomedical Press, Amsterdam: pp 161-166.

Maliga, P., Menczel, L., Sidorov, V., Márton L., Cséplő, A., Medgyesy, P., Dung, T.M., Lázár, G., and Nagy, F. 1982, Cell culture mutants and their uses, in : "Plant Improvement and Somatic Cell Genetics', I.K. Vasil, K.J. Frey, and W.R. Scowcroft eds., Academic Press, New York : in press.

Márton, L., Dung, T.M., Mendel, R.R., Maliga, P., 1982, Nitrate reductase deficient cell lines from haploid protoplast cultures of *Nicotiana plumbaginifolia*, Mol. Gen. Genet., in press.

Melchers, G., 1975, Genetik und Pflanzenzüchtung mit mikrobiologischen Methoden, Planta Medica, Suppl., Hippokrates Verlag, Stuttgart: pp 5-34.

Meyer, Y. and Cooke, R., 1979, Time course of hormonal control of the first mitosis in tobacco mesophyll protoplasts cultivated in vitro, Planta, 147: 181-185.

Miflin, B.J., 1969, The inhibitory effects of various amino acids on the growth of barley seedlings, J. exp. Bot., 20: 810-819.

Miflin, B.J., 1973, Amino acid biosynthesis and its control in plants, in: "Biosynthesis and its control in plants", B.V. Milborrow ed., Academic Press, New-York: pp 49-68.

Müller, A.J. and Grafe, R., 1978, Isolation and characterization of cell lines of *Nicotiana tabacum* lacking nitrate reductase. Mol. Gen. Genet., 161: 67-76.

Murashige, T. and Nakano, R., 1967, Chromosome complement as a determinant of the morphogenic potential of tobacco cells, Am. J. Bot., 54: 963-970.

Nagata, T. and Takebe, I., 1971, Plating of isolated tobacco mesophyll protoplasts on agar medium, Planta, 99: 12-20.

Nasim, A., Hannan, M.A., and Nestmann, E.R., 1981, Pure and mosaic clones - A reflection of differences in mechanisms of mutagenesis by different agents in *Saccharomyces cerevisiae*, Can. J. Genet. Cytol., 23: 73-79

Negrutiu, I., 1981, Improved conditions for large-scale culture, mutagenesis, and selection of haploid protoplasts of *Nicotiana plumbaginifolia* Viviani, Z. Pflanzenphysiol., 104: 431-442

Nitsch, J.P. and Nitsch, C., 1969, Haploid plants from pollen grains, Science, 163: 85-87.

Nitsch, J.P. and Ohyama, K., 1971, Obtention de plantes à partir de protoplastes haploïdes cultivés in vitro, C.R. Acad. Sc. Paris, sér. D, 273: 801-804.

Ogura, H., 1976, The cytological chimeras in original regenerates from tobacco tissue cultures and in their offsprings, Jap. J. Genet., 51: 161-174.

Pandey, K.K., 1978. Gametic gene transfer in *Nicotiana* by means of irradiated pollen, Genetica, 49: 53-69.

Pandey, K.K., 1980, Further evidence for egg transformation in *Nicotiana*, Heredity, 45: 15-29.

Pental, D., Cooper-Bland, S., Harding, K., Cocking, E.C., and Müller, A.J. 1982, Cultural studies on nitrate reductase deficient *Nicotiana tabacum* mutant protoplasts, Z. Pflanzenphysiol., 105: 219-227.

Pfahler, P.L. and Linskens, H.F., 1977, Ultraviolet irradiation of maize (*Zea mays* L.) pollen grains. II. Pollen genotype effects on plant characteristics, Theor. Appl. Genet., 50 : 17-21.

Rashid, A. and Street H.A., 1974, Growth, embryogenic potential and stability of a haploid cell culture of *Atropa belladonna* L., Plant Sci. Lett., 2: 89-94.

Schieder, O., 1976, Isolation of mutants with altered pigments after irradiating haploid protoplasts from *Datura innoxia* Mill. with X-rays. Mol. Gen. Genet., 149: 251-254.

Shillito, R.D., Street, H.E., and Schilperoort, R.A., 1981, Model system studies of the use of 5-bromo-2'-deoxyuridine for selection of deficient mutants in plant cell suspension and protoplast cultures, Mutation Res., 81: 165-175.

Sidorov, V.A., Menczel, L., and Maliga, P., 1981, Isoleucine-requiring *Nicotiana* plant deficient in threonine deaminase, Nature, 294: 87-88.

Sidorov, V.A. and Maliga, P., 1982, Fusion-complementations analysis of auxotrophic and chlorophyll-deficient lines isolated in haploid *Nicotiana plumbaginifolia* protoplast cultures, Theor. Appl. Genet., in press.

Smith, H.H., 1968, Recent cytogenetic studies in the genus *Nicotiana* Adv. Genet., 14: 1-54.

Smith, S. and Street H.E., 1974, The decline of embryogenic potential as callus and suspension cultures of carrot (*Daucus carota* L.) are serially subcultured, Ann. Bot., 38: 223-241.

Stadler, L.J. and Sprague, G.F., 1936. Genetic effects of ultraviolet radiation in maize, Proc. Natl. Acad. Sci.U.S., 22: 572-591.

Steinberg, R.A., 1959, Comparison of daylength and temperature responses in *Nicotiana* and its taxonomic sections, Am. J. Bot., 46: 261-268.

Stines, B.J. and Mann, T.J., 1960, Diploidization in *Nicotiana tabacum*. A study of the yellow burley character, J. Hered., 51: 222-227.

Strauss, A., Bucher, F., and King, P.J., 1981, Isolation of biochemical mutants using haploid mesophyll protoplasts of *Hyoscyamus muticus* I. A NO_3^- non-utilizing clone, Planta, 153: 75-80.
Sunderland, N., 1973, Nuclear cytology, in: "Plant Tissue and Cell Culture", H.E. Street ed., Blackwell Scientific Publications, Oxford : pp 161-190.
Sung, Z.R., 1976, Mutagenesis of cultured plant cells, Genetics, 84: 51-57.
Thomas, E., King, P.J., and Potrykus, I., 1979, Improvement of crop plants via single cells in vitro, Z. Pflanzenzüchtg. 82: 1-30.
Umbarger, H.E., 1969, Regulation of the biosynthesis of the branched-chain amino acids, Curr. Top. Cell Regul. 1: 57-76.
Vanzulli, L., Magnien, E., and Olivi, L., 1980, Caryological stability of *Datura innoxia* calli analysed by cytophotometry for 22 hormonal combinations, Plant Sci. Lett., 17: 181-192.
White, D.W.R., and Vasil, I.K., 1979, Use of amino acid analogue-resistant cell lines for selection of *Nicotiana sylvestris* somatic cell hybrids, Theor. Appl. Genet., 55: 107-112.
Widholm, J., 1976, Selection and characterization of cultured carrot and tobacco cells resistant to lysine, methionine, and proline analogs, Can. J. Bot., 54: 1523-1529
Widholm, J., 1977a, Selection and characterization of amino acid analog resistant plant cell cultures, Crop Sci., 17: 597-600.
Widholm, J.M., 1977b, Selection and characterization of biochemical mutants, in: "Plant Tissue Culture and its Biotechnological Application". W. Barz, E. Reinhard and M.H. Zenk eds., Springer-Verlag, Berlin and New York: pp 112-122.
Widholm, J.M., 1977c, Isolation of biochemical mutants of cultured plant cells. in: "Molecular genetic modification of eucaryotes" I. Rubenstein, R.L. Phillips, C.E. Green and R. Desnick eds. Academic Press, New York: pp 57-64.
Withers, L.A. and Cocking, E.C., 1972, Fine structural studies on spontaneous and induced fusion of higher plant protoplasts, J. Cell Sci., 11: 59-75.
Wright, L.A. and Murphy, T.M., 1978, Ultraviolet radiation-stimulated efflux of 86-rubidium from cultured tobacco cells, Plant Physiol., 61: 434-436.
Yeoman, M.M. and Street, H.E., 1973. General cytology of cultured cells, in : "Plant Tissue and Cell Culture", H.E. Street ed., Blackwell Scientific Publications, Oxford: pp 121-160.
Zelcer, A. and Galun, E., 1980, Culture of newly isolated tobacco protoplasts: cell division and precursor incorporation following a transient exposure to coumarin, Plant Sci. Lett., 18: 185-190.

NITRATE REDUCTASE GENES AS SELECTABLE MARKERS FOR PLANT CELL TRANSFORMATION

A. Kleinhofs, J. Taylor, T. M. Kuo, D. A. Somers and
R. L. Warner

Department of Agronomy and Soils and
Program in Genetics and Cell Biology
Washington State University
Pullman, Washington 99164-6420

Plant cell transformation, when finally established, will probably differ little from other eukaryotic systems such as fungi and animal cells. Assuming the accuracy of this statement, we presumed that the major factors delaying the establishment of a reliable plant cell transformation system are the lack of suitable selectable markers and the corresponding gene(s) in appropriate vectors. In order to rectify this situation, we undertook the establishment of a plant cell transformation system using nitrate reductase as the central component.

There are both advantages and disadvantages to the use of nitrate reductase (NR) as a model for plant cell transformation. The major advantage of this system is the availability of conditional lethal mutants and the major disadvantage is the lack of cloned and characterized NR genes. When we initiated this work, NR-deficient higher plant mutants had been described only in *Arabidopsis thaliana* (Oostindier-Braaksma, 1973). Today such mutants have been described in at least seven different higher plant species (Table 1) and should be possible in most higher plants. In this paper we describe in some detail our work with the *Hordeum vulgare* NR-deficient mutants and briefly review the NR mutants from other species. However, there has been only limited progress in the cloning of NR genes. A few of the *Escherichia coli* NR genes have been cloned but have not yet been fully characterized. We also report herein our work with the *chlM* (previously *chlA* in mutant SA493) gene cloned from *E. coli*. This gene codes for a still undefined activity in the NR molybdenum cofactor (MoCo) synthesis or function.

Table 1

Nitrate reductase-deficient mutants isolated in higher plants.

Genus species	References
Arabidopsis thaliana	Oostindier-Braaksma and Feenstra, 1973
Hordeum vulgare	Warner et al., 1977; Tokarev and Shumny, 1977; Kleinhofs et al., 1980
Nicotiana tabacum	Mendel and Müller, 1976
Pisum sativum	Kleinhofs et al., 1978; Feenstra and Jacobsen, 1980; Warner et al., 1982
Datura innoxia	King and Khanna, 1980
Nicotiana plumbaginifolia	Marton et al., 1982a
Hyoscyamus muticus	Strauss et al., 1981

Nitrate Reductase Structure

Nitrate reductase catalyzes the initial controlling step in nitrate assimilation, reducing nitrate to nitrite. Nitrite is reduced to ammonium by nitrite reductase and ammonium is assimilated into amino acids. Our first objective was to purify and characterize the NR from *H. vulgare* (Kuo et al., 1980; Somers et al., 1982a). Barley NR has a native molecular weight of 221,000 and can use NADH, $FMNH_2$ and reduced methyl viologen but not NADPH as electron donors for nitrate reduction. It also possesses a NADH-cytochrome c reductase activity. Although it was possible to obtain small amounts of pure NR by affinity chromatography, preparative scale isolation resulted in contaminated preparations. Among the 5-6 protein bands resolved by native polyacrylamide gel electrophoresis, a major slow running protein band was identified as NR by staining for reduced methyl viologen NR activity, NO_2^- production and diaphorase activity (Fig. 1A, band 1). Second dimension SDS-polyacrylamide gel electrophoresis (PAGE) of the native gel or excision of the NR band followed by SDS-PAGE demonstrated a single protein band of 110kDa (Fig. 1B). These data show that the barley NR subunit molecular weight is 110,000 daltons and that the native polyacrylamide purified NR is homogeneous. Thus, barley NR appears to be composed of two identical subunits and is similar to *Neuro-*

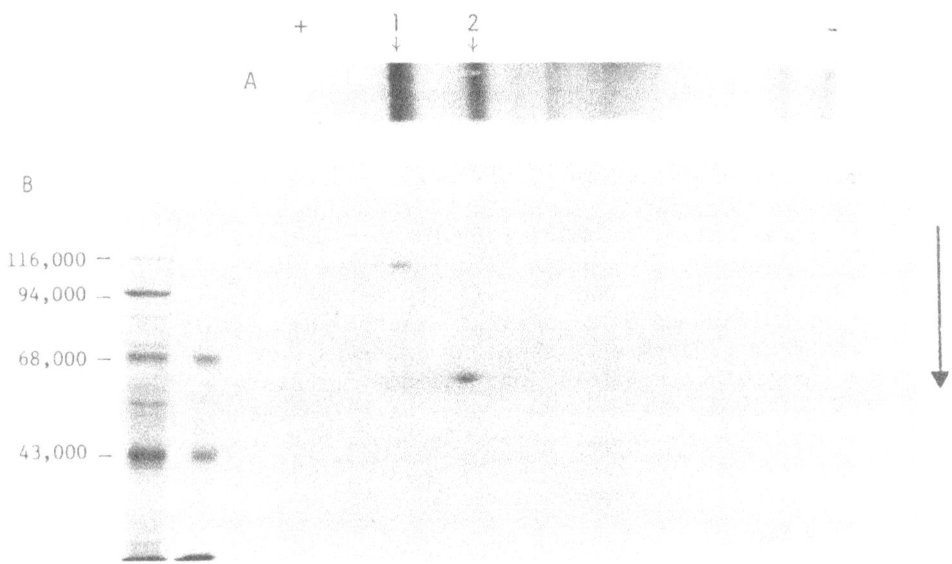

Figure 1. A. Affinity purified barley NR was separated by native gel electrophoresis and stained for MVH-NR, NO_2^- production, diaphorase activity and protein. Protein band 1 was associated with all three enzymatic activities while protein band 2 was stained positive only for diaphorase activity. B. Second dimension SDS gel electrophoresis of an activity stained native gel electrophoresis slice. The molecular weight markers were: ß-galactosidase, 116,000; phosphorylase b, 94,000; bovine serum albumin, 68,000; ovalbumin, 43,000; carbonic anhydrolase, 30,000.

spora crassa (Pan and Nason, 1978) and Rhodotorula glutinis (Guerrero and Gutierrez, 1977) NRs.

It has been suggested by others that NR is made up of multiple subunits (Small and Wray, 1980; Notton and Hewitt, 1979; Downey and Steiner, 1979) but our data and that of others argue for a single NR subunit (Solomonson et al., 1975; Giri and Ramadoss, 1979; De la Rosa et al., 1981; Pan and Nason, 1978; Guerrero and Gutierrez, 1979). The genetic analyses performed with numerous organisms (to be discussed later) also argues for a single NR subunit. Some of the observed protein subunit heterogeneity is probably due to either contaminating proteins or due to proteolytic breakdown of NR. To differentiate between these possibilities in preparations of affinity purified barley NR containing multiple bands on SDS-PAGE, we submitted the various protein bands resolved by SDS-PAGE to Cleveland mapping analysis (Kuo et al., 1982). The data clearly showed that the other protein bands are not related to NR and, therefore, are contaminants rather than NR breakdown products.

The purification of the barley NR to homogeneity was important for the preparation of monospecific antiserum (Kuo et al., 1981; Somers et al., 1982b). Monospecificity of the antiserum was demonstrated by the formation of a single rocket when either affinity gel purified NR or crude barley seedling extracts were subjected to crossed immunoelectrophoresis and stained for protein (Fig. 2A and B). This antiserum was used to study the NR antigen in NR-deficient mutants and to study the relationship among NRs from diverse higher plant species.

Molybdenum Cofactor

The existence of a molybdenum cofactor (MoCo) common to the molybdoenzymes, NR and xanthine dehydrogenase, was first postulated by Pateman et al. (1964). This work was extended by Nason's group who showed that the MoCo obtained from various sources, except nitrogenase (Pienkos et al., 1977; Kiss et al., 1979), could be used to reconstitute NR activity in the *nit-1* *Neurospora crassa* MoCo mutant extracts (Nason et al., 1970, 1971; Ketchum et al., 1970). The *N. crassa* *nit-1* NR reconstitution provides a convenient assay for the biological activity of MoCo. This has been exploited to study MoCo from the *E. coli* wild type and *chl* mutants (Amy and Rajogopalan, 1979; Amy, 1981), and from the *Nicotiana tabacum* *cnx* 68 mutant (Mendel et al., 1981). We have adapted this assay to investigate the *E. coli* *chl* mutant MoCos by NR reconstitution in the *N. tabacum* mutant *cnx* 68 (discussed later).

In spite of the biological characterization of the MoCo, the actual nature of the MoCo is still unclear. It appears to be a low molecular weight (ca. 1000) molecule (Lee et al., 1974; Amy and Rajagopalan, 1979) that is highly sensitive to oxygen (Pienkos et al., 1977). The low molecular weight molecule is insensitive to trypsin, but is associated with a carrier molecule, presumably a protein, of ca. 40 kDa from which it is easily removed by dialysis. The carrier molecule provides protection of the cofactor from inactivation by heat or oxygen (Amy and Rajagopalan, 1979). Johnson et al. (1980) identified the structural component of the cofactor as a novel pteridine.

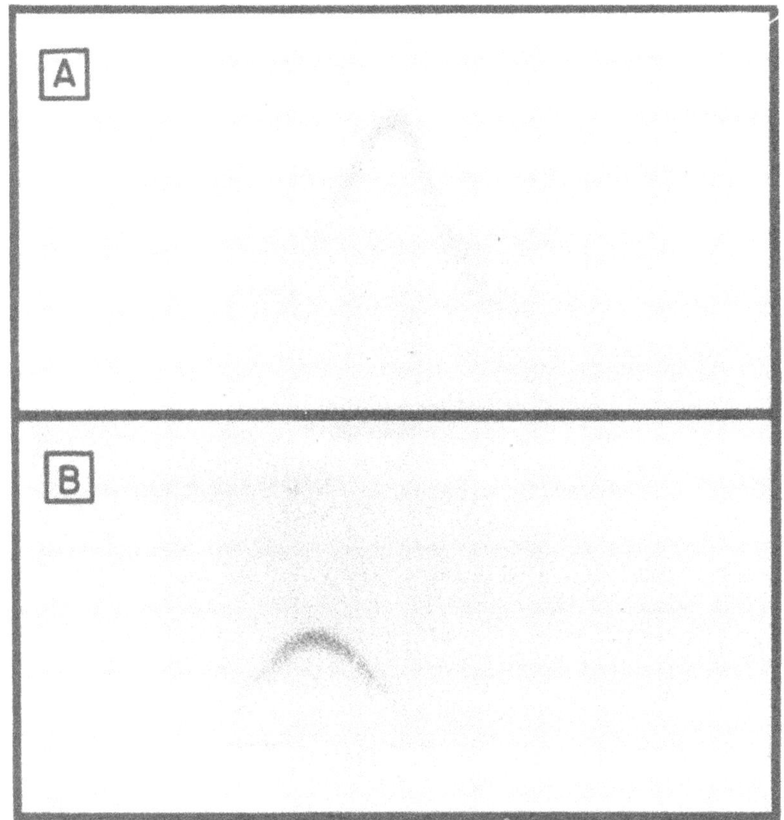

Figure 2. Barley NR was separated by electrophoresis in 1% agarose, immunoelectrophoresed in the second dimension in 0.8% agarose gels containing antiserum (0.3% in A and 0.4% in B) and stained for protein. A. Affinity purified barley NR (0.006 units NR). B. Crude wild type barley extract (0.005 units NR).

Some insight into the MoCo has been gained from genetic studies. MoCo mutants are typically characterized as such if they show a pleiotropic loss of two or more molybdoenzyme activities. Three loci have been identified in E. coli (Amy, 1981), five in A. nidulans (Cove, 1979), and four in N. crassa (Tomsett and Garrett, 1980) that affect MoCo functions. These mutants seem to be involved with the MoCo synthesis, activation or insertion. Other functions are also possible. In A. nidulans, the cnx H MoCo mutant has been implicated as contribution to the structure of the NR protein based on its temperature sensitive nature and the production of an unstable NR (MacDonald and Cove, 1974).

Nitrate Reductase-Deficient Mutants in Higher Plants

The first NR-deficient mutants in higher plants were obtained by Oostindier-Braaksma and Feenstra (1973) in *Arabidopsis*. Ethylmethane sulfonate or N-nitro-N-methyl-guanosine mutagenized M_2 seedlings were selected in petri dishes on 2.2 mM chlorate. Among the chlorate resistant seedlings were mutants defective in nitrate reductase and mutants that had lost their ability to take up chlorate. To date, ten chlorate resistant NR-defective mutants have been partially characterized (Braaksma, 1982). These mutants represent seven different loci located on three different chromosomes. Mutants B25 and B73 are probably MoCo mutants while B2-1 and B29 have been suggested as possible structural gene mutants. Mutants B36 and B40 have almost 50% of wild type NR activity and their biochemical nature is not understood at this time.

In our laboratory we have isolated NR-deficient mutants in azide mutagenized barley (Kleinhofs et al., 1978) by a rapid in vivo assay procedure on M_2 seedlings (Warner et al., 1977; Kleinhofs et al., 1980). In this procedure seedling leaves or leaf pieces are vacuum infiltrated with a nitrate containing buffer and incubated in the dark for 30 min. The presence of nitrite is detected by the standard colorimetric assay. Wild-type seedlings produce bright purple-red color while NR-deficient mutant seedlings fail to give a color reaction due to the absence of nitrite.

We have extensively characterized ten mutants which represent two loci (Table 2). Nine mutants are allelic and were assigned the gene designation *nar* 1. The remaining mutant was designated *nar* 2. Since *nar* 2 lacks xanthine dehydrogenase activity as well as NR activity, it is presumed to be a MoCo mutant. Three additional NR-deficient barley mutants isolated by Tokarev and Shumny (1977) after ethylmethane sulfonate mutagenesis and selection for chlorate resistance have been investigated. The mutants Xno 18 and Xno 19 are allelic to one another (Shumny and Tokarev, 1982) and not allelic to *nar* 1 or *nar* 2, therefore, we propose this locus be designated *nar* 3. These mutants are also xanthine dehydrogenase deficient and therefore, MoCo mutants (Somers et al., 1982b). The mutant Xno 29 is allelic to *nar* 1 and constitutes the tenth allele at this locus and is designated *nar* 1j. The NR, NR associated catalytic activities ($FMNH_2$-NR and NADH-cytochrome c reductase), xanthine dehydrogenase and nitrite reductase activities of these mutants and the two parent wild types are summarized in Table 2. Some of the interesting things to note are that all of the mutants, except Xno 29 (*nar* 1j) have elevated nitrite reductase activities and that there is substantial variability in the NR-associated catalytic activities among the *nar* 1 alleles. Particularly exceptional are the mutants *nar* 1d (very high NADH CR activity) and *nar* 1h (high $FMNH_2$ NR activity). The presence of these NR-associated activities in some *nar* 1 alleles suggested to us that

Table 2

Characteristics of nitrate reductase-deficient barley mutants.

Selection Number	Gene Designation	NR* NADH	NR* $FMNH_2$	CR*	NiR*	XDH*
		% of Control				
Az 12	nar 1a	0.8	0	7	174	+
Az 13	nar 1b	0.7	0	61	174	+
Az 23	nar 1c	0.9	0	16	164	+
Az 28	nar 1d	1.5	0	227	193	+
Az 29	nar 1e	1.1	0	13	119	+
Az 30	nar 1f	1.6	0	8	191	+
Az 31	nar 1g	2.5	0	68	147	+
Az 32	nar 1h	1.7	167	10	156	+
Az 33	nar 1i	1.0	0	71	180	+
Xno 29	nar 1j	12.0	0	38	104	+
Az 34	nar 2a	5.5	0	64	170	-
Xno 18	nar 3a	5.3	0	86	127	-
Xno 19	nar 3b	4.3	0	93	128	-
		μmoles, gfw^{-1}, h^{-1}				
Steptoe		33.1	29.8	278	261	+
Viner		29.9	35.4	270	227	+

*NR, nitrate reductase; CR, cytochrome c reductase; NiR nitrite reductase; XDH, xanthine dehydrogenase.

a protein defective in NADH NR must be present in these mutants. This was confirmed by antigenicity studies (Kuo et al., 1981; Somers et al., 1982b). Data obtained with either NR protection assay (Kuo et al., 1981) or direct rocket immunoelectrophoresis (Somers et al.,

1982) showed that all of the mutants had NR antigen present although some (nar 1a, nar 1e, nar 1f) had very low levels (Table 3). Based upon the rocket immunoelectrophoresis data, the mutants could be subdivided into two discrete groups, i.e. those that produced rockets directly and those that produced rockets only when small quantities of partially purified NR was added to the mutant extracts (+NR). We interpret this to indicate that those mutants requiring added NR to produce a precipitate with the NR antiserum must possess a structurally altered antigen. Note that all of the mutants fitting into this category are nar 1 alleles. These data, taken together, led us to conclude that nar 1 is the barley NR structural gene. Further support for the structural role of the nar 1 locus is provided by our preliminary data indicating that the nar 1d NADH CR contains a glutamic acid substitution when compared to the wild-type NR by Cleveland mapping using Streptococcus aureus V8 protease.

Table 3

Antigenicity and nitrate reductase crossreacting materials (NR CRM) in nitrate reductase-deficient barley mutants. NR CRM was determined by rocket immunoelectrophoresis in the presence (+NR) and absence (-NR) of wild-type NR. Antigenicity reflects the relative ability of crude extracts to prevent the inactivation of wild-type NR by NR specific antiserum.

Selection Number	Gene Designation	NR CRM -NR	NR CRM +NR	Antigenicity
Group I				
Az 12	nar 1a	0	11	4
Az 13	nar 1b	0	38	64
Az 23	nar 1c	0	29	18
Az 29	nar 1e	0	8	3
Az 30	nar 1f	0	8	4
Az 31	nar 1g	0	46	77
Az 33	nar 1i	0	28	49
Group II				
Az 28	nar 1d	136	128	138
Az 32	nar 1h	128	137	125
Az 34	nar 2a	32	43	46
Xno 18	--	54	67	--
Xno 19	--	51	47	--
Xno 29	--	20	20	--

Physiology of NR-Deficient Barley Mutants

The NR-deficient structural gene (nar 1) mutants in barley examined to date grow perfectly well in soil in the field or greenhouse; or in aseptic culture (Table 4) with nitrate as the sole source of nitrogen (Oh et al., 1980; Warner and Kleinhofs, 1981). These data demonstrate the presence of alternate pathway(s) for nitrate reduction in barley. One possible alternative pathway was indicated by the discovery that the nar 1 mutants contain low levels of a NAD(P)H bispecific NR (Dailey et al., 1982a). This enzyme was not found in the wild-type barley seedlings (Dailey et al., 1982b). To further characterize this system, we have attempted to select NADPH NR-deficient mutants. Mutant nar 1a seed were treated with sodium azide and M_2 seedlings completely devoid of NR activity were selected. To date, we have confirmed and partly characterized three mutants. These mutants grow very poorly on nitrate as the sole nitrogen source and are deficient in xanthine dehydrogenase activity, thus they are probably MoCo mutants. It is noteworthy that the MoCo mutants in general do not grow well on nitrate as the sole nitrogen source. This is particularly true with these new mutants and with mutants Xno 18 (nar 3a) and Xno 19 (nar 3b) (Shumny and Tokarev, 1982). The nar 2a mutant does grow on nitrate, but not as well as the wild type nor nar 1 mutants, which is probably due to its somewhat leaky nature. We have observed that nar 2a will develop increased NR activity with age perhaps due to accumulation of MoCo with time. The failure of MoCo mutants to grow on nitrate as the sole nitrogen source is consistant with the hypothesis that the NAD(P)H bispecific NR

Table 4

Growth in sterile culture of isolated embryos from wild type and nitrate reductase-deficient mutants with nitrate as the nitrogen source.

Genotype	Nitrate (mM) 0	2	5	10	60
	dry wt./seedling*				
Steptoe	5.5	12.4	18.5	21.0	24.6
nar 1a	8.5	8.8	10.7	19.2	25.7
nar 1b	6.1	13.2	13.2	17.8	24.9

*Seedlings were grown for 21 days at 20°C and 16 hr photoperiod (Warner and Kleinhofs, 1981).

accounts for the nitrate reduction observed in the nar 1 mutants and the presumption that all NRs would use the same MoCo.

Cell Culture NR-Deficient Mutants

The whole plant mutants investigated by Braaksma (1982) in Arabidopsis and by our laboratory in barley are very suitable for genetic and physiological studies. However, present day technology for DNA transfer to plant cells is dependent upon the use of protoplasts. It has not been possible to culture Hordeum protoplasts to date. Fortunately, Müller and coworkers have isolated NR-deficient mutants in an amphihaploid Nicotiana tabacum cell culture line using chlorate as a selective agent (Müller and Grafe, 1978; Mendel and Müller, 1979). Two types of mutants, i.e. nia and cnx, presumed NR structural gene and MoCo mutants respectively, have been characterized. These mutant cells do not grow on nitrate as the sole nitrogen source and thus provide strict selection for nitrate utilization (Glimelius et al., 1978). Additional NR-deficient mutants have been produced in N. tabacum by S. Evola (personal communication) and in N. plumbaginifolia by Maliga and coworkers (Marton et al., 1982a, b and these proceedings) and in Hyoscyamus muticus by (King and Khanna, 1980; Shillito, these proceedings). These mutants represent the NR structural gene and several MoCo-deficient genes and promise to be highly useful for future gene transfer experiments.

We have investigated the potential for the transfer of an E. coli MoCo gene(s) to the N. tabacum cell culture mutant cnx 68. As discussed previously, it has been known for some time that the MoCo from widely divergent phylogenic sources can function to restore NR activity in the N. crassa nit-1 mutant extracts. Therefore, we presumed that the E. coli MoCo should function to restore the NR activity in the N. tabacum cnx68 mutant. In order to test this hypothesis and to determine which E. coli chl gene was the desired one, we performed in vitro reconstitution experiments using the E. coli wild type and chl mutant extracts with the N. tabacum cnx 68 mutant extract. The data confirmed that the E. coli MoCo can function with the plant NR apoprotein in vitro to produce an active NR complex. We also identified chlA as the most likely gene to perform the critical function lacking in the cnx 68 mutant (Table 5).

Cloning and Characterization of the E. coli chlA gene

The E. coli chlA gene was cloned on a large cosmid and selected for its ability to revert the mutant SA493 to NR^+. This plasmid, designated pJT1, was subcloned by Hae II deletion to a 10.8 kb plasmid designated pJT13 (Fig. 3). Characterization of the pJT13 clone showed that it was able to restore wild type functions to the chlA mutant SA493 but not to the chlA mutant JP382. These data

Table 5

Molybdenum cofactor activity in the soluble extracts of aerobically grown *Escherichia coli* K12 wild type and *chl* mutants as determined by in vitro reconstitution of plant specific nitrate reductase activity in extracts of *Nicotiana tabacum* mutant *cnx* 68 and *Hyoscyamus muticus* mutant MA-2 cells.

Plant Extract Source	Bacterial Extract Source	NADH-nitrate reductase activity (nmoles NO_2^-/hr/mg protein)
cnx 68	3000 wild type	54.9
	SA493 *chlA*	<0.1
	JP382 *chlA*	<0.1
	FC442 *chlB*	1.9
	JP426 *chlC*	11.0
	JRG97 *chlD*	6.6
	JF1130 *chlG*	1.6
MA-2	3000 wild type	68.8
	SA493 *chlA*	<0.1
	JP382 *chlA*	<0.1
	FC442 *chlB*	3.9
	JP426 *chlC*	7.1
	JRG94 *chlD*	14.3
	JRG97 *chlE*	2.6
	JF1130 *chlG*	4.8

indicated that the *chlA* locus is divisible into two components. The presence of a second gene within the *chlA* locus was confirmed by subcloning a Hind III fragment of pJT1 into pBR322 to obtain a 10.5 kb plasmid that restores the wild type functions to the *chlA* mutant JP382 (to be described elsewhere). Based on this evidence, the *chlA* locus was designated *chlM* (represented by mutant SA493) and *chlN* (represented by mutant JP382).

The plasmid pJT14 was generated from pJT13 (Fig. 3) by deletion of the Bgl II fragment from the vector. The two Bcl I sites in the insert were used to excise that fragment and insert it into pBR322 Bam HI site. Two plasmids designated pFG2 and pFG3 were isolated with the insert in opposite orientation. The observation that both plasmids produced functional *chlM*$^+$ product (as tested by transformation of mutant SA493) indicated that the gene was active from its own promoter. This fact was exploited to identify the *chlM*$^+$ product as a ca. 15,000 molecular weight protein by maxicell and minicell in vivo translation procedures. In accordance with these data, a 800 kb insert was constructed by insertion of pFG1 Tag I

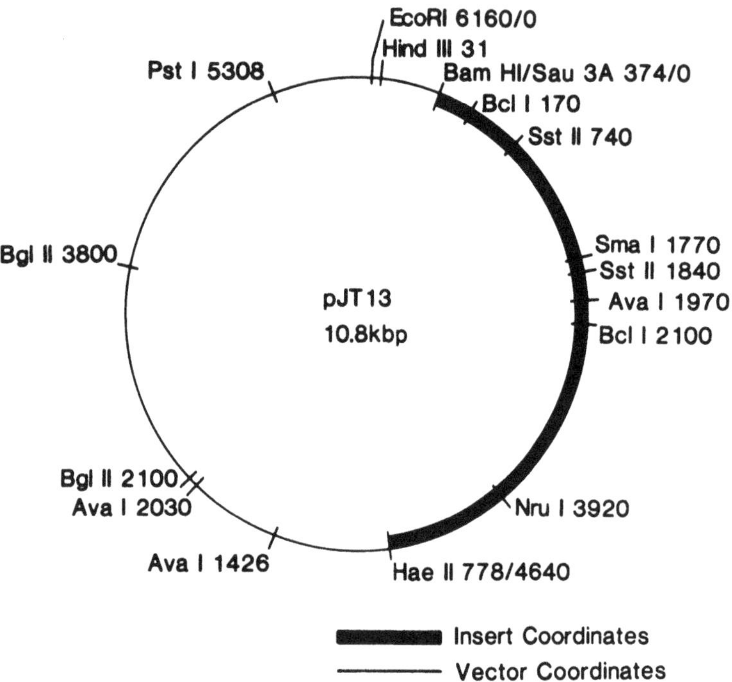

Figure 3. Restriction enzyme map of the chl M subclone pJT13.

fragments in the Cla I site of pBR322. The plasmid pFG1 was obtained by Ava I deletion of pJT14. The derivation of these plasmids is outlined in Fig. 4.

SUMMARY

Considerable progress has been made in developing the nitrate reductase system for plant cell transformation work. Our work with the Hordeum vulgare nitrate reductase indicates that the protein consists of two large (110,000) molecular weight subunits. The genetic and in vitro reconstitution experiments indicate that higher plant nitrate reductase apoproteins are associated with a molybdenum cofactor. The molybdenum cofactor structure and association with apoprotein is not yet clearly characterized. Genetic analyses indicate that higher plant molybdenum cofactor functions are controlled by several genes as has been shown in Escherichia coli, Aspergillus nidulans and Neurospora crassa. Data presented here suggest that if the right E. coli chl gene is matched up with

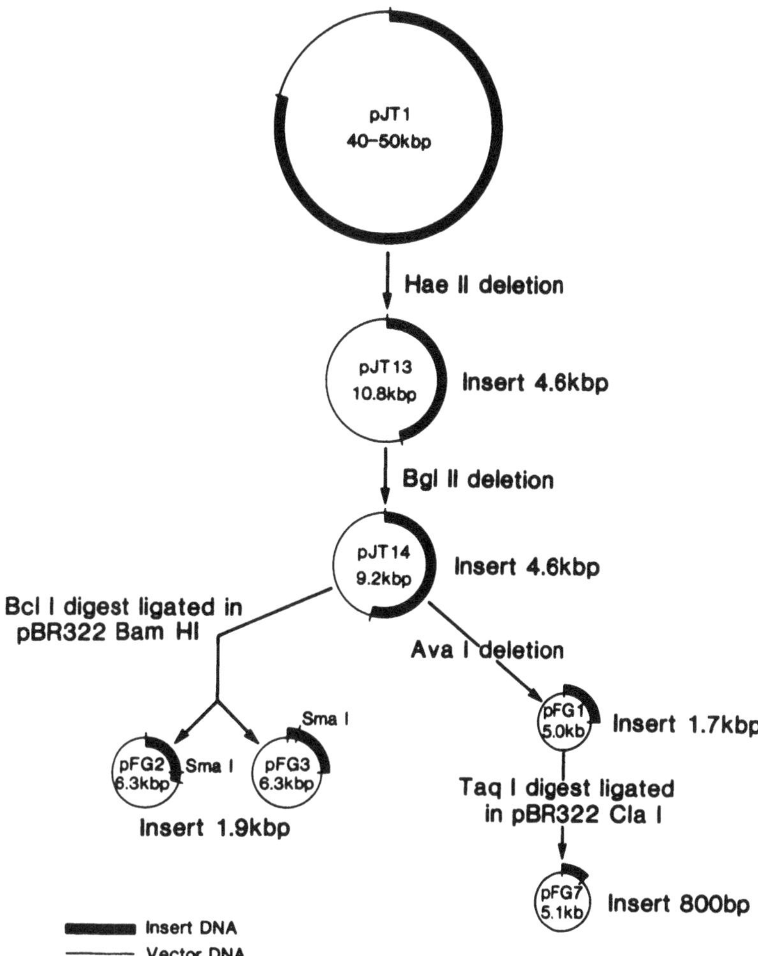

Figure 4. Derivation of the various chlM subclones from the cosmid pJT1.

the correct plant molybdenum cofactor mutant, and if expression of the E. coli gene can be obtained then an active nitrate reductase should be produced. It should be possible to select this event with high efficiency even if it is a very rare event. Thus, it should be possible to develop an effective plant cell transformation model using the NR system. The cloning of the E. coli chlM and chlN genes will facilitate this work.

REFERENCES

Amy, N. K., 1981, Identification of the molybdenum cofactor in chlorate-resistant mutants of Escherichia coli, J. Bacteriol., 148:274-282.
Amy, N. K., and Rajagopalan, K. V., 1979, Characterization of molybdenum cofactor from Escherichia coli, J. Bacteriol., 140:114-124.
Braaksma, F., 1982, Genetic control of nitrate reduction in Arabidopsis thaliana, Ph.D. Dissertation, University of Groningen, Haren, The Netherlands.
Cove, D. J., 1979, Genetic studies of nitrate assimilation in Aspergillus nidulans, Biol. Rev. 54:291-327.
Dailey, F. A., Warner, R. L., Somers, D. A., and Kleinhofs, A., 1982a, Characteristics of a nitrate reductase in a barley mutant deficient in NADH nitrate reductase, Plant Physiol., 69:1200-1204.
Dailey, F. A., Kuo, T., and Warner, R. L., 1982b. Pyridine nucleotide specificity of barley nitrate reductase, Plant Physiol., 69:1196-1199.
De la Rosa, M. A., Vega, J. M., and Zumft, W. G., 1981, Composition and structure of assimilatory nitrate reductase from Ankistrodesmus braunii, J. Biol. Chem., 256:5814-5819.
Downey, R. J., and Steiner, F. X., 1979, Further characterization of the reduced nicotinamide adenine dinucleotide phosphate: Nitrate oxidoreductase in Aspergillus nidulans, J. Bacteriol., 137:105-114.
Feenstra, W. J. and Jacobsen, E., 1980, Isolation of a nitrate reductase deficient mutant of Pisum sativum by means of selection for chlorate resistance, Theor. Appl. Genet., 58: 39-42.
Giri, L., and Ramadoss, C. S., 1979, Physical studies on assimilatory nitrate reductase from Chlorella vulgaris, J. Biol. Chem., 254:11703-11712.
Glimelius, K., Eriksson, T., Grafe, R., and Müller, A. J., 1978, Somatic hybridization of nitrate reductase-deficient mutants of Nicotiana tabacum by protoplast fusion, Physiol. Plant., 44:273-277.
Guerrero, M. G., and Gutierrez, M., 1977, Purification and properties of the NAD(P)H: Nitrate reductase of the yeast Rhodotorula glutinis, Biochim. Biophys. Acta, 482:272-285.
Johnson, J. L., Hainline, B. E., and Rajagopalan, K. V., 1980, Characterization of the molybdenum cofactor of sulfite oxidase, xanthine oxidase, and nitrate reductase, J. Biol. Chem., 255:1783-1786.

Ketchum, P. A., Cambier, H. Y., Frazier, W. A., III, Madansky, C. H., and Nason, A., 1970, In vitro assembly of Neurospora assimilatory nitrate reductase from protein subunits of a Neurospora mutant and the xanthine oxidizing or aldehyde oxidase systems of higher animals, Proc. Natl. Acad. Sci. USA, 66:1016-1023.

King, J., and Khanna, V., 1980, A nitrate reductase-less variant isolated from suspension cultures of Datura innoxia (Mill.), Plant Physiol., 66:632-636.

Kiss, G. B., Vincze, E., Kálmán, Z., Forrai, T., and Kondorosi, A., 1979, Genetic and biochemical analysis of mutants affected in nitrate reduction in Rhizobium meliloti, J. Gen. Microbiol., 113:105-118.

Kleinhofs, A., Warner, R. L., Muehlbauer, F. J., and Nilan, R. A., 1978, Induction and selection of specific gene mutations in Hordeum and Pisum, Mutation Res., 51:29-35.

Kleinhofs, A., Kuo, T., and Warner, R. L., 1980, Characterization of nitrate reductase-deficient barley mutants, Molec. Gen. Genet., 177:421-425.

Kuo, T., Kleinhofs, A., Somers, D., and Warner, R. L., 1981, Antigenicity of nitrate reductase-deficient mutants in Hordeum vulgare L., Molec. Gen. Genet., 181:20-23.

Kuo, T., Kleinhofs, A., and Warner, R. L., 1980, Purification and partial characterization of nitrate reductase from barley leaves, Plant Sci. Lett. 17:371-381.

Kuo, T. M., Somers, D. A., Kleinhofs, A., and Warner, R. L., 1982, NADH-nitrate reductase in barley leaves: Identification and animo acid composition of subunit protein, Biochim. Biophys. Acta, 708:75-81.

Lee, K.-Y., Pan, S.-S., Erickson, R., and Nason, A., 1974, Involvement of molybdenum and iron in the in vitro assembly of assimilatory nitrate reductase utilizing Neurospora mutant nit-1, J. Biol. Chem., 249:3941-3952.

MacDonald, D. W., and Cove, D. J., 1974, Studies on temperature-sensitive mutants affecting the assimilatory nitrate reductase of Aspergillus nidulans, Eur. J. Biochem., 47:107-110.

Marton, L., Dung, T. M., Mendel, R. R., and Maliga, P., 1982a, Nitrate reductase deficient cell lines from haploid protoplast cultures of Nicotiana plumbaginifolia, Molec. Gen. Genet., 182:301-304.

Marton, L., Sidorov, V., Biasini, G., and Maliga, P., 1982b, Complementation in somatic hybrids indicates four types of nitrate reductase deficient lines in Nicotiana plumbaginifolia, Molec. Gen. Genet., 187:1-3.

Mendel, R.-R., and Müller, A. J., 1976, A common genetic determinant of xanthine dehydrogenase and nitrate reductase in Nicotiana tabacum, Biochem. Physiol. Pflanzen, 170: 538-541.

Mendel, R. R., and Müller, A. J., 1979, Nitrate reductase-deficient mutant cell lines of Nicotiana tabacum. Further biochemical characterization, Molec. Gen. Genet., 177, 145-153.
Mendel, R. R., Alikulov, Z. A., Lvov, N. P., and Müller, A. J., 1981, Presence of the molybdenum-cofactor in nitrate reductase-deficient mutant cell lines of Nicotiana tabacum, Molec. Gen. Genet., 181:395-399.
Müller, A. J., and Grafe, R., 1978, Isolation and characterization of cell lines of Nicotiana tabacum lacking nitrate reductase, Molec. Gen. Genet., 161, 67-76.
Nason, A., Antoine, A. D., Ketchum, P. A., Frazier, W. A., III, and Lee, D. K., 1970, Formation of assimilatory nitrate reductase by in vitro inter-cistronic complementation in Neurospora crassa, Proc. Natl. Acad. Sci. USA, 65:137-144.
Nason, A., Lee, K.-Y., Pan, S.-S., Ketchum, P. A., Lamberti, A., and DeVries, J., 1971, In vitro formation of assimilatory reduced nicotinamide adenine dinucleotide phosphate: Nitrate reductase from a Neurospora mutant and a component of molybdenum-enzymes, Proc. Natl. Acad. Sci. USA, 68:3242-3246.
Notton, B. A., and Hewitt, E. J., 1979, Structure and properties of higher plant nitrate reductase, especially Spinacea oleracea, in: "Nitrogen Assimilation of Plants," E. J. Hewitt and C. V. Cutting, eds., Academic Press, New York.
Oh, J. Y., Warner, R. L. and Kleinhofs, A., 1980, Effect of nitrate reductase deficiency upon growth, yield, and protein in barley, Crop Sci., 20:487-490.
Oostindier-Braaksma, F. J., and Feenstra, W. J., 1973, Isolation and characterization of chlorate-resistant mutants of Arabidopsis thaliana, Mutation Res., 19:175-185.
Pan, S.-S., and Nason, A., 1978, Purification and characterization of homogeneous assimilatory reduced nicotinamide adenine dinucleotide phosphate-nitrate reductase from Neurospora crassa, Biochim. Biophys. Acta, 523:297-313.
Pateman, J. A., Cove, D. J., Rever, B. M., and Roberts, D. B., 1964, A common co-factor for nitrate reductase and xanthine dehydrogenase which also regulates the synthesis of nitrate reductase, Nature, 201:58-60.
Pienkos, P. T., Shah, V. K., and Brill, W. J., 1977, Molybdenum cofactors from molybdoenzymes and in vitro reconstitution of nitrogenase and nitrate reductase, Proc. Natl. Acad. Sci. USA, 74:5468-5474.
Shumny, V. K., and Tokarev, B. I., 1982, Genetic control of nitrate reductase activity in barley, Proc. IV Internatl. Barley Symp., (in press).
Small, I. S., and Wray, J. L., 1980, NADH nitrate reductase and related NADH cytochrome c reductase species in barley, Phytochemistry, 19:387-394.

Solomonson, L. P., Lorimer, G. H., Hall, R. L., Borchers, R., and Bailey, J. L., 1975, Reduced nicotinamide adenine dinucleotide-nitrate reductase of Chlorella vulgaris, J. Biol. Chem., 250:4120-4127.

Somers, D. A., Kuo, T., Kleinhofs, A., and Warner, R. L., 1982a, Barley nitrate reductase contains a functional cytochrome b_{557}, Plant Sci. Lett., 24:261-265.

Somers, D. A., Kuo, T. M., Kleinhofs, A., and Warner, R. L., 1982b, Nitrate reductase-deficient mutants in barley. Immunoelectrophoretic characterization, Plant Physiol., (in press).

Strauss, A., Bucher, F., and King, P. J., 1981, Isolation of biochemical mutants using haploid mesophyll protoplasts of Hyoscyamus muticus. I. A NO_3^- non-utilizing clone, Planta, 153:75-80.

Tokarev, B. I., and Shumny, V. K., 1977, Detection of barley mutants with low level of nitrate reductase activity after the seed treatment with ethylmethanesulphonate, Genetika, Moskva, 13:2097-2103.

Tomsett, A. B., and Garrett, R. H., 1980, The isolation and characterization of mutants defective in nitrate assimilation in Neurospora crassa, Genetics, 95:649-660.

Warner, R. L., and Kleinhofs, A., 1981, Nitrate utilization by nitrate reductase-deficient barley mutants, Plant Physiol., 67:740-743.

Warner, R. L., Kleinhofs, A., and Muehlbauer, F. J., 1982, Characterization of nitrate reductase-deficient mutants in pea, Crop Sci., 22:389-393.

Warner, R. L., Lin, C. J., and Kleinhofs, A., 1977, Nitrate reductase-deficient mutants in barley, Nature, 269:406-407.

REGENERATION OF PLANTS FROM SINGLE CELLS OF CEREALS AND GRASSES

Indra K. Vasil

Department of Botany
University of Florida
Gainesville, FL 32611
U.S.A.

INTRODUCTION

A variety of novel methods have been developed in recent years for the genetic modification of plant cells. These include the techniques of protoplast and cytoplast fusion, uptake of cell organelles, and molecular techniques involving the uptake and integration of foreign DNA. Each of these aspects is adequately covered elsewhere in this volume.

The widespread enthusiasm for the potentials of genetic modification techniques is based on a few instances of success in the somatic hybridization of plants following protoplast fusion (Schieder and Vasil, 1980) and the integration and expression of T-DNA in model plant species like tobacco and petunia (Marton et al., 1979; Chilton et al., 1980; Davey et al., 1980; Willmitzer et al., 1980).

The success achieved in these pioneering attempts has demonstrated the impressive power and potentials of the techniques of cellular and molecular biology. Much of the scientific, government and corporate interest and support for research in this area is based on the assumption that the developing techniques will lead to the genetic modification and improvement of important crop plants. Yet the fact remains that almost all of the attempts so far have been limited to model plant species which have traditionally proven amenable to experimental manipulation, and very little serious effort has been directed at major groups of crop plants, namely the cereals/grasses and legumes.

The development of plants from single cells is one of the most important requirements for the success of genetic modification experiments. This is now routinely done in plants like petunia, carrot, tobacco and jimsonweed (Vasil and Vasil, 1980). Most of the transformation experiments are also, therefore, limited to similar plants. In order to derive maximum benefits from the new biotechnology these pioneering successes must now be extended to crop plant species. A major problem that must be overcome before this becomes a reality is the refractory nature of cereal/grass and legume species to regeneration from single cells in vitro.

Important progress has been made recently in the regeneration of plants form single cells of many species of cereals and grasses. These encouraging developments toward the establishment of suitable single cell systems for this important group of crop plants are chronicled and discussed in this brief report. More detailed accounts can be found elsewhere (Vasil, 1982 a, b, c).

MEHTODS OF PLANT REGENERATION IN VITRO

There are two principal methods of plant regeneration in vitro: (i) Shoot morphogenesis, and (ii) Somatic embryogenesis.

Shoot morphogenesis takes place either by the development of axillary shoot buds or the de novo organization of shoot meristems in callus tissues. Formation of axillary buds is promoted by plant growth regulators like cytokinins. This method is now widely used in the commercial propagation of many horticultural plants and some species of fruits and vegetables. Plants obtained by this method are generally identical to the original donor, and the incidence of chimeras or genetically abnormal plants is rather low. This is because the cells that participate in the organization of axillary buds are very close to the shoot meristem, are still a part of the active meristematic tissue, are undifferentiated, and are cytologically stable.

New shoot meristems can also be induced in callus cultures by the use of cytokinins and other plant growth substances. Such tissues contain mostly vacuolated cells, are highly differentiated, and are mixoploid in nature. Plants regenerated from such tissue cultures not only show genetic variability, which is a reflection of their source of origin, but many of the regenerated plants are also chimeras because of their multicellular origin.

The risks of chimeral or genetically variable plants can be minimised or eliminated by obtaining plants from single cells, protoplasts, or somatic embryos. Somatic embryos, like their zygotic counterparts, arise from single cells either directly or after the formation of a proembryonal complex of cells (Haccius, 1978).

Apomictic development of embryos from gametic as well as somatic cells takes place in a wide variety of plants (Maheshwari, 1950; Maheshwari and Sachar, 1963). Artificially induced formation of embryos from somatic cells in tissue cultures was first described in Daucus carota (Reinert, 1958; Steward et al., 1958), and has since been reported in many other angiosperms (Tisserat et al., 1979).

Plant propagation by somatic embryogenesis is advantageous not only because of the single cell origin of plants, but also because plants can be produced rapidly and in very large numbers, and the embryogenic competence of the cultures can be maintained for long periods of time. Shoot morphogenesis, in comparison, is slower and can yield only a limited number of plants. Furthermore, the shoot forming ability of callus cultures is of limited duration.

Plant regeneration from gametic cells (androgenesis from cultured anthers or microspores) has been reported in many species of the Gramineae (Vasil, 1980). Plants are formed by shoot morphogenesis or somatic embryogenesis, although rigorous evidence of the formation of somatic embryos is not always available. Plant regeneration from gametic cells is not included in this review.

PLANT REGENERATION IN TISSUE CULTURES OF CEREALS AND GRASSES

It is now possible to regenerate plants from callus cultures of most of the important species of cereals and grasses (Green, 1978; Vasil et al., 1979). However, regeneration is often sporadic, short-lived, limited to a few genotypes, and results in the formation of only a few plants.

Plant Regeneration in Callus Cultures by Shoot Morphogenesis

In most cases of plant regeneration from tissue cultures of the Gramineae (Table 1), regeneration is believed to take place by the derepression of presumptive shoot primordia which proliferate adventitiously in vitro producing the so-called microtillering effect (King et al., 1978; Dunstan et al., 1979; Thomas et al., 1979). In many instances, specially where the calli are derived from more mature explants, the cultures consist predominantly of root primordia (Cure and Mott, 1978; Mott and Cure, 1978; King et al., 1978). Only in rare instances has the de novo origin of shoot meristems been reported in callus tissues (Springer et al., 1979).

Table 1. Plant regeneration in vitro by shoot morphogenesis in cereal and grass species.

Species	Reference
Agropyron	Lo et al. (1980)
Andropogon gerardii	Chen et al. (1977)
Avena sativa	Carter et al. (1967), Cummings et al. (1976), Lorz et al. (1976)
Dactylis glomerata	Conger and Carabia (1978), Dale (1977)
Eleusine coracana	Rangan (1976)
Festuca arundinacea	Dale (1977), Low and Conger (1979)
Hordeum jubatum	Orton (1979)
Hordeum vulgare	Cheng and Smith (1975), Dale and Deambrogio (1979), Orton (1979)
Hordeum vulgare x H. jubatum	Orton (1979)
Lolium multiflorum	Dale (1977)
Lolium multiflorum x L. perenne	Ahloowalia (1975, 1976)
Lolium multiflorum x Festuca arundinacea	Kasperbauer et al. (1979)
Oryza sativa	Nishi et al. (1968, 1973), Kawata and Ishihara (1968), Tamura (1968), Yan and Zhao (1982)
Panicum miliaceum	Rangan (1974)
Paspalum scrobiculatum	Rangan (1976)
Pennisetum americanum	Rangan (1976)
Pennisetum purpureum	Bajaj and Dhanju (1981)
Phleum pratense	Dale (1977)

Table 1. Continued

Phragmites communis	Sangwan and Gorenflot (1975)
Saccharum officinarum	Barba and Nickell (1969) Heinz and Mee (1969, 1971), Nadar and Heinz (1977)
Saccharum officinarum x Zea mays	Sreenivasan and Jalaja (1982)
Sorghum bicolor	Masteller and Holden (1970), Gamborg et al. (1977)
Secale cereale	Rybczynski (1980)
Sorghastrum nutans	Chen et al. (1979)
Triticale	Sharma et al. (1981), Nakamura and Keller (1982 a, b)
Triticum aestivum	Shimada et al. (1969), Dudits et al (1975), Shimada (1978), Gosch-Wackerle et al. (1979)
Triticum crassum	Nakamura et al. (1981)
Triticum crassum x Hordeum vulgare	Nakamura et al. (1981)
Triticum dicoccum	Shimada et al. (1969)
Triticum durum	Bennici and D'Amato (1978)
Triticum longissimum	Gosch-Wackerle et al. (1979)
Triticum monococcum	Shimada et al. (1969)
Zea mays	Green and Phillips (1975), Freeling et al. (1976), Harms et al. (1980)

The organization of shoot meristems is considered to be multicellular in origin (Crooks, 1933; Vasil and Hilderbrandt, 1966; Steffensen, 1968; Coe and Neuffer, 1978; Bennici and D'Amato, 1978; Bennici et al., 1979; Lupi et al., 1981; Ogihara, 1981). Plants of multicellular origin arising from heterogenous cell populations can not always be genetically uniform, and may indeed be chimeras (Sacristan and Melchers, 1969; Yamabe and Yamada, 1973; Novak and Vyskot, 1975; Ogura, 1976; Sree Ramulu et al., 1976; Bennici and D'Amato, 1978; Mix et al., 1978; Bennici, 1979). Such plants are unsuitable for mutation breeding, genetic analyses, propagation of selected genotypes, etc.

Plant Regeneration in Callus Cultures by Somatic Embryogenesis

In several species of the Gramineae apomictic embryos are formed from somatic as well as gametic cells in vivo (Tisserat et al., 1979). But the phenomenon of somatic embryogenesis in tissue cultures of cereal and grass species was considered until quite recently to be rare. Norstog (1970) first described the formation of atypical embryoids on the scutellum of cultured young barley embryos. The embryoids neither survived long in culture nor developed into plants. In cultured immature embryos of maize scutellar bodies and scutellum-like structures were observed, but no somatic embryos were formed (Green and Phillips, 1975; Freeling et al., 1976). Embryo-like structures were also found in tissue cultures derived from cultured embryos of sorghum, but plant regeneration was said to take place primarily by the process of "micro-tillering" (Thomas et al., 1977; Dunstan et al., 1978, 1979). We first described the formation of typical grass embryos in protoplast-derived callus cultures of *Pennisetum americanum* (Vasil and Vasil, 1980), and have since provided extensive morphological and histological evidence of somatic embryogenesis in a variety of species of the Gramineae (Vasil and Vasil, 1982a, b; Vasil et al., 1982; Table 2). The embryoids are formed in compact embryogenic callus tissues, comprised of small, richly cytoplasmic cells with prominent nuclei, and storage starch, by internal segmenting divisions in single embryogenic cells (Vasil and Vasil, 1982b; Ho and Vasil, 1982; Botti and Vasil, 1982).

Immature embryos, young inflorescences and young leaves are ideal sources for the initiation of embryogenic callus cultures. The developmental and physiological stages of the donor tissues are also critical for the initiation of stable embryogenic cultures. Mature and differentiated tissues of the Gramineae generally do not give rise to shoot forming or embryogenic cultures.

Embryogenic competence is attained in the presence of 2,4-D during the early period of cell proliferation. The embryogenic cells have a strong tendency to enlarge, become vacuolated,

Table 2. The formation of somatic embryos and plants in callus cultures of the Gramineae.

Dactylis glomerata	McDaniel et al. (1982)
Lolium multiflorum	Dale (1980), Dale et al. (1981)
Oryza sativa	Wernicke et al. (1981)
Panicum maximum	Lu and Vasil (1981a, 1982a)
Panicum miliaceum	Rangan and Vasil (1982)
Panicum miliare	Rangan and Vasil (1982)
Pennisetum americanum	Vasil and Vasil (1981a)
Pennisetum purpureum	Haydu and Vasil (1981), Wang and Vasil (1982)
Pennisetum americanum x P. purpureum	Vasil and Vasil (1981a)
Saccharum officinarum	Ho and Vasil (1982)
Sorghum arundinaceum	Boyes and Vasil (unpublished)
Sorghum bicolor	Thomas et al. (1977), Dunstan et al. (1978, 1979), Wernicke and Brettell (1980)
Triticum aestivum	Ozias-Akins and Vasil (1982)
Zea mays	Lu et al. (1982)

lose their starch reserves and become non-embryogenic. This irreversible change is apparently caused by decreasing levels of 2,4-D. Regular sub-culture to fresh nutrient media can ensure the maintenance of embryogenic competence for long periods of time. Some non-embryogenic cells are always present in the cultures, and must be physically excluded during sub-culture to avoid overwhelming the embryogenic tissues by rapid rates of growth.

The formation of somatic embryos has recently been described in _Dacylis glomerata_ (McDaniel et al., 1982), _Panicum miliaceum_ (Rangan and Vasil, 1982), _Pennisetum americanum_ (=_P. typhoideum_, Vasil and Vasil, 1981a), _P. purpureum_ (Haydu and Vasil, 1981; Wang and Vasil, 1982), _Saccharum officinarum_ (Ho and Vasil, 1982), _Sorghum bicolor_ (Brettell et al., 1980), _Triticum aestivum_ (Ozias-Akins and Vasil, 1982) and _Zea mays_ (Lu et al., 1982). Earlier investigators had described only shoot morphogenesis in these species (Heinz and Mee, 1969; Rangan, 1974, 1976; Freeling et al., 1976; Dale, 1977; Gamborg et al., 1977; Conger and Carabia, 1978; Gosch-Wackerle et al., 1979; Shimada and Yamada, 1979; Bajaj and Dhanju, 1981). It is likely that in many of the earlier studies also compact and slow-growing embryogenic tissues were formed, but these were either inadvertently or deliberately discarded in favor of the more common, relatively faster growing, and friable non-embryogenic tissues. In other instances the phenomenon of somatic embryogenesis was either not recognised or was misinterpreted. The general absence of typical and well organized embryoids added to the confusion.

There are many accounts of the appearance of green leafy structures followed by the formation of multiple shoot buds (Tamura, 1968; Green and Phillips, 1975; Nakano and Maeda, 1979). Such green leafy structures have now been interpreted to be the enlarged scutella of precociously germinating embryoids (Ozias-Akins and Vasil, 1982; Vasil and Vasil, 1982a, b; Wang and Vasil, 1982), which develop an expanded organogenetic zone where multiple shoot meristems are organized. Even in those instances where micro-tillering has been proposed to be the principal means of propagation (Dunstan et al., 1978, 1979), somatic embryos are likely formed first, followed by the de novo development of multiple shoot meristems as well as axillary shoot buds in precociously germinating somatic embryos. The tillering response is thus secondary in nature.

Plant Regeneration in Cell Suspension Cultures by Somatic Embryogenesis

Establishment of stable cell suspension cultures in cereal and grass species has generally proved to be difficult (King et al., 1978). In most instances the cultures consist of tissue masses that are kept in suspension because of rapid agitation during which large, vacuolated and non-dividing cells are sloughed off from their surface. The cultures represent rapidly proliferating roots or root meristems, and have no other organogenetic capacity except to form roots under certain conditions. Such cultures can not be truly described as suspensions and are not useful for most cell culture and somatic cell genetics studies.

There is an early report of the formation of only albino plantlets by somatic embryogenesis from cell suspension cultures of Bromus inermis (Gamborg et al., 1970). However, the recent availability of embryogenic callus cultures of the Gramineae has encouraged attempts to isolate stable embryogenic cell suspension cultures capable of plant regeneration. Vasil and Vasil (1981b) first reported the regeneration of plants by somatic embryogenesis from cell suspension cultures of Pennisetum americanum. Similar results were obtained in Panicum maximum (Lu and Vasil, 1981b) and Saccharum officinarum (Ho and Vasil, 1982). Embryogenic cell suspensions have also been isolated in Pennisetum purpureum (Wang et al., 1982) and Zea mays (Lu et al., 1982; Lu and Vasil, 1982b).

Embryogenic cell suspensions can be initiated from callus tissues derived from immature embryos (Vasil and Vasil, 1981b; Lu and Vasil, 1981b), young inflorescences (Lu and Vasil, 1981b; Vasil and Vasil, 1982a), or young leaves (Ho and Vasil, 1982; Wang et al., 1982). The suspensions contain both embryogenic and non-embryogenic cells. Cultures comprising predominantly embryogenic cells can be obtained by manipulating the dilution rations at the time of sub-culture and the length of each sub-culture (Vasil and Vasil, 1982a).

Somatic embryos do not develop beyond the globular or the early scutellar stage in suspension. Further development is assured when the suspensions are plated onto agar nutrient media. Although the cultures may contain as many as 15-20 million cells/ml and also form hundreds of globular or early scutellar embryoids, only a few of the embryoids actually reach maturity and germinate to form plants. This problem must be overcome and the number of plants formed must be maximised.

Stable embryogenic cell suspension cultures are difficult to establish. Nevertheless, they have been repeatedly isolated from diverse sources in a number of species showing that it is not a random or isolated event, but is reproducible and predictable. Availability of good embryogenic callus cultures is critical for their isolation. After the embryogenic calli have been placed in liquid media, a gradual but deliberate enrichment of the cultures with embryogenic cells must be achieved through physical and physiological manipulation of the cultures (Vasil and Vasil, 1981b, 1982a). Failure to do so results in the rapid and irreversible conversion of the cultures to non-embryogenic suspensions.

Plant Regeneration in Protoplast Cultures by Somatic Embryogenesis

Mesophyll protoplasts isolated from leaf tissues have been extensively used in Solanaceous species for the regeneration of plants (Vasil and Vasil, 1980). Similar protoplasts can be isolated from leaves of many species of the Gramineae, but exhaustive efforts to culture them have not been successful (Potrykus et al., 1976; Potrykus, 1980). Protoplasts of the Gramineae in general have been found to be extremely recalcitrant to culture (Vasil and Vasil, 1980), leading to the erroneous conclusion that they suffer from a mitotic block and "are constitutionally incapable of sustained division" (Flores et al., 1981).

Protoplasts isolated from cell cultures have been cultured successfully in *Hordeum vulgare* (Koblitz, 1976), *Lolium multiflorum* (Jones and Dale, 1982), *Oryza sativa* (Deka and Sen, 1976; Cai et al., 1978), *Pennisetum americanum* (Vasil and Vasil, 1979), *Saccharum officinarum* (Maretzki and Nickell, 1973), *Sorghum bicolor* (Brar et al., 1980), *Triticum monococcum* (Nemet and Dudits, 1977), and *Zea mays* (Potrykus et al., 1979). No organized growth into shoots, embryoids or plants took place in the calli derived from the protoplasts.

In *Pennisetum americanum* (Vasil and Vasil, 1980) and *Panicum maximum* (Lu et al., 1981), embryoids, embryogenic calli and plantlets were obtained reproducibly and repeatedly from protoplasts isolated from embryogenic cell suspension cultures. Recently, we have cultured similar protoplasts isolated from *Pennisetum purpureum* (Wang et al., 1982) and *Zea mays* (Lu and Vasil, 1982b), and have obtained embryogenic calli and embryoids. Protoplast derived plantlets were not grown to maturity. This serious deficiency, and the relatively low plating efficiency of the protoplasts, must be resolved.

GENETIC STABILITY/VARIABILITY OF REGENERATED PLANTS

Cytological variability is a common feature of plant tissue cultures (Bayliss, 1980). At least some of the variability found in cell cultures is reflected in the regenerated plants, and has been used advantageously in some species for the selection of agronomically or horticulturally superior plants (D'Amato, 1978; Skirvin, 1978). Uncontrolled introduction of variability during culture can become a serious problem in those instances where true clonal propagation of a selected and improved cultivar or genotype is desired.

There are several reports of genetically variant plants regenerated from tissue cultures of the Gramineae: *Avena sativa* (McCoy et al., 1982), *Hordeum* sp. (Mix et al., 1978; Orton, 1980),

Oryza sativa (Oono, 1978), *Saccharum* sp. (Heinz et al., 1977), *Triticum durum* (Bennici and D'Amato, 1978; Lupi et al., 1981), and *Zea mays* (Edallo et al., 1981). On the other hand, significant genetic stability was found in tissue cultures and regenerated plants of *Zea mays* (McCoy and Phillips, 1982).

In our experience with regeneration of plants from many species of cereals and grasses (Vasil et al., 1982), we have not encountered any instances of polyploidy or aneuploidy in the regenerated plants, nor any noticeable phenotypic changes. This remarkable genetic stability is considered to be the result of regeneration by somatic embryogenesis. It has been argued that only those cells that are cytologically normal retain the capacity to develop into embryoids (Vasil, 1982a,b, c). This argument implies that cytologically atypical cells may continue to maintain their competence to organize into shoot meristems while altered embryogenic cells lose their capacity for embryogenesis. Cells which undergo major cytological changes neither have the capacity to organize into shoot meristems nor into embryoids.

Further detailed studies of plants regenerated from tissue cultures of the Gramineae need to be carried out to understand the genetic variability or stability variously reported. The possible correlation between the mode of plant regeneration - shoot morphogenesis versus somatic embryogenesis - and genetic stability/variability must also be determined. In most studies only a small number of plants is used for cytological analyses that are limited to root tip mitoses. These have been found to be inadequate. As shown by McCoy et al. (1982), meiotic chromosome analyses of a larger population of plants may provide more definitive information.

CONCLUSIONS

Somatic embryogenesis has been shown to be a reliable and efficient method for the regeneration of plants from cereal and grass species in vitro. Plants derived from somatic embryos are of single cell origin and more suitable for mutation breeding, isolation of mutants, genetic analyses, etc. than plants formed by shoot morphogenesis which are cytologically atypical and often chimeras. Embryogenic callus cultures have allowed the establishment of stable cell suspension cultures which have proved to be the only source of graminaceous protoplasts from which embryogenic calli, embryoids and plantlets can be produced. Although much further work needs to be carried out, the progress made so far has clearly brought us closer to the establishment of model single cell systems for the genetic manipulation of cereal and grass species.

REFERENCES

Ahloowalia, B.S. 1975. Regeneration of ryegrass in tissue culture. Crop Sci. 15:449-452.

Ahloowalia, B.S. 1976. Chromosomal changes in parasexually produced ryegrass. In "Current Chromosome Research", K. Jones and P.E. Brandham, eds. Elsevier/North-Holland Amsterdam.

Bajaj, Y.P.S. and Dhanju, B.S. 1981. Regeneration of plants from callus cultures of Napier grass (Pennisetum purpureum). Pl. Sci. Let. 20:343-345.

Barba, R. and Nickell, L.G. 1969. Nutrition and organ differentiation in tissue cultures of sugarcane, a monocotyledon. Planta 89:299-302.

Bayliss, M.W. 1980. Chromosomal variation in plant tissues in culture. In: "Perspectives in Plant Cell and Tissue Culture", I.K. Vasil, ed. Int. Rev. Cytol. Suppl. XIA. Academic Press, New York.

Bennici, A. 1979. Cytological chimeras in plants regenerated from Lilium longiflorum tissues grown in vitro. Z. Pflanzenzuchtg. 82:349-353.

Bennici, A. and D'Amato, F. 1978. In vitro regeneration of Durum wheat plants. I. Chromosome numbers of regenerated plantlets. Z. Pflanzenzuchtg. 81:305-311.

Bennici, A., Baroncelli, S. and D'Amato, F. 1979. Cytogenetics of Durum wheat plants regenerated in vitro. In: "Proc. Israeli-Italian Joint Meeting on Genetics and Breeding of Crop Plants". Instituto Sperimentale per la Cerealicolture, Roma.

Botti, C. and I. K. Vasil. 1982. Somatic embryogenesis and plant regeneration from inflorescence segments of Pennisetum americanum. I. Ontogeny of somatic embryos. In preparation.

Brar, D.S., Rambold, D., Constabel, F. and Gamborg, O.L. 1980. Isolation, fusion and culture of Sorghum and corn protoplasts. Z. Pflanzenphysiol. 96:269-275.

Brettell, R.I.S., Wernicke, W. and Thomas, E. 1980. Embryogenesis from cultured immature inflorescences of Sorghum bicolor. Protoplasma 104:141-148.

Cai, Q., Quain, Y., Zhou, Y. and Wu, S. 1978. A further study on the isolation and culture of rice (Oryza sativa L.) protoplasts. Acta Bot. Sin. 20:97-102.

Carter, O., Yamada, Y. and Takahashi, E. 1967. Tissue culture of oats. Nature 214:1029-1030.

Chen, C.H., Lo, P.F. and Ross, J.G. 1979. Regeneration of plantlets from callus cultures of Indian grass. Crop Sci. 19:117-118.

Chen, C.H., Stenberg, N.E. and Ross, J.G. 1977. Clonal propagation of big bluestem by tissue culture. Crop Sci. 17:847-850.

Cheng, T. and Smith, H.H. 1975. Organogenesis from callus culture of Hordeum vulgare. Planta 123:307-310.

Chilton, M.D., Saiki, R.K., Yadav, N. Gordon, M.P. and Quetier, F. 1980. T-DNA from Agrobacterium Ti plasmid is in the nuclear DNA fraction of crown gall tumor cells. Proc. Nat. Acad. Sci. U.S.A. 77:4060-4064.

Coe, E.H., Jr. and Neuffer, M.G. 1978. Embryo cells and their destinies in the corn plant. In: "The Clonal Basis of Development", S. Subtelny and I.M. Sussex, eds. Academic Press, New York.

Conger, B.V. and Carabia, J.V. 1978. Callus induction and plantlet regeneration in orchardgrass. Crop Sci. 18:157-159.

Crooks, D.M. 1933. Histological and regenerative studies on the flax seedling. Bot. Gaz. 95:209-239.

Cummings, D.P., Green, C.E. and Stuthman, D.D. 1976. Callus induction and regeneration in oats. Crop Sci. 16:465-470.

Cure, W.W. and Mott, R.L. 1978. A comparative anatomical study of organogenesis in cultured tissues of maize, wheat and oats. Physiol. Pl. 42:91-96.

D'Amato, F. 1978. Chromosome number variation in cultured cells and regenerated plants. In: "Frontiers of Plant Tissue Culture 1978", ed. T. A. Thorpe. University of Calgary, Canada.

Dale, P.J. 1977. Meristem tip culture in Lolium, Festuca, Phleum and Dactylis. Pl. Sci. Let. 9:333-338.

Dale, P.J. 1980. Embryoids from cultured immature embryos of Lolium multiflorum. Z. Pflanzenphysiol. 100:73-77.

Dale, P.J. and Deambrogio, E. 1979. A comparison of callus induction and plant regeneration from different explants of Hordeum vulgare. Z. Pflanzenphysiol. 94:65-77.

Dale, P.J., Thomas, E., Brettell, R.I.S. and Wernicke, W. 1981. Embryogenesis from cultured immature inflorescences and nodes of Lolium multiflorum. Pl. Cell Tiss. Org. Cult. 1:47-55.

Davey, M.R., Cocking, E.C., Freeman, J., Pearce, N. and Rudor, I. 1980. Transformation of Petunia protoplasts by isolated Agrobacterium plasmids. Pl. Sci. Let. 18:307-313.

Deka, P.C. and Sen, S.K. 1976. Differentiation in calli originated from isolated protoplasts of rice (Oryza sativa L.) through plating technique. Mol. Gen. Genet. 145:239-243.

Dudits, D., Nemet, G. and Haydu, Z. 1975. Study of callus growth and organ formation in wheat (Triticum aestivum) tissue cultures. Canad. J. Bot. 53:957-967.

Dunstan, D.I., Short, K.C. and Thomas E. 1978. The anatomy of secondary morphogenesis in cultured scutellum tissues of Sorghum bicolor. Protoplasma 97:251-260.

Dunstan, D.I., Short, K.C., Dhaliwal, H. and Thomas, E. 1979. Further studies on plantlet production from cultured tissues of Sorghum bicolor. Protoplasma 101:355-351.

Edallo, S., Zucchinali, C., Perenzin, M. and Salamini, F. 1981. Chromosomal variation and frequency of spontaneous mutation associated with in vitro culture and plant regeneration in

maize. Maydica 26:39-56.
Flores, H.E., Kaur-Sawhney, R. and Galston, A.W. 1981. Protoplasts as vehicles for plant propagation and improvement. Adv. Cell. Cult. 1:241-279.
Freeling, M., Woodman, J.C. and Cheng, D.S.K. 1976. Developmental potentials of maize tissue cultures. Maydica 21:97-112.
Gamborg, O.L., Constabel, F. and Miller, R.A. 1970. Embryogenesis and production of albino plants from cell cultures of Bromus inermis. Planta 95:355-358.
Gamborg, O.L., Shyluk, J.P., Brar, D.S. and Constabel, F. 1977. Morphogenesis and plant regeneration from callus of immature embryos of sorghum. Pl. Sci. Let 10:67-74.
Gosch-Wackerle, G., Avivi, L. and Galun, E. 1979. Induction, culture and differentiation of callus from immature rachises, seeds and embryos of Triticum. Z. Pflanzenphysiol. 91:267-278.
Green, C.E. 1978. In vitro plant regeneration in cereals and grasses. In: "Frontiers of Plant Tissue Culture 1978", T.A. Thrope, ed. University of Calgary, Canada.
Green, C.E. and Phillips, R.L. 1975. Plant regeneration from tissue cultures of maize. Crop. Sci. 15:417-421.
Haccius, B. 1978. Question of unicellular origin of non-zygotic embryos in callus cultures. Phytomorphology 28:74-81.
Harms, C.T., Lorz, H. and Potrykus, I. 1976. Regeneration of plantlets from callus cultures of Zea mays L. Z. Pflanzenzuchtg. 77:347-351.
Haydu, Z. and Vasil, I.K. 1981. Somatic embryogenesis and plant regeneration from leaf tissues and anthers of Pennisetum purpureum. Theoret. Appl. Genet. 59:269-273.
Heinz, D.J. and Mee, G.W.P. 1969. Plant differentiation from callus tissue of Saccharum species. Crop. Sci. 9:346-348.
Heinz, D.J. and Mee, G.W.P. 1971. Morphologic, cytogenetic and enzymatic variation in Saccharum species hybrid clones derived from callus tissue. Amer. J. Bot. 58:275-262.
Heinz, D.J., Krishnamurthi, M., Nickell, L.G. and Maretzki, A. 1977. Cell, tissue and organ culture in sugarcane improvement. In: "Plant Cell, Tissue and Organ Culture", J. Reinert and Y.P.S. Bajaj, eds. Springer-Verlag, New York.
Ho, W. and Vasil, I.K. 1982. Somatic embryogenesis in callus and cell suspension cultures of sugarcane. In preparation.
Jones, M.G.K. and Dale, P.J. 1982. Reproducible regeneration of callus from suspension culture protoplasts of the grass Lolium multiflorum. Z. Pflanzenphysiol. 105:267-274.
Kasperbauer, M.J., Beckner, R.C. and Bush, L.P. 1979. Tissue culture of annual ryegrass x tall fescue F_1 hybrids: callus establishment and plant regeneration. Crop. Sci. 19:457-460.
Kawata, S. and Ishihara, A. 1968. The regeneration of rice plant, Oryza sativa L., in the callus derived from the seminal root. Proc. Japan Acad. 44:549-553.

King, P.J., Potrykus, I. and Thomas E. 1978. In vitro genetics of cereals: problems and perspectives. Physiol. Veg. 16: 381-399.

Koblitz, H. 1976. Isolation and cultivation of protoplasts from callus cultures of barley. Biochem. Physiol. Pflanz. 170: 287-293.

Lo, P.F., Chen, C.H. and Ross, J.G. 1980. Vegetative propagation of temperate grasses through callus culture. Crop. Sci. 20:363-367.

Lorz, H., Harms, C.T. and Potrykus, I. 1976. Regeneration of plants from callus in Avena sativa. Z. Pflanzenzuchtg. 77: 257-259.

Lowe, K.W. and Conger, B.V. 1979. Root and shoot formation from callus cultures of tall fescue. Crop. Sci. 19:397-400.

Lu, C. and Vasil, I.K. 1981a. Somatic embryogenesis and plant regeneration from leaf tissues of Panicum maximum Jacq. Theoret. Appl. Genet. 59:275-280.

Lu, C. and Vasil, I.K. 1981b. Somatic embryogenesis and plant regeneration from freely suspended cells and cell groups of Panicum maximum in vitro. Ann. Bot. 47:543-548.

Lu, C. and Vasil, I.K. 1982a. Somatic embryogenesis and plant regeneration in tissue cultures of Panicum maximum Jacq. Amer. J. Bot. 69:77-81.

Lu, C. and Vasil, I.K. 1982b. Somatic embryogenesis in cell suspension and protoplast cultures of Zea mays L. In preparation.

Lu, C., Vasil, I.K. and Ozias-Akins, P. 1982. Somatic embryogenesis in Zea mays L. Theoret. Appl. Genet. 62:109-112.

Lu, C., Vasil, V. and Vasil, I.K. 1981. Isolation and culture of protoplasts of Panicum maximum Jacq. (Guinea grass): somatic embryogenesis and plantlet formation. Z. Pflanzenphysiol. 104:311-318.

Lupi, M.C., Bennici, A., Baroncelli, S., Gennari, D. and D'Amato, F. 1981. In vitro regeneration of Durum wheat plants. II. Diplontic selection of aneusomatic plants. Z. Pflanzenzuchtg. 87:167-171.

Maheshwari, P. 1950. An Introduction to the Embryology of Angiosperms. McGraw Hill, New York.

Maheshwari, P. and Sachar, R.C. 1963. Polyembryony. In: "Recent Advances in the Embryology of Angiosperms", P. Maheshwari, ed. Int. Assoc. Pl. Morphol., Delhi.

Maretzki, A. and Nickell, L.G. 1973. Formation of protoplasts from sugarcane cell suspensions and the regeneration of cell cultures from protoplasts. Colloq. Internat. C.N.R.S. 212:51-63.

Marton, L., Williams, G.J., Molendijk, L. and Schilperoort, R.A. 1979. In vitro transformation of cultured cells from Nicotiana tabacum by Agrobacterium tumefaciens. Nature 277:129-131.

Masteler, V.J. and Holden, D.J. 1970. The growth of and organ formation from callus tissue fo sorghum. Pl. Physiol. 45: 362-364.
McCoy, T.J. and Phillips, R.L. 1982. Chromosome stability in maize (Zea mays L.) tissue cultures and sectoring among regenerated plants. Canad. J. Genet. Cytol. In press.
McCoy, T.J., Phillips, R.L. and Rines, H.W. 1982. Cytogenetic analysis of plants regenerated from oat (Avena sativa) tissue cultures: high frequency of partial chromosomal loss. Canad. J. Genet. Cytol. 24:37-50.
McDaniel, J.K., Conger, B.V. and Graham, E.T. 1982. A histological study of tissue proliferation, embryogenesis, and organogenesis from tissue cultures of Dactylis glomerata L. Protoplasma 110:121-128.
Mix, G., Wilson, H.W. and Foroughi-Wehr, B. 1978. The cytological status of plants of Hordeum vulgare L. regenerated from microspore callus. Z. Pflanzenzuchtg. 80:89-99.
Mott, R.L. and Cure, W.W. 1978. Anatomy of maize tissue cultures. Physiol. Plant. 42:139-145.
Nadar, H.M. and Heinz, D.J. 1977. Root and shoot development from sugarcane callus tissue. Crop Sci. 17:814-816.
Nakamura, C. and Keller, W.A. 1982a. Callus proliferation and plant regeneration from immature embryos of hexaploid triticale. Z. Pflanzenzuchtg. 88:137-160.
Nakamura, C. and Keller, W.A. 1982b. Plant regeneration from inflorescence cultures of hexaploid triticale. Pl. Sci. Let. 24:275-280.
Nakamura, C., Keller, W.A. and Fedak, G. 1981. In vitro propagation and chromosome doubling of a Triticum crassum x Hordeum vulgare intergeneric hybrid. Theoret. Appl. Genet. 60:89-96.
Nakano, H. and Maeda, E. 1979. Shoot differentiation in callus of Oryza sativa L. Z. Pflanzenphysiol. 93:449-458.
Nemet, G. and Dudits, D. 1977. Potential of protoplast, cell and tissue culture research in cereal research. In: "Use of Tissue Cultures in Plant Breeding", F.J. Novak, ed. Czechoslovak Academy of Sciences, Institute of Experimental Botany, Praha.
Nishi, T., Yamada, Y. and Takahashi, E. 1968. Organ redifferentiation and plant restoration in rice callus. Nature 219: 508-509.
Nishi, T., Yamada, Y. and Takahashi, E. 1973. The role of auxins in differentiation of rice tissues cultured in vitro. Bot. Mag. 86:183-188.
Norstog, K. 1970. Induction of embryo-like structures by kinetin in cultured barley embryos. Dev. Biol. 23:665-670.
Novak, F.J. and Vyskot, B. 1975. Karyology of callus cultures derivied from Nicotiana tabacum L. haploids and ploidy of regenerants. Z. Pflanzenzuchtg. 75:62-70.

Ogihara, Y. 1981. Tissue culture in Haworthia. IV. Genetic characterization of plants regenerated from callus. Theoret. Appl. Genet. 60:353-363.
Ogura, H. 1976. Cytological chimeras in original regenerates from tobacco tissue cultures and their offsprings. Jap. J. Genet. 51:161-174.
Oono, K. 1978. Test tube breeding of rice by tissue culture. Tróp. Agric. Res. Series 11:109-123.
Orton, T.J. 1979. A quantitative analysis of growth and regeneration from tissue cultures of Hordeum vulgare, H. jubatum and their interspecific hybrid. Environ. Exp. Bot. 19:319-335.
Orton, T.J. 1980. Chromosomal variability in tissue cultures and regenerated plants of Hordeum. Theoret. Appl. Genet. 56: 101-112.
Ozias-Akins, P. and Vasil, I.K. 1982. Plant regeneration from cultured immature embryos and inflorescences of Triticum aestivum L. (wheat): evidence for somatic embryogenesis. Protoplasma 110:95-105.
Potrykus, I. 1980. The old problem of protoplast cutlure: cereals. In: "Advances in Protoplast Research", L. Ferenczy, G. L. Farkas, and G. Lazar, eds. Akademiai Kiado, Budapest.
Potrykus, I., Harms, C.T. and Lorz, H. 1976. Problems in culturing cereal protoplasts. In: "Cell Genetics in Higher Plants", D. Dudits, G.L. Farkas and P. Maliga, eds. Akademiai Kiado, Budapest.
Potrykus, I., Harms, C.T. and Lorz, H. 1979. Callus formation from cell culture protoplasts of corn (Zea mays L.). Theoret. Appl. Genet. 54:209-214.
Rangan, T.S. 1974. Morphogenic investigations on tissue cultures of Panicum miliaceum. Z. Pflanzenphysiol. 72:456-459.
Rangan, T.S. 1976. Growth and plantlet regeneration in tissue cultures of some Indian millets: Paspalum scrobiculatum L., Eleusine coracana Gaertn., and Pennisetum typhoideum Pers. Z. Pflanzenphysiol. 78:208-216.
Rangan, T.S. and Vasil, I.K. 1982. Somatic embryogenesis and plant regeneration from cultured inflorescence segments of Panicum miliaceum and P. miliare. In preparation.
Reinert, J. 1958. Untersuchungen uber die morphogenese in gewebekulturen. Ber. Dtsch. Bot. Ges. 71:15.
Rybczynski, J.J. 1980. In vitro culture of Secale cereale L. explants - callus formation and organ differentiation. Acta Soc. Bot. Polon. 49:155-160.
Sacristan, M.D. and Melchers, G. 1969. The karyological analysis of plants regenerated from tumorous and other callus cultures of tobacco. Mol. Gen. Genet. 105:317-333.
Sangwan, R.S. and Gorenflot, R. 1975. In vitro culture of Phragmites tissues. Callus formation, organ differentiation and cell suspension culture. Z. Pflanzenphysiol. 75:256-259.

Schieder, O. and Vasil, I.K. 1980. Protoplast fusion and somatic hybridization. In: "Perspectives in Plant Cell and Tissue Culture", I.K. Vasil, ed. Int. Rev. Cytol. Suppl. XIB. Academic Press, New York.

Sharma, G.C., Bello, L.L., Sapra, V.T. and Peterson, C.M. 1981. Callus initiation and plant regeneration from triticale embryos. Crop. Sci. 21:113-118.

Shimada, T. 1978. Plant regeneration from the callus induced from wheat embryo. Jap. J. Genet. 53:371-374.

Shimada, T., Sasakuma, T. and Tsunewaki, K. 1969. In vitro culture of wheat tissues. I. Callus formation, organ differentiation and single cell culture. Canad. J. Genet. Cytol. 11:294-304.

Shimada, T. and Yamada, Y. 1979. Wheat plants regenerated from embryo cell cultures. Jap. J. Genet. 54:379-385.

Springer, W.D., Green C.E. and Kohn, K.A. 1979. A histological examination of tissue culture initiation from immature embryos of maize. Protoplasma 101:269-281.

Sreenivasan, T.V. and Jalaja, N.C. 1982. Production of subclones from the callus culture of Saccharum-Zea hybrid. Pl. Sci. Let. 24:255-259.

Sree Ramulu, K., Devreux, M., Ancora, G. and Laneri, U. 1976. Chimerism in Lycopersicum peruvianum plants regenerated from in vitro cultures of anthers and stem internodes. Z. Pflanzenzuchtg. 76:299-319.

Steffensen, D.M. 1968. A reconstruction of cell development in the shoot apex of maize. Amer. J. Bot. 55:354-369.

Skirvin, R.M. 1978. Natural and induced variation in tissue culture. Euphytica 27:241-266.

Steward, F.C., Mapes, M.O. and Mears, K. 1958. Growth and organized development of cultured cells. II. Organization in cultures from freely suspended cells. Amer. J. Bot. 45:705-708.

Tamura, S. 1968. Shoot formation in calli originated from rice embryo. Proc. Jap. Acad. 44:544-548.

Thomas, E., King, P.J. and Potrykus, I. 1977. Shoot and embryo-like structure formation from cultured tissues of Sorghum bicolor. Naturwiss. 64:587.

Thomas, E., King, P.J. and Potrykus, I. 1979. Improvement of crop plants via single cells in vitro - an assessment. Z. Pflanzenzuchtg. 82:1-30.

Tisserat, B., Esan, E. and Murashige, T. 1979. Somatic embryogenesis in angiosperms. Hort. Rev. 1:1-78.

Torne, J. M., Santos, M.A., Pons, A. and Blanco, M. 1980. Regeneration of plants from mesocotyl tissue cultures of immature embryos of Zea mays L. Pl. Sci. Let. 17:339-344.

Vasil, I.K. 1980. Androgenetic haploids. In: "Perspectives in Plant Cell and Tissue Culture", I.K. Vasil, ed. Int. Rev. Cytol. Suppl. XIA. Academic Press. New York.

Vasil, I.K. 1982a. Plant cell culture and somatic cell genetics of cereals and grasses. In: "Plant Improvement and Somatic Cell Genetics", I.K. Vasil, W.R. Scowcroft and K.J. Frey, eds. Academic Press, New York.

Vasil, I.K. 1982b. Toward the development of a single cell system for grasses. In: "Cell and Tissue Culture for Cereal Crop Improvement." Science Press, Peking. In press.

Vasil, I.K. 1982c. Somatic embryogenesis and plant regeneration in cereals and grasses. In" Proc. Vth Int. Congr. Plant Cell and Tissue Culture, Tokyo, Japan. In press.

Vasil, I.K., Ahuja, M.R. and Vasil, V. 1979. Plant tissue cultures in genetics and plant breeding. Adv. Genet. 20: 127-215.

Vasil, I.K. and Hildebrandt, A.C. 1966. Variations of morphogenetic behaviour in plant tissue cultures. I. Cichorium endivia. Amer. J. Bot. 53:860-869.

Vasil, I.K., Vasil, V., Lu, C., Ozias-Akins, P., Haydu, Z. and Wang, D. 1982. Somatic embryogenesis in cereals and grasses. In: "Plant Regeneration and Genetic Variability", E. Earle, ed. Praeger Press, New York.

Vasil, I.K. and Vasil, V. 1980. Isolation and culture of protoplasts. In: "Perspectives in Plant Cell and Tissue Culture", I.K. Vasil, ed. Int. Rev. Cytol. Suppl. XIB. Academic Press, New York.

Vasil, V. and Vasil, I.K. 1979. Isolation and culture of cereal protoplasts. I. Callus formation from pearl millet (Pennisetum americanum) protoplasts. Z. Pflanzenphysiol. 92:379-383.

Vasil, V. and Vasil, I.K. 1980. Isolation and culture of cereal protoplasts. II. Embryogenesis and plantlet formation from protoplasts of Pennisetum americanum. Theoret. Appl. Genet. 56:97-99.

Vasil, V. and Vasil, I.K. 1981a. Somatic embryogenesis and plant regeneration from tissue cultures of Pennisetum americanum, and P. americanum x P. purpureum. Amer. J. Bot. 68:864-872.

Vasil, V. and Vasil, I.K. 1981b. Somatic embryogenesis and plant regeneration from suspension cultures of pearl millet (Pennisetum americanum). Ann. Bot. 47:669-678.

Vasil, V. and Vasil, I.K. 1982a. Characterization of an embryogenic cell suspension culture derived from inflorescences of Pennisetum americanum (Pearl millet, Gramineae). Amer. J. Bot. 69: In Press.

Vasil, V. and Vasil, I.K. 1982b. The ontogeny of somatic embryos of Pennisetum americanum (L.)K. Schum. I. In cultured immature embryos. Bot. Gaz. In Press.

Wang. D. and Vasil, I.K. 1982. Somatic embryogenesis and plant regeneration from inflorescence segments of Pennisetum purpureum Schum. (Napier or elephant grass). Pl. Sci. Let. 25:147-154.

Wang, D., Vasil, V. and Vasil, I.K. 1982. Somatic embryogenesis in cell suspension and protoplast cultures of _Pennisetum purpureum._ In preparaiton.

Wernicke, W. and Brettell, R. 1980. Somatic embryogenesis from _Sorghum bicolor_ leaves. Nature 287:138-139.

Wernicke, W., Brettell, R., Wakizuka, T. and Potrykus, I. 1981. Adventitious embryoid and root formation from rice leaves. Z. Pflanzenphysiol. 103:361-365.

Willmitzer, L., de Benckeleer, M., Lemmers, M., Van Montagu, M. and Schell, J. 1980. DNA from Ti plasmid present in nucleus and absent from plastids of crown gall plant cells. Nature 287:359-360.

Yamabe, M. and Yamada, T. 1973. Studies on differentiation in cultured cells. II. Chromosomes of _Haworthia_ callus and of the plants grown from the callus. La Kromosome (Tokyo) 94: 2923-2931,

Yan, C. and Zhao, Q. 1982. Callus induction and plantlet regeneration from leaf blade of _oryza sativa_ L. subsp. _indica._ Pl. Sci. Let. 25:187-192.

AUXOTROPH COMPLEMENTATION VIA PROTOPLAST FUSION IN HYOSCYAMUS MUTICUS AND NICOTIANA TABACUM

I. Potrykus, R.D. Shillito, J. Jia, and G.B. Lazar

Friedrich Miescher-Institut

P.O. Box 2543, CH-4002 Basel, Switzerland

SUMMARY

Routine plant regeneration from haploid protoplasts of *Hyoscyamus muticus* (egyptian henbane) has been established as basis for auxotroph selection (Lörz et al., 1979; Wernicke et al., 1979). A series of four histidine-, one tryptophan-, three nicotinamide-, and one leucine-requiring auxotrophs of four nitrate nonutilizing lines and of two temperature-sensitive clones have been recovered (Strauss et al., 1981; Gebhardt et al., 1981). Protoplast fusion and subsequent selection by complementation led to the recovery of wild-type clones in various combinations, e.g., his^- + trp^-, nic^- + nic^-, nic^- + NR^-, ts + ts, ts + trp^-, ts + his^-. Intergeneric combination of one of the NR^- auxotrophs of *Hyoscyamus muticus* with both the defined NR^- mutants nia-115 and cnx-68 of *Nicotiana tabacum* (Müller and Grafe, 1978) yielded wild-type clones with the apoenzyme mutant exclusively. Intergeneric combination of one of the nic^- clones of *Hyoscyamus* and the NR^- mutant cnx-68 of *Nicotiana* gave wild-type clones with high morphogenetic potential producing a variety of different morphological types including flowering and fertile plants. Crossing analysis and anther culture analysis of these plants is in progress.

With efficient fusion methods available, the limiting step in somatic hybridization is selection. The ideal selection procedure is auxotroph complementation, which allows for a tight and continuous selective pressure for hybrid clones. It was of interest to test whether this principle would function not only in intraspecific fusion combinations but also in interspecific hybridization, and we will discuss two successful experiments along these lines. However, somatic hybridization among the auxotrophs was of interest also for a different reason: although shoots could be regenerated from the majority of the auxotrophs, none of these shoots developed far enough to produce flowers. Complementation to wild type was expected to facilitate production of flowering plants for crossing analysis and anther culture analysis, and we will report on one example. Independent auxotrophic clones with similar phenotypes, e.g., the four histidine-requiring lines or the three nicotinamide-requiring lines, provided interesting material for somatic cell genetic analysis by both intra- and interspecific

TABLE 1

Phenotype and clone number	Culture stage reached	Biochemical characterization
his^- VA5	shoots	Appears to be blocked in pathway between IGP and histidinol phosphate
his^- IIIE3	callus	Precursor feeding pattern identical to VA5 above
his^- PO3	shoots	Precursor feeding pattern identical to VA5 above
his^- XIIIB5	callus	Precursor feeding pattern identical to VA5 above
trp^- VIIIB9	shoots	Probably A reaction of tryptophan synthetase
nic^- IVH2	grafted shoots	Growth on nicotinamide, nicotinic acid, or quinolinic acid
nic^- III2F10	shoots	Precursor feeding pattern as for IVH2 above
nic^- XE1	shoots	Growth on nicotinamide and nicotinic acid but not on quinolinic acid
NR^- MA-2	shoots	No constitutive or induced NR and no XDH
NR^- I2D12	shoots	As for MA-2 above
NR^- VIC2	shoots	As for MA-2 above
NR^-leu^- XIVE9	callus	As for MA-2 above; has an absolute requirement for leu
ts VG10	callus	No growth at 32°C (growth at 26°C)
ts XIIB2	plants	On transfer to 32°C the cell cultures lose chlorophyll and accumulate brown, insoluble pigment; growth is little affected

TABLE 2

Phenotype and clone number	Culture stage reached	Biochemical characterization
NR^- nia-115	callus	Altered NR apoenzyme, analogous in its properties to nia-63 (Mendel et al., 1981)
NR^- cnx-68	callus	Defective in the molybdenum containing cofactor, no xanthine dehydrogenase activity (Müller and Grafe, 1978; Mendel et al., 1982)

fusion, and we will present two examples of such analyses. Finally, auxotrophs for which the biochemical lesion has been characterized are very valuable material for transformation experiments, and we refer to our separate communication on transformation.

AUXOTROPHIC AND TEMPERATURE-SENSITIVE CLONES USED IN THE SOMATIC HYBRIDIZATION STUDIES

Hyoscyamus muticus: The clones listed in Table 1 have been isolated from haploid mesophyll protoplasts. The phenotypes are stable and tight under rigid retesting. All clones are independent isolates. The isolation procedure and part of the clones have been published (Gebhardt et al., 1981; Strauss et al., 1981).

Nicotiana tabacum: The defined nitrate reductase-deficient mutants nia-115 and cnx-68 have kindly been supplied by A.J. Müller, Gatersleben. Their characteristics are given in Table 2.

INTERSPECIFIC COMPLEMENTATION

Hyoscyamus muticus nic^-IVH2 + *Nicotiana tabacum* NR^-cnx-68

Hyoscyamus muticus clone nic^-IVH2 has an absolute requirement for nicotinic acid or nicotinamide. It grows on AA culture medium (Müller and Grafe, 1978) supplemented with 5 mg/liter nicotinic acid. Protoplasts isolated from suspension cultures grow with plating efficiencies around 5% in the same culture medium.

Nicotiana tabacum clone NR^-cnx-68 has an absolute requirement for reduced nitrogen. It grows on AA culture medium. Protoplasts isolated from suspension cultures grow with plating efficiencies around 10% in the same culture medium. Protoplast-derived microcolonies of nic^-IVH2 stop proliferating and die upon transfer into nicotinic acid-free culture medium. Protoplast-derived microcolonie of NR$^-$cnx-68 die upon transfer into culture medium containing nitrat as sole nitrogen source.

The protocol for protoplast fusion was modified from that of Glimelius et al. (1978). Protoplast populations were mixed to give a final population density of 2.5 x 10^5/ml of both fusion partners. The mixed population was pipetted into 6-cm-diameter plastic Petri dishes to give 8 regularly arranged 100-µl drops, and the protoplast were allowed to sediment onto the plastic surface. Thereafter 100 µl of 25% PEG 4000 dissolved in osmoticum was added to each drop and left for 3 minutes. Washing solution at pH 8 was then gently added 3 times at 10 minute intervals. Finally the Petri dishes were fille with 10 ml of culture medium to dilute out the PEG, and the excess was removed to leave 3 ml culture medium per Petri dish. The dishes were incubated at 26°C in the dark.

In each experiment half of the parental protoplast populations were used for the following control experiments: (1) mixing and coculture of the parental types to study possible cross-feeding effects, (2) homologous fusion of both parental types separately to study possible PEG effects, (3) culture of untreated parental types to study plating efficiency and possible reversion.

All protoplast populations were cultured for 10-14 days under nonselective conditions (AA culture medium supplemented with 5 mg pe liter nicotinic acid). Transfer into selective conditions (AA culture medium with KNO_3 as sole nitrogen source according to Glimelius et al. (1978) and without nicotinic acid was by sequential dilution which also included a reduction in the osmotic pressure. Following two dilutions with "minimal" medium, protoplast-derived cell cultures were collected by sedimentation, resuspended in selection medium, plated over agar-solidified selection medium, and further incubated at 27°C, 12 hours light. Proliferating clones were transferred onto fresh selection medium every two weeks. Shoot and root differentiation was approached by reducing the auxin concentration and maintaining the cytokinin concentration, or by omitting the growth regulators completely from the culture medium. The cultures were maintained throughout the experiment under strict selective conditions. The experiments were repeated three times and the results were reproducible.

Results

(a) Control experiments

(1) nic$^-$IVH2 protoplasts and NR$^-$cnx-68 protoplasts grew under non-selective conditions with plating efficiencies (% of the originally plated protoplasts forming macrocolonies) of not less than 5%.

(2) PEG nontreated mixtures of nic$^-$IVH2 and NR$^-$cnx-68 grew in nonselective medium with similar plating efficiencies.
(3) nic$^-$IVH2 protoplasts, NR$^-$cnx-68 protoplasts, and PEG non-treated mixtures of both did not grow in selective medium.
(4) nic$^-$IVH2 protoplasts treated with PEG developed to macro-colonies in nonselective medium, and did not proliferate further in selective medium.
(5) NR$^-$cnx-68 protoplasts treated with PEG developed to macro-colonies in nonselective medium, and did not proliferate further in selective medium.
(6) Microcolonies (4-50 cells) grown within the first 10-14 days and thereafter gradually transferred into selective medium did not proliferate further.
(7) Macrocolonies (larger than 500 cells) grown within four weeks did not develop further when transferred into selective medium.
(8) nic$^-$IVH2- and NR$^-$cnx-68-derived clones grown under non-selective conditions did not form shoots.

(b) Somatic hybridization treatment

(9) In those Petri dishes where mixtures of nic$^-$IVH2 protoplasts and NR$^-$cnx-68 protoplasts had been treated with PEG, colonies continued to develop further under selective conditions and numerous macrocolonies developed in a background of dying microcolonies. The hybridization frequency (% of originally plated protoplasts forming macrocolonies under selective conditions) has not been established and only a sample of the presumptive hybrid clones was further subcultured.
(10) Proliferation of these clones on minimal medium was far more rapid than that of either parental clone on complete medium.
(11) Transfer to selection medium with reduced auxin or to hormone-free medium resulted in the formation of numerous shoots from individual clones; however, not all clones produced shoots.
(12) There was considerable variation in morphological character between clones and relative homogeneity within clones. The variation ranged from nonmorphogenetic white and green clones, over different types of teratomata-producing clones, to clones which differentiated "normal" shoots, however with differently formed leaves.
(13) The majority of the clones tested were hormone-independent in their proliferation, and root differentiation was not possible with the routine techniques. Only recently, in four cases so far, has it been possible to induce roots on shoots in vitro. These plants are growing in soil.
(14) Routine further development of the shoots was possible, however, via grafting. Shoots were grafted onto *Nicotiana tabacum* and onto *Hyoscyamus muticus*. They took exclusively on *N. tabacum*,

where they developed to flowering and fertile shoots with predominantly *Hyoscyamus* morphology. Genetic crossing analysis and anther culture analysis of selected clones is in progress.

(15) Shoots which upon grafting had developed vigorous shoot systems have been rooted with commercial rooting powder, and numerous subclones are growing in soil.

(16) Amylase isoenzyme analysis revealed bands from both parental plants in the presumptive hybrid clones.

The results strongly support the hypothesis that the clones which proliferated under continuous selective conditions are indeed intergeneric somatic fusion hybrid clones between *Hyoscyamus muticus* nic$^-$IVH2 and *Nicotiana tabacum* NR$^-$cnx-68. In addition to the conclusions possible on the basis of the control experiments, support is provided by the results of the isoenzyme analysis, the more vigorous growth (hybrid vigor?), the hormone-independent growth (genetic tumor?), the unique morphogenetic potential which exceeds dramatically that of both parental clones. Final proof will, however, be available only from the crossing analysis and anther culture analysis. Chloroplast DNA restriction analysis and Fraction I protein analysis are in progress and will also contribute to the final decision as to whether auxotroph complementation selection is a safe method for intergeneric fusion hybrids. Chromosome analysis has not been attempted yet and will be difficult due to the lack of clear marker chromosomes.

H. muticus NR$^-$MA-2 + *N. tabacum* NR$^-$nia-115 and NR$^-$cnx-68

The auxotrophs isolated from haploid *Hyoscyamus* protoplasts also included a series of nitrate nonutilizing clones. With the two defined NR$^-$ mutants available from *Nicotiana tabacum* two questions could be asked directly: (1) can auxotroph complementation be applied to select for intergeneric fusion hybrids, and (2) can somatic hybridization be used to identify biochemical defects via complementation analysis not only within one species but also among unrelated species.

Hyoscyamus muticus clone NR$^-$MA-2 is deficient in nitrate reductase activity. *Nicotiana tabacum* clone NR$^-$nia-115 has an altered (nonfunctional) NR-apoenzyme, clone cnx-68 is defective in the molybdenum containing cofactor and also lacks activity of the molybdenum cofactor-requiring xanthine dehydrogenase. All three clones and their protoplasts grow in AA culture medium (Glimelius et al., 1978) containing amino acid mixture as nitrogen source, and do not grow on NO_3 medium (Müller and Grafe, 1978) which contains KNO_3 as sole nitrogen source. If intergeneric complementation is possible via protoplast fusion, hybridization between MA-2 and nia-115 or cnx-68 should enable one to (a) identify the nature of the nitrate reductase defect in MA-2 (apoenzyme or cofactor) and (b) select for intergeneric fusion hybrids.

Protoplasts isolated from suspension cultures were adjusted to a population of density of 10^5 per ml. Depending upon the number of protoplasts available, 3-7 independent fusion treatments were done from the same population as well as the control experiments, which included homologous fusion of both parental types separately, mixing and coculture without PEG treatment, and culture of both parental protoplasts without PEG treatment.

In a standard fusion procedure equal volumes of protoplast suspensions were mixed, subdivided into 1 ml aliquots pipetted into plastic Petri dishes in 100 µl drops, treated with an equal volume of 50% PEG 4000 for 10 minutes, and thereafter gradually diluted with washing solution at pH 9. The protoplasts were then carefully washed twice with the nonselective AA culture medium and incubated in this medium for 10-14 days at 24°C in the dark. Thereafter NO_3 culture medium with reduced osmotic pressure was gradually added over a further 7 days. The protoplast-derived clones were then washed with selective medium and plated onto agar-solidified selective medium.

Results

(1) In 8 independent fusion treatments of MA-2 + MA-2 (10^5 protoplasts per treatment) no nitrate-utilizing colonies could be recovered.
(2) In 8 independent fusion treatments of nia-115 + nia-115 no nitrate-utilizing colonies could be recovered.
(3) In 8 independent fusion treatments of cnx-68 + cnx-68 no nitrate-utilizing colonies could be recovered.
(4) In 24 independent fusion treatments of MA-2 + cnx-68 no nitrate-utilizing clone could be recovered.
(5) From 9 independent fusion treatments of nia-115 + cnx-68, 206 nitrate-utilizing clones have been recovered with a complementation frequency ranging from 1.5×10^{-4} to 1.9×10^{-3}.
(6) From 18 independent fusion treatments of MA-2 + nia-115, 200 nitrate-utilizing clones have been recovered with complementation frequencies ranging from 0 to 1.3×10^{-3}.

These results are consistent with the assumption that MA-2 is a molybdenum cofactor mutant (complementation exclusively with the apoenzyme mutant of *Nicotiana*), that complementation via fusion between the *Nicotiana* apoenzyme mutant and the *Hyoscyamus* cofactor mutant is not disturbed by intergeneric incompatibilities (similar complementation frequencies between MA-2 + nia-115 and between cnx-68 + nia-115), and that the nitrate-utilizing clones are intergeneric hybrid clones between *H. muticus* and *N. tabacum*.

(7) As xanthine dehydrogenase shares a common molybdenum cofactor with the nitrate reductase (Mendel and Müller, 1976), MA-2 should also lack xanthine dehydrogenase activity if it is a

molybdenum cofactor mutant. nia-115, *H. muticus* wild type, and three selected clones from the putative hybrids were positive for xanthine dehydrogenase, while MA-2 and cnx-68 did not show any activity.

(8) The hybrid nature of some selected putative hybrid clones was confirmed by results from alcohol dehydrogenase isoenzyme analysis. MA-2 and nia-115 cultures produce one band each, differing in electrophoretic mobility. The putative hybrid clones produced both parental bands plus an additional band with intermediate mobility.

(9) In vivo nitrate reductase activity could be detected in the hybrid clones and in *H. muticus* wild type only after induction on NO_3 medium and on similar levels. Neither MA-2 nor nia-115 has measurable activity under inductive or noninductive conditions.

(10) In contrast to the *H. muticus* nic^-IVH2 + *N. tabacum* NR^-cnx-68 hybrid described above, the *H. muticus* MA-2 + *N. tabacum* NR^-nia-115 hybrid clones did not express any morphogenetic potential.

INTRASPECIFIC COMPLEMENTATION

Following the same experimental scheme and including the controls as given for the intergeneric hybridization experiments described above, a series of intraspecific fusion experiments has been performed to study complementation within *Hyoscyamus muticus* and to combine the defective genotypes in complementing wild-type clones for subsequent plant regeneration for crossing and anther culture analysis.

Hyoscyamus muticus nic^-XE1 + NR^-MA-2

From PEG treated mixtures of protoplasts of the nicotinic acid-requiring clone XE1 and of the nitrate reductase-deficient clone MA-2, and from none of the control treatments, presumptive hybrid clones could be selected and maintained on minimal medium. Besides white and green nonmorphogenic clones, numerous clones which produced shoots with fleshy and recallusing leaves developed on hormone-free medium or under shoot-inductive conditions. So far four "normalized" shoots have grown out spontaneously from the recallusing clones. Three of these have been lost after transfer to soil, but one is growing vigorously in soil and will, we hope, produce flowers.

Hyoscyamus muticus trp^-VIIIB9 + his^-VA5

Protoplasts from the tryptophan-requiring clone VIIIB9 and from the histidine-requiring clone VA5 yielded, following mixing and PEG treatment, a number of clones which proliferate vigorously on minimal medium. Clones which grow on minimal medium could not be recovered from the controls. The putative hybrid clones did not, so far, respond with plant regeneration to a variety of treatments aimed at shoot induction.

Hyoscyamus muticus nic$^-$IVH2 + nic$^-$XE1 + nic$^-$III2F10

Complementation among the three independent nicotinamide-requiring clones was studied. However, since clone III2F10 has not yet been established as rapidly growing suspension, and since good suspensions are a prerequisite for the isolation of large enough populations of protoplasts to include all controls in each experiment, these complementation studies are incomplete and only preliminary. So far complementation leading to wild-type clones was observed only in the combination of clone IVH2 + clone XE1.

Hyoscyamus muticus ts VG10 + ts XIIB2

The temperature-sensitive clones differ in their phenotype, and therefore complementation was to be expected. VG10 does not grow at 32°C whereas XIIB2 grows as well at 32°C as at 27°C but accumulates a brown insoluble pigment and loses chlorophyll at the higher temperature. Fusion combination of both temperature-sensitive clones restored wild-type phenotype, and ca. 30 clones are growing under restrictive conditions. Shoot induction from these clones has not yet been achieved. No wild-type clones were recovered from the control experiments. In this experiment division could not be induced in the XIIB2 protoplasts cultured alone with or without PEG treatment. This fusion therefore also represents a rescue of the XIIB2 genome by the VG10 cells. However, XIIB2 was not rescued by either VA5 or VIIIB9.

Hyoscyamus muticus trp$^-$VIIIB9 + ts VG10

This combination of the tryptophan-requiring clone VIIIB9 and the temperature-sensitive clone VG10 was established as a "satellite" control experiment in the ts-complementation test, set up to check that any lack of complementation of the ts mutants was not due to an inability to survive fusion or to divide. Of a total of 173 clones tested, 21 proliferate under continuous restrictive conditions. No wild-type clones were recovered from the control experiments. Plant regeneration has not yet been achieved.

The series of fusion experiments among the auxotrophs and temperature-sensitive clones from *Hyoscyamus muticus* and between some of these auxotrophs and the nitrate reductase-deficient mutants of *Nicotiana tabacum* has shown that:

(a) auxotroph complementation selection provides an efficient method for the isolation of somatic hybrids even in intergeneric combinations,

(b) complementation analysis by protoplast fusion provides a method for the characterization of metabolic defects even in intergeneric combinations,

(c) recovery of wild type phenotype by auxotroph complementation does not necessarily restore the morphogenetic response of the original wild type. It will have to be seen in future combinations of *N. tabacum* NR$^-$cnx-68 with other *Hyoscyamus* auxotrophs whether or not the intensive shoot regeneration response from the hybrid clones *N. tabacum* NR$^-$cnx-68 + *H. muticus* nic$^-$IVH2 is a unique phenomenon or is to be found in other crosses of this type.

ACKNOWLEDGMENT

Isolation and characterization of the auxotrophs and temperature sensitive clones as well as part of the characterization of some of the putative hybrid clones, e.g., ts + ts, ts + trp, ts + his, MA-2 + cnx-68, is the work of P.J. King's group at the FMI, including Drs. C. Gebhardt, H. Fankhauser, and K. Shimamoto.

LITERATURE

Gebhardt, C., Schnebli, V., and King, P.J. (1981), Isolation of biochemical mutants using haploid mesophyll protoplasts of *Hyoscyamus muticus*. II. Auxotrophic and temperature-sensitive clones. Planta 153, 81-89.

Glimelius, K., Eriksson, T., Grafe, R., and Müller, A.J. (1978), Somatic hybridization of nitrate reductase-deficient mutants of *Nicotiana tabacum* by protoplast fusion. Physiol. Plant. 44, 273-277

Lörz, H., Wernicke, W., and Potrykus, I. (1979), Culture and plant regeneration of *Hyoscyamus* protoplasts. Planta Medica 36, 21-29.

Mendel, R.-R., and Müller, A.J. (1979), Nitrate reductase-deficient cell lines of *Nicotiana tabacum*. Further biochemical characterization. Molec. gen. Genet. 177, 145-153.

Mendel, R.-R., Alikulov, Z.A., and Müller, A.J. (1982), Molybdenum cofactor in nitrate reductase-deficient tobacco mutants, II. Release of cofactor by heat treatment. Plant Science Letters, 25, 67-72.

Mendel, R.-R., Alikulov, Z.A., Lvov, N.P., and Müller, A.J. (1981), Presence of the molybdenum cofactor in nitrate reductase-deficient mutant cell lines of *Nicotiana tabacum*. Molec. gen. Genet. 181, 395-399.

Müller, A.J., and Grafe, R. (1978), Isolation and characterization of cell lines of *Nicotiana tabacum* lacking nitrate reductase. Molec. gen. Genet. 161, 67-76.

Strauss, A., Bucher, F., and King, P.J. (1981), Isolation of biochemical mutants using haploid mesophyll protoplasts of *Hyoscyamus muticus*. I. A NO_3-non-utilising clone. Planta 153, 75-80.

Wernicke, W., Lörz, H., and Thomas, E. (1979), Plant regeneration from leaf protoplasts of haploid *Hyoscyamus muticus* produced via anther culture. Plant Science Letters 15, 239-249.

APPROACHES TO PLANT PROTOPLAST TRANSFORMATION USING DRUG RESISTANCE AND AUXOTROPH COMPLEMENTATION AS SELECTIVE MARKERS

R.D. Shillito, G. Lazar, J. Paszkowski, K. Shimamoto, Z. Nicola-Koukolikova, B. Hohn, T. Hohn, and I. Potrykus

Friedrich Miescher-Institut
P.O. Box 2543, CH-4002 Basel
Switzerland

SUMMARY

The factors involved in building a successful plant protoplast transformation system are discussed, with particular reference to the methods of delivery, choice of markers and expression of introduced DNA. Experiments aimed at transforming protoplasts with resistance and other genes are described.

INTRODUCTION

Research on DNA mediated transformation of higher plants is still in the technical phase of development, focused on the setting up of systems for introducing and expressing foreign DNA in plant cells.

There are a number of approaches available:

a: Introduction of DNA sequences via integration into the T-DNA region of the Ti plasmid of Agrobacterium tumefaciens and in-planta or in-vitro bacterial mediated transformation (piggy-back method). This is a reliable method of introducing DNA and ensuring its integration (see other contributions to this meeting) but has not as yet led to expression of any markers other than those of T-DNA itself. Similar methods using the Ti plasmid of *A. rhizogenes* will probably be developed in the near future.

b: Naked DNA transformation of protoplasts. This includes methods using liposomes and bacterial spheroplasts (packaged DNA) and microinjection. In this case plant protoplasts are treated with DNA in uptake-promoting conditions (or injected), but success has only been reported when whole Ti plasmid was used as the vector (Davey et al. 1980; Krens et al. 1981). This method requires the use of some suitable marker for selection of transformants that occur at a low frequency; in the Ti plasmid experiments this is typically 10^{-5}. A number of authors have reported transformation of plant cells with naked DNA in-planta (Ledoux et al. 1974; Korohoda and Strzalka, 1979; Hess, 1981), but these experiments appear difficult to reproduce in other laboratories.

c: Transformation with plant viruses carrying inserts. This route for introducing DNA is particularly interesting as it may allow the maintenance of independent replicons in plant cells. The gemini and caulimoviruses are possible candidates for adaptation to this role, being the only two known groups of plant DNA viruses The cauliflower mosaic virus (CaMV) is particularly well studied in this respect (see reviews of Hohn et al. 1982; and Howell et al. 1980).

In this paper we deal mainly with those systems involving use of protoplasts as recipients of DNA.

THE REQUIREMENTS FOR PLANT PROTOPLASTS TRANSFORMATION

Successful transformation depends upon the uptake of intact genetic material, its integration or autonomous replication, correct transcription, processing and translation, and upon the gene product being able to function in its new genetic background. Finally, the protoplasts used must divide and form colonies with a reproducibly high plating efficiency.

Choice of vector

Vectors to be employed in transformation studies should be chosen so as to allow rapid DNA production, afford protection from degradation during and after entry into the cells, promote integration and/or autonomously replicate, contain a selectable marker and not interfere with the expression of inserted genetic material. All vectors so far used have been cloned and multiplied in *E. coli*, on small multicopy plasmids. Incorporation of the chosen material into viral- or T-DNA sequences may or may not afford some degree of protection. In general, integration into the plant genome by illegitimate recombination has been relied upon. The occurrence of this may be increased by some unknown properties of the T-DNA end fragments. Incorporation of pieces of repeated DNA sequences from plants to provide a region of homology with the plant genome may be a further way of increasing the chance of integration.

Autonomously replicating plasmids have facilitated greatly the study of genes in bacteria, yeasts and fungi. It may be that DNA viruses of the gemini or caulimo type can be used as a source of origins for autonomous replication in plant cells. If they are to become useful as vectors in their own right then pathogenic functions must be mapped and eliminated and space created for insertion of foreign material. It has been shown recently (Gronenborn et al. 1981) that small pieces of foreign DNA can be propagated through virus particles of CaMV in the plant. For a review of this field see Howell, 1982).

Delivery of DNA to protoplasts

A number of groups have investigated the uptake of DNA by higher plant protoplasts (Behki and Lesley, 1979; Kado and Kleinhofs, 1980). The protocols generally employed are those that have proved successful for virus transfection or are based on the treatments promoting fusion. Davey (pers. comm.) has investigated a number of these methods for transforming *Petunia hybrida* protoplasts with Ti plasmid and concluded that the polyethylene-glycol (PEG) based method was the most efficient, although poly-L-ornithine treatment has proved better for the algae *Chlamydomonas* (Rochaix, 1982). The PEG method has been employed in successful transformation of protoplasts with Ti plasmid (Davey et al. 1980; Krens et al. 1982).

Packaging experiments with liposomes are being carried out in a number of laboratories and the delivery of their contents into cells investigated (Uchimiya, 1981; Lurquin, 1982; Rollo et al. 1981). This system has given high transformation frequencies with fungal and animal cells (Fraley et al. 1980; Radford et al. 1981) but has yet to be proven useful for plant cells. Fusion of bacteria with eukaryotic cells has been successful as a means of gene transfer in a number of cases (Schaffner, 1980; Rassoulzadegan et al. 1982). *A. tumefaciens* spheroplasts carrying Ti plasmid have been reported to be taken up by and to transform *Vinca rosea* protoplasts (Hasezawa et al. 1981). However, transformants were also obtained in similar treatments using whole bacteria and we have ourselves never been able to repeat this spheroplast work using conditions which preclude whole bacteria-mediated transformation.

Although microinjection is a certain way of delivering DNA (Diacumakos et al. 1970; Anderson et al. 1980), there are a number of unsolved problems in using this method with plant cells, including the holding of cells or protoplasts and avoidance of the vacuole. No successes with this method have been reported for plants.

Choice of Markers

There are no reported cases of the combination of a cloned plant gene and a fully developed mutant cell culture system that allows selection. A number of laboratories including our own are investigating the use of dominant drug-resistance markers in transformation experiments. Two drugs that are particularly useful in this respect are G-418, an aminoglycoside antibiotic (Daniels, 1973; Davies and Jimenez, 1980; Ursic et al. 1981), and methotrexate, both of which are toxic for a wide range of organisms including plant cells.

G-418: Bacterial phosphotransferases from transposons Tn5 and Tn903 can be introduced into yeast where they are expressed and confer resistance to G-418 (Jimenez and Davies, 1980; J.P. and Z.N-K. unpub.). The Tn903 appears to be expressed from sequences upstream of the coding region while the Tn5 gene has to be provided with a yeast promotor. The latter gene has also been expressed from appropriate promotors in animal cells (Colbere-Gerapin et al. 1981; Southern and Berg, 1982).

Methotrexate: The target enzyme for methotrexate is dihydrofolate reductase (DHFR). In this case the gene for a methotrexate resistant DHFR from an *Escherichia coli* plasmid is available (Fling and Elwell, 1980) and when expressed from the SV40 early promoter can confer methotrexate resistance on mouse fibroblasts (O'Hare et al. 1981).

These genes that have been expressed in other eukaryotes may be selectable in plant cells. A further source of selectable genes is the T-DNA of Ti plasmid e.g. the area coding for hormone independence. The nopaline and octopine synthesis genes would make good markers to confirm the identity of transformants and may themselves be selectable (van Slogteren et al. 1982). A further approach is the use of Ti plasmid together with other DNA in co-transformation. The advantage of this method over the normal crown gall route is that a wide range of foreign DNAs can be tested without the need to insert them into T-DNA. It should be possible to separate the tumourous and the non-selected genes by segregation.

The availability of plant mutants such as nitrate reductase mutants (Müller & Grafe, 1978), Adh$^{1-0}$ or the recently produced auxotrophs (Gebhardt et al. 1981; Savage et al. 1979; Sidorov and Maliga, 1982) which show little or no reversion offers the possibility of correcting mutants using complementary genes from other sources.

Expression

Once DNA sequences have been introduced into plant cells and are maintained by integration or autonomous replication, then expression of the genes may be still a problem. Many transformation studies rely on expression of the chosen gene for selection of transformants. However, in no case where foreign genes have been inserted into plant cells via the crown gall method have the genes been shown to be expressed faithfully, except those of T-DNA itself. Constructions in the T-DNA designed to give accurate fusion between the gene to be expressed and known plant transcriptional and translation signals are now being tested in several laboratories. Testing of such 'engineered' genes without insertion into the T-DNA can also be carried out, but selection would rely on expression of the desired phenotype.

While it is possible that a number of genes may be expressed from their own signals, it will be generally necessary to link the chosen gene to promotion sequences giving a high level of expression in plants, such as from opine synthesis and other genes of T-DNA or from the genes of CaMV. A third approach is to search for plant promotors by shotgun cloning of plant or other DNA sequences upstream of a selectable gene deprived of its own promotor. In addition one might add splicing and stop signals to the end of the gene as has been done in animal cell systems (eg: O'Hare et al. 1981). The polyadenylation site of the nopaline dehydrogenase gene of T-DNA is being used by a number of people for this purpose.

EXPERIMENTS AT THE FRIEDRICH MIESCHER-INSTITUT, BASEL

Studies of plant transformation with naked DNA are being carried out at our Institute using protoplasts as recipients. Experiments with CaMV based vectors were carried out using nia 115 tobacco and 2A2A carrot suspension culture protoplasts as these systems produce large numbers of uniform protoplasts. Tobacco (SR_1) leaf protoplasts were used for promoter search and co-transformation experiments as it was known that they were transformable, at least with Ti plasmid.

In designing our experiments, we have concentrated on the following lines of approach based on considerations discussed above. Only a small proportion of the 100 or more experiments gave results suggesting that transformation occurred. These experiments were of four types:

1) Attempts to use CaMV as a vector to offer the possibility of independent replication or short term protection of the introduced gene.

2) Use of a yeast gene in attempts to correct a cell line auxotrophic for tryptophan.

3) Shotgun promoter search experiments.

4) Co-transformation.

1) CaMV vectors

The concept of using CaMV as a vector was investigated in the following ways:

a) The unmodified aminoglycoside phosphotransferase I (APH I) from Tn903 (Grindley and Joyce, 1980) was inserted into a cloned CaMV and the hybrid plasmids obtained were offered to tobacco and carrot cell-line protoplasts. Cultures were selected for resistance to G-418. Only tobacco protoplasts gave a differential response after DNA treatment.

b) The eukaryotic expression vector of O'Hare et al. (1981) carrying a methotrexate resistance gene was offered to carrot protoplasts either unmodified or as a cointegrate with CaMV and the cultures selected for resistance to the drug.

a) Tobacco cell transformation with CaMV vectors carrying the APH I gene

The first CaMV vector used contained the complete APH I gene, including the sequences thought to promote expression in yeast (Jimenez and Davies, 1980). This gene was introduced into three different EcoRI sites of cloned CaMV DNA. *Nia* 115 protoplasts were treated with the three vectors as calcium phosphate co-precipitates in the presence of PEG. After washing out of the PEG with a high pH washing medium (pH 9.0), the protoplasts were cultured for 2 weeks and then plated into solid medium containing 5 mg/l G-418. Resistant colonies from each plate were transferred into medium containing 10 mg/l G-418. In this way 5 lines were recovered showing stable resistance to the drug at a concentration of 32 mg/l. Such lines were only recovered from protoplasts treated with the vector containing the APH I gene inserted downstream from the CaMV gene VI promoter. Control cultures treated with the other 2 constructs or with carrier DNA alone were sensitive to 5 mg/l G-418.

Sequences hybridising to CaMV DNA were not found in the resistant material. However, on probing of a blot of EcoRl cut DNA, faint bands with a size of around 4 kb were found hybridising to the APH I gene at the limit of resolution, corresponding to about 0.1 copies per haploid genome. The cells are on average decaploid, so that if these bands represent foreign DNA then it must be present at about a single copy per cell. As the gene was inserted originally into the vector as an EcoRl fragment of 1200 base pairs, recombination must have occurred within this fragment to give the higher molecular weight bands. The doublet of bands suggested that the culture tested was chimeric and cell cloning via protoplasts was carried out. Lines resistance to 32 mg/l G-418 were recovered and are now being probed for the presence of the gene.

b) Carrot protoplast transformation with a eukaryotic expression vector

The pHG expression vector is able to confer methotrexate resistance on mouse fibroblasts (O'Hare et al. 1981) via expression of a methotrexate insensitive DHFR gene derived from an *E. coli* plasmid (Fling and Elwell,

1980). This vector was used at the F.M.I. either as received or as a cointegrate with CaMV. Carrot protoplasts were treated with the DNA and then washed with a high pH medium as described above. Dimethylsulphoxide was included in the first 5 minute wash at 1% as this has been advantageous in transformation of bacterial and avian cells (Orlova et al. 1978; Graf, 1975). After 2 weeks culture without the selective drug, the cells were plated out in solid medium containing 5 mg/l methotrexate and 10 mg/l dihydrofolate (DHF). The latter was included to reduce toxicity of the methotrexate to the plant cells due to the inhibition of folic acid reductase by methotrexate. The drug is inhibitory to cells at a lower concentration in the absence of DHF. In experiments carried out with selection on methotrexate alone, no differences between treated and control cultures were ever observed. Two colonies were recovered following treatment of 8 x 10^6 protoplasts with the original vector and four colonies after treatment of the same number with the cointegrate vector. None were recovered from control protoplasts (16 x 10^6), although resistant lines could be recovered at a low frequency following plating of large numbers of cells in the lower level of 2 mg/l methotrexate in the presence of DHF. The putative transformant lines were resistant to 100 mg/l methotrexate in the absence of DHF, whereas the wild type was inhibited completely by 1 mg/l. The resistant phenotype was stable in the absence of the drug for a period of 4 months (15-20 cell generations). Measurement of DHFR activity in the lines suggested that a small percentage of the activity is insensitive to methotrexate, whereas the activity in extracts of wild type cells was completely inhibited by 5 µg/l of the drug.

Probing of this material has not detected any CaMV or other foreign DNA sequences. In a repeat of the experiment using only the cointegrate vector, clones resistant to methotrexate were recovered again from treated cells at a frequency 8 times that found in the controls.

Great care must be taken in interpreting the results since in animal cells endogenous DHFR genes tend to be amplified in response to selective pressure for methotrexate resistance (eg: Alt et al. 1978). Final characterisation of the carrot cell lines will require unambiguous southern blots and the reisolation of the gene.

2) Attempted auxotroph transformation to prototrophy

Complementation of the *H.muticus* tryptophan auxotroph (VIIIB9) isolated by Gebhardt et al. (1982) has been attempted. No revertants of this line have been observed and the defect has been identified as the absence of the A-reaction of tryptophan synthetase (H. Fankhauser, unpub.). Cloned yeast tryptophan synthetase gene was used in preliminary attempts to transform this line using treatment of protoplasts with DNA in the presence of PEG. No prototrophs were recovered from 5 x 10^7 treated protoplasts. Work is in progress to contruct a vector carrying plant transcriptional signals linked to the tryptophan synthetase structural gene to be applied using naked DNA/PEG or the *Agrobacterium* Ti plasmid insertion method.

3) Transformation with a shotgun promoter search vector

Plasmids have been constructed in which the gene for the aminoglycoside phosphotransferase II from Tn5 (APH II) has been deprived of its promoter and where a unique BglII site exists just in front of the structural part of the gene. This construction has been used to recover sequences promoting high levels of expression of the gene marker in yeast using shotgun insertion of a partial Sau3A digest of yeast DNA into this site (J.P. and Z.N-K. unpub.).

Three G-418 resistant clones were obtained following transformation of tobacco protoplasts with a family of 600 plasmids obtained using CaMV and T-DNA as the source of DNA for the partial Sau3A digest. Selection of possible transformants was carried out on 10 mg/l of the drug and the lines actually survive on 32 mg/l. Wildtype cultures are sensitive to 5 mg/l and we were not able to isolate lines resistant to the higher levels of the drug by any method other than the DNA treatment. These lines are being characterised further and their DNA probed for presence of the APH II structural gene.

4) Co-transformation

Co-transformation is used routinely to transfer non-selectable DNA sequences into animal cells (eg: Wigler et al 1978). We have made use of the repeatable Ti plasmid naked DNA transformation to attempt insertion of some of our drug resistance vectors into tobacco cells (in collaboration with Drs. F. Krens of the University of Leiden, Holland). Selection for hormone autotrophy was carried out and preliminary results in one clone so far analysed suggest that DNA from the non-selected vectors is indeed integrated into the DNA of the cells (F. Krens). The drug resistance of these cells has not yet been determined.

IN CONCLUSION

There is, as yet no unambiguous proof that any of the drug resistant cell lines obtained at the F.M.I. is a true transformant, although their phenotypes strongly suggest this to be the case. However, the experiments to date have been helpful for understanding the problems inherent in selecting possible transformants from DNA-treated protoplast populations and they have indicated the advantages of using non-revertant auxotrophs in place of the leaky resistance phenotypes.

The vectors used were of crude construction or were not made specifically for plant work. The way forward lies in constructing precise, plant-oriented vectors containing transcriptional and translational signals derived from genes known to be expressed in plant cells.

CaMV-based vectors were not seen to replicate autonomously for long periods in the systems tested, although some replication may have occurred in the initial phase. Recent advances in the culture of Brassica napus protoplasts will allow the CaMV approach to be investigated more fully as replication at the whole plant level is known to occur in this species.

We expect that one or a combination of these approaches will lead to the expression of foreign genes in plant cells in the not too distant future. The extension of this step to useful genetic engineering of plants requires the identification and the long-term study of the genes governing desirable traits in plants.

Literature

Alt, F.W., R.E. Kellems, J.R. Bertino and R.T. Schimke, 1978: J. Biol. Chem. 253, 1357-1370.
Anderson, W.F., L. Killos, L. Sanders-Haigh, P.J. Kretschmer and E.G. Diacumakos, 1980: Proc. Natl. Acad. Sci. USA., 77, 5399-5403.
Behki, R.M. and S.M. Lesley, 1979: In Vitro, 15, 851-856.
Colbere-Garapin, F., F. Horodniceanu, P. Kourilsky and

A.C. Garapin, 1981: J. Mol. Biol., 150, 1-14.
Daniels, P.J.L., A.S. Yehaskel and J.B. Morton, 1973: Proc. 13th Interscience Conf. on Antimicrobial Agents and Chemotherapy, Washington, 1973, Abs. 137.
Davey, M.R., E.C. Cocking, J. Freeman, N. Pearce and I. Tudor, 1980: Plant Sci. Lett., 18, 307-313.
Davies, J. and A. Jimenez, 1980: Am. J. Trop. Med. 29 suppl., 1089-1092.
Diacumakos, E.G., S. Holland and P. Pecora, 1970: Proc. Natl. Acad. Sci. USA., 65, 911-918.
Fling, M.E. and L.P. Elwell, 1980: J. Bacteriol., 141, 779-785.
Fraley, R.T., C.S. Fornani and S. Kaplan, 1979: Proc. Natl. Acad. Sci. USA., 76, 3348-3352.
Gebhardt, C., V. Schnebli and P.J. King, 1981: Planta, 153, 81-89.
Graf, T., 1975: Z. Naturforsch., 30c, 847-849.
Grindley, N.D.F. and C.M. Joyce, 1980: Proc. Natl. Acad. Sci. USA., 77, 7176-7180.
Gronenborn, B., R.C. Gardner, S. Schaefer and R.J. Shephard, 1981: Nature, 294, 773-776.
Hasezawa, S., T. Nagata and S. Syono, 1981: Mol. Gen. Genet., 182, 206-210.
Hohn, T., K. Richards and G. Lebeurier, 1982: Current Topics in Microbiology and Immunology, 96, 193-236.
Howell, S.H., L.L. Walker, R.K. Dudley, 1980: Science, 208, 1265-1267.
Howell, S.H., 1982: Ann. Rev. Plant Physiol., 33, 609-650.
Jimenez, A. and J. Davies, 1980: Nature, 287, 869-871.
Kado, C.I. and A. Kleinhofs, 1980: Int. Rev. Cytol. suppl. 11B, 47-80.
Korohoda, J. and K. Strzalka, 1979: Z. Pflanzenphysiol., 94, 95-99.
Krens, F.A., L. Molendijk, G.J. Wullems and R.A. Schilperoort, 1982: Nature, 296, 72-74.
Ledoux, L., R. Huart and M. Jacobs, 1974: Nature, 249, 17-21.
Lurquin, P.F., 1981: Plant Sci. Lett. 21, 31-40.
Müller, A.F. and R. Grafe, 1978: Mol. Gen. Genet. 161, 67-76.
O'Hare, K., C. Benoist and B. Breathnach, 1981: Proc. Natl. Acad. Sci. USA., 78, 1527-1531.
Orlova, E.B., L.G. Stolyarova, O.S. Perevenzentseva and V.A. Drozhennikov, 1978: Bull. Exp. Biol. Med., 86, 1467-1469.
Radford, A., S. Pope, A. Sazci, M.J. Fraser and J.H. Parish, 1981: Mol. Gen. Genet. 184, 567-569.
Rassoulzadegan, M., B. Binetruy and F. Cuzin, 1982: Nature, 295, 257-259.

Rochaix, J-D. and J. van Dillewijn, 1982: Nature, 296, 70-72.
Rollo, F., M.G. Galli and B. Parisi, 1981: Plant Sci. Lett., 20, 347-354.
Savage, A.D., J. King and O.L. Gamborg, 1979; Plant Sci. Lett., 16, 367-376.
Schaffner, W., 1980: Proc. Natl. Acad. Sci. USA., 77, 2163-2167.
Sidorov, V.A. and P. Maliga, 1982: Mol. Gen. Genet., 186, 328-332.
Southern, P.J. and P. Berg, 1982: J. Mol. Appl. Genet., 1, 327-341.
Uchimiya, H., 1981: Plant Physiol., 67, 629-632.
Ursic, D., J. Kemp and J.P. Helgeson, 1981: Biochem. Biophys. Res. Comm. 101, 1031-1037.
Van Slogteren, G.M.S., P.J.J. Hooykaas, K. Planqué and B. de Groot, 1982: Plant Mol. Biol., 1, 133-142.
Wigler, M., R. Sweet, G.K. Sim, B. Wold, A. Pellicer, E. Lacy, T. Maniatis, S. Silverstein and R. Axel, 1979: Cell, 16, 777-785.

CONTRIBUTORS

M. J. Adang
Department of Bacteriology and Biochemistry
University of Idaho
Moscow, ID 83843

M. R. Altherr
Department of Genetics
University of California
Davis, CA 95616

J. P. Bourgin
Laboratoire de Biologie Cellulaire
Institut National de la Recherche Agronomique
F-78000 Versailles, France

M. Case
Program in Genetics
Department of Zoology
University of Georgia
Athens, GA 30602

T. J. Close
Department of Genetics
University of California
Davis, CA 95616

E. C. Cocking
Department of Botany
University of Nottingham
University Park, Nottingham
NG7 2RD England

F. Colbère-Garapin
Biologie Moleculaire du Gene
Institute Pasteur
75724 Paris Cedex 15, France

D. E. Cress
Plant Physiology Institute
United States Dept. of Agriculture
Beltsville, MD 20705

H. De Greve
Laboratory for Genetics
University of Ghent, Belgium

T. Diener
Plant Virology Laboratory
USDA-ARS, Building 011A
DARC-West
Beltsville, MD 20705

A. Garapin
Institut Pasteur
ER CNRS 201 - SC INSERM 20
28, Rue Du Docteur Roux
7524 Paris Cedex 15, France

M. Gordon
Department of Microbiology and Immunology, SC-42
School of Medicine
University of Washington
Seattle, WA 98195

C. M. Gorman
Laboratory of Molecular Biology
Building 37, Room 2E10
National Institutes of Health
Bethesda, MD 20205

M. Hagiya
Department of Plant Pathology
University of California
Davis, CA 95616

J. P. Hernalsteens
Laboratory for Genetical
Virology
University of Brussels, Belgium

B. Hohn
Friedrich Miescher Institute
P.O. Box 273
Basel, Switzerland 4002

T. Hohn
Friedrich Miescher Institute
P.O. Box 273
Basel, Switzerland 4002

F. Horodniceanu
Biologie Moleculaire du Gene
Institut Pasteur
75724 Paris Cedex 15, France

B. Howard
Laboratory of Molecular Biology
Building 37, Room 2E10
National Institutes of Health
Bethesda, MD 20205

J. Jia
Friedrich Meischer Institut
P.O. Box 273
Basel, Switzerland 4002

C. I. Kado
Department of Plant Pathology
University of California
Davis, CA 95616

A. Kleinhofs
Program in Genetics and Cell
Biology, and Department of
Agronomy and Soils
Washington State University
Pullman, WA 99164-6420

P. Kourilsky
Biologie Moleculaire du Gene
Institut Pasteur
75724 Paris Cedex 15, France

G. B. Lazar
Friedrich Miescher Institut
P.O. Box 273
Basel, Switzerland 4002

J. Leemans
Laboratory for Genetical Virology
University of Brussels, Belgium

R. C. Lundquist
Department of Plant Pathology
University of California
Davis, CA 95616

P. Lurquin
Program in Genetics and Cell
Biology
Washington State University
Pullman, WA 99164-4350

T. Manzara
Program in Genetics and Cell
Biology
Washington State University
Pullman, WA 99164-4350

E. W. McBride
National Cancer Institute
National Institutes of Health
Bethesda, MD 20205

L. Miller
Department of Bacteriology and
Biochemistry
University of Idaho
Moscow, ID 83843

D. W. Miller
Department of Bacteriology and
Biochemistry
University of Idaho
Moscow, ID 83843

Z. Nicola-Koukolikova
Friedrich Miescher Institute
P.O. Box 273
Basel, Switzerland 4002

L. Otten
Max-Planck Institute
D-5000 Köln 30
Federal Republic of Germany

R. A. Owens
Plant Virology Laboratory
USDA-ARS, Building 011A
DARC-West
Beltsville, MD 20705

R. Padmanabhan
Laboratory of Molecular Biology
Building 37, Room 2E10
National Institutes of Health
Bethesda, MD 20205

J. Paszkowski
Friedrich Miescher Institute
P.O. Box 273
Basel, Switzerland 4002

J. L. Peterson
Laboratory of Biochemistry
National Cancer Institute
National Institutes of Health
Bethesda, MD 20205

I. Potrykus
Friedrich Miescher Institute
P.O. Box 273
Basel, Switzerland 4002

L. A. Quinn
Department of Genetics
University of California
Davis, CA 95616

R. Reeves
Program in Genetics and Cell
Biology, and Program in
Biochemistry and Biophysics
Washington State University
Pullman, WA 99164-4350

R. L. Rodriguez
Department of Genetics
University of California
Davis, CA 95616

F. Rollo
Istituto di Microbiologie e
Fisiologia Vegetale
Universita di Pavia
27100 Pavia, Italy

J. Schell
Max-Planck Institute
D-500 Köln 30

R. Shillito
Friedrich Miescher Institute
P.O. Box 273
Basel, Switzerland 4002

K. Shimamoto
Friedrich Miescher Institute
P.O. Box 273
Basel, Switzerland 4002

R. C. Tait
Department of Plant Pathology
University of California
Davis, CA 95616

J. Taylor
Program in Genetics and Cell
Biology
Washington State University
Pullman, WA 99164-6419

D. Tepfer
INRA
Laboratoire de Biologie
Cellulaire, CNRA
78000 Versailles, France

M. Van Montaga
Laboratory for Genetical Virology
University of Brussels, Belgium

I. Vasil
Department of Botany
220 Bartram Hall East
University of Florida
Gainesville, FL 32611

V. Williamson
ARCO Plant Cell Research Institute
6560 Trinity Courty
Dublin, CA 94566

A. Wöstemeyer
Max-Planck Institut für Züchtungsforschung
Cologne, Federal Republic of Germany

INDEX

www.ingramcontent.com/pod-product-compliance
Ingram Content Group UK Ltd.
Pitfield, Milton Keynes, MK11 3LW, UK
UKHW051127260726
13967UKWH00010B/2900

* 9 7 8 1 4 6 8 4 4 4 9 4 0 *